Nursing in the European Union

Nursing in the European Union

The World of Work

Volume 2

Sondra Z. Koff

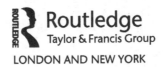

Routledge
Taylor & Francis Group

LONDON AND NEW YORK

First published 2016 by Transaction Publishers

Published 2017 by Routledge
4 Park Square, Milton Park, Abingdon, Oxon OX14 4RN
605 Third Avenue, New York, NY 10017

First issued in paperback 2022

Routledge is an imprint of the Taylor & Francis Group, an informa business

Library of Congress Catalog Number: 2016010382

Library of Congress Cataloging-in-Publication Data

Names: Koff, Sondra Z., author.
Title: Nursing in the European Union / Sondra Z. Koff.
Description: New Brunswick : Transaction Publishers, [2016]- |
    Includes bibliographical references and index.
Identifiers: LCCN 2016010382 (print) | LCCN 2016011155 (ebook) |
    ISBN 9781412863124 (hardcover : alk. paper) | ISBN 9781412863520
    (eBook)
Subjects: | MESH: European Union. | Nursing | Education, Nursing |
    Europe
Classification: LCC RT10 (print) | LCC RT10 (ebook) | NLM WY 16
    GA1 | DDC 610.730947--dc23
LC record available at http://lccn.loc.gov/2016010382

ISBN 13: 978-1-03-247707-7 (pbk)
ISBN 13: 978-1-4128-6395-7 (hbk)

DOI: 10.4324/9781315125435

STEVE More for you with love

Contents

List of Abbreviations

CJEU	Court of Justice of the European Union
EFN	European Federation of Nurses Associations
EP	European Parliament
EU	European Union
EU15	Number of Member States prior to the accession of ten nations in 2004
FEPI	European Council of Nursing Regulators
ICN	International Council of Nurses
ILO	International Labor Organization
RN4 CAST	Registered Nurse Forecasting Study
WHO	World Health Organization

List of European Union Institutions and Processes

The Commission—An executive organ consisting of one person from each Member State, who has responsibility for a particular area of policy. The Commission acts as sole initiator of European Union legislative proposals for consideration by the Council and the Parliament and has major executive responsibilities focused on monitoring and coordinating functions.

Council of Ministers—This body is composed of Member States' ministers in different formations depending on the issue under discussion. The unit decides on proposals developed by the Commission.

European Parliament—This is the only body directly elected by the citizens of the Member States. Over the years it has accrued more legislative authority. The structure exercises influence via legislative and budgetary processes and control and supervision of the executive organ.

Court of Justice of the European Union—This is the supreme judicial organ of the European Union consisting of one judge from each Member State.

Regulation—This instrument grants rights and obligations to be observed by all Member States and other actors, whether they be corporations, individuals, and so forth. It is automatically embodied into national legal systems.

Directive—This is a binding document as to the objective to be achieved by a certain date. Member State authorities may choose appropriate methods to do so.

Decision—This instrument is binding on all addressees, who are not necessarily Member States.

Recommendations and Opinions—These tools lack binding force and they are often used to clarify perspectives and issues.

Open Method of Coordination—A decision-making mechanism adopted in the late 1990s which avoids reliance on formal regulatory instruments. It supplements the legislative and financial tools of social policy. Based on voluntary cooperation between the Member States, the European Union assumes a strong coordinating role, while the former formally retain their authority in social policy. Decision-making includes exchange of best practices, benchmarking, national- and regional-level target setting, and periodic reporting.

Social Dialogue—Primarily concerned with social policy, this process obliges the Commission to consult labor and management when formulating such policy.

List of European Union Member States and Year of Entry

Austria (1995)
Belgium (1952)
Bulgaria (2007)
Croatia (2013)
Cyprus (2004)
Czech Republic (2004)
Denmark (1973)
Estonia (2004)
Finland (1995)
France (1952)
Germany (1952)
Greece (1981)
Hungary (2004)
Ireland (1973)

Italy (1952)
Latvia (2004)
Lithuania (2004)
Luxembourg (1952)
Malta (2004)
Netherlands (1952)
Poland (2004)
Portugal (1986)
Romania (2007)
Slovakia (2004)
Slovenia (2004)
Spain (1986)
Sweden (1995)
United Kingdom (1973)

1

Employment

Introduction

In the health-care sector, a human resources–intensive domain, the production of an adequate workforce is a major challenge. In spite of its significance, this matter, over time, has not occupied a place at the top of many policy agendas and, in fact, has often been viewed as a burden, rather than an asset. Consequently, today, many Member States have to deal with complex human resource problems, especially in the nursing sector. A vibrant health-care workforce represents an investment not only in the present, but in the future as well. It reaps multiple advantages for many sectors.

Health labor markets have been described as complex, fluid, and dynamic (World Health Organization: Europe 2006). The employment of nursing professionals is contextual and has been influenced by social and economic trends. The workforce challenge has felt the effects of the recent recession which brought about significant decreases in health-care spending in several Member States of the European Union (EU). At the same time, there has been an increase in the demand for health-care services. The most important demand-inducing trend has been demographic evolution, featuring overall aging of the population, which has generated an augment in the consumption of health-care and social services. Developments related to medical technologies, chronic conditions, pathologies, consumer expectations, care systems, and sites of practice, among other elements, have borne implications for the employment of nursing professionals, required skills, the types of services they can perform, the structures in which they offer them, the organization of their work, the division of labor, and boundaries between professional groups.

Health-care labor markets not only operate within each Member State, but their context is also regional and international in nature, given the objective of the EU as stated in the Preamble of the Treaty

1

of Rome to realize "an ever closer union among the peoples of Europe" and other factors. Professional nurses' responsibilities cover a broad continuum, ranging from the prevention of ill-health to palliative care when cure is impossible. The central thrust of nursing practice is the provision of holistic, patient-centered care, consisting of assessment and monitoring, diverse treatments and medications, education for patients and their families, and participation in an interdisciplinary team. Nurses provide services to individuals and families in all facets of the health and wellness continuum and leadership in health-care delivery systems and academia (Institute of Medicine of the National Academies 2011). In essence, nurses' role consists of practice, education, training and development, quality and service development, leadership, management, and supervision. In the Member States, professional nurses execute their role in a variety of structures. This role, like any other, has three facets: the ideal role, consisting of the socially prescribed or consensual rights and responsibilities affiliated with it; the perceived role, consisting of the vision of how it should be performed, held by the person who exercises it; and the performed role, meaning what the role incumbent actually does (Blais et al. 2006).

Initial Employment—The First Position

Over time, in many places, many new entrants to the profession have not encountered major hurdles in their search for employment after completion of training, although there have been some exceptions to this rule of thumb. For example, in France, 87 percent of new graduates have tended to find work in less than a month. It has also been reported that in Denmark, Finland, Sweden, and the United Kingdom, a large majority, meaning 75 percent or more, of new graduates have generally found employment as nurses within three months of having completed training (*Formation et trajectoires* 2011; International Council of Nurses Workforce Forum 2013; Marquier and Idmachiche 2006). On the other hand, the situation has been different elsewhere. In Spain, not all new nurses find jobs and so they are forced to emigrate to nations with shortages. In Ireland, the situation has been termed bleak. New graduates have been offered short-term contracts or part-time employment. Recognizing that these people have financial obligations related to their studies and the need for experience, the Irish Nurses Organisation succeeded in persuading the government to provide each new graduate with a two-year contract. In Lithuania, recent graduates have had difficulties in finding employment because many practitioners for economic reasons continue working beyond retirement age (Kapborg 2000; McConaghy 2007; *Surplus of Spanish Nurses* n.d.).

The global economic crisis has drastically changed the employment scene for all nurses, including new graduates, adding to the cited examples. Austerity measures, closure of health-care institutions and departments, curtailment of service, and reconfiguration of skill mix, among other policies, have caused the reduction of nursing posts, meaning that more often recent graduates remain unemployed. This has been the case in Slovenia, Portugal, Greece, Ireland, and now Denmark, to cite some examples. In Denmark, unemployment has recently struck one-quarter of new graduates and in Greece, one-third. Reaction to a similar scenario in Portugal has included the offer to work on a voluntary basis in order to gain experience. In short, the economic crisis has impacted the stock of nursing practitioners, their mobility, and compensation, as well as other elements (Dussault, Buchan, and Wismar 2013; European Federation of Nurses Associations [EFN] 2012; "New Report" 2012; Thomson et al. 2014).

Although later in their careers, they will most likely be employed in another site, a large majority of newly qualified nurses prefer to work in the hospital setting, usually in the public sector, perhaps because this is the one with which they are most familiar. Research has indicated that the selection of site of employment has been based, to a large extent, on the type of patients to be nursed, possibilities to utilize knowledge obtained during training, and professional advancement opportunities. Least consideration has been assigned to the types of shift work involved and qualities of institutional leadership (Palese, Tosatto, and Mesaglio 2009).

In terms of popularity, geriatric units, nursing homes, and psychiatric nursing seem to enjoy little with newly qualified practitioners. Reluctance to work in elderly care is particularly evident. This phenomenon is distressing, given the growth in the aged component of most societies and its implications for health care. A study (Lambrinou et al. 2009) undertaken in Greece evaluated the influence of education on trainees' knowledge of and attitudes toward older citizens. It was determined that attitudes were more positive and knowledge of their health better in the last year of training. A difference was found in both elements between the initial and final years, indicating that nursing education impacts knowledge of and attitudes toward senior citizens. It should serve as a signal to nurse educators that they can be instrumental in enhancing the possibilities for change in trainees' preferences for working with older people.

3

When new registrants assume their first position, often, they encounter "reality shock," their reaction to a work situation for which they find themselves unprepared. Job satisfaction is of extreme importance to these professionals in this stage of their career. Turnover rates and lack of commitment to the profession are especially elevated within this cohort. Such does not aid the general nursing shortage, the replacement of retiring practitioners, or efforts in the direction of cost efficiency. Very often, these practitioners are overwhelmed by the breadth and magnitude of the workload. They are also stunned by the fact that it can involve less patient contact and more nonnursing tasks than anticipated. Moreover, the extent of in-depth knowledge expected combined with new responsibilities and the relatively limited clinical experience acquired to date do not make for an easy entry into the world of employment. Study after study (Mooney 2007; "Preserving the Nursing Workforce" 2008; Weinberg 2003; Whitehead 2001) conclude that these elementary practitioners, for all intents and purposes, are lacking in confidence and control over their practice.

They also have concerns pertaining to organization and priority setting, communication with physicians, the work environment, dependency on others, and the road to becoming an independent practitioner. There is a paucity of literature on military nursing in the Member States. However, it has been noted that for the military practitioner, the transition from trainee to staff nurse is even more challenging because there are military as well as nursing demands to be met under the constant possibility of being deployed overseas which adds another dimension of anxiety (Moore 2006). The novices' employment situation is not always congruent with their expectations. They face many hurdles to be overcome. In the words of Brown and Kirpal (2004):

> The novice will need to negotiate . . . major learning challenges involving successful engagement with major work activities; successful learning from experience, alignment of professional and personal values; commitment to continuing professional development and coping with demands for flexibility, transferability and work intensification in the workplace (p. 230).

In short, novices must be socialized to the world of work and to the specific institution in which they are employed. They must acquire the necessary knowledge, skills, attitudes, and comportment for adaptation to the work role (Wanberg 2012). Organizational socialization is important to the structure involved as well as the newcomer.

Evaluations of various scenarios have concluded that effective support programs are vital to the transition from student to professional nurse and to the tempering of "reality shock" and the high turnover rates among recent graduates.

Such arrangements can help ensure that these practitioners are prepared for and sustained in their professional role. These programs, when available, differ in terms of their main features. The national development program for all newly qualified nurses in the National Health Service Scotland is entitled Flying Start NHS (National Health Service). Its purpose is to build confidence during the first year of employment and to make the transition period easier via a range of learning activities related to daily practice. The program focuses on communication and clinical skills, teamwork, safe practice, research for practice, equality and diversity policy, reflective practice, professional development, and career pathways. The scope is broad and intended to meet the needs of newly qualified practitioners working in any National Health Service setting. In addition to using online resources, participants work with a mentor, peers, and multidisciplinary team colleagues.

Extensive use has been made of mentors or preceptors, especially in the United Kingdom and Scandinavia. These figures, experienced nurses, help novices to evaluate their knowledge and skills, elevate their confidence, and garner professional satisfaction. They orient them to the specific nursing unit, teach them any necessary skills, and further socialize them to the profession. Essentially, they serve as role models, advisers, and points of reference for newly qualified practitioners. Evidence shows that mentor programs perform a key role. Improvement in patient care has, in part, been attributed to them. They have aided recent graduates in the development of their clinical skills and with their support have positively influenced workforce retention. Equally important is the fact that most newly qualified nurses have sanctioned mentorships. In addition, mentors themselves have expressed satisfaction with the arrangement. They have benefitted from helping others, furthering their own knowledge, and developing their teaching competences as a result of participation in such a program. On the negative side, it has been found that frequently, they have not received adequate preparation for their role (England: Department of Health, Professional Leadership-CNO's Directorate 2011; Robinson and Griffiths 2009).

Mentorships are congruent with the notion that current preregistration programs do not completely prepare trainees for the practice conditions affiliated with the fast-paced and fast-changing environment of health service delivery. Thus, often there is a need to refine and further develop some facets of preregistration curricula in the interests of facilitating the initial transition to staff nurse. As instruments of transition-to-practice, the development of nurse residency programs has been proposed (Institute of Medicine of the National Academies 2011). The rationale for this arrangement is that nurses, like physicians, require a period of apprenticeship or extended orientation after completion of their formal education to help them master the complexities of actual practice.

Job satisfaction is particularly important in one's early career. Most newly qualified practitioners require time to become confident and satisfied with their employment. In general, up to a year is necessary. Often, a low point is reached at six months or soon after. Evidently, a nurse, after completion of preregistration training, acquires skills in identifiable stages. During training the aspiring practitioner is a novice. In initial employment, the professional becomes a beginner. From there, passage takes place to the stage of competent, then to proficient, and finally, to expert. Not every nurse arrives at the final stage. When it happens, the entire process after graduation usually requires five years (Gordon 2005). It could be that the aforementioned support programs might curtail the time needed to travel through each phase.

The Hospital

Most nurses in the EU are employed in health-care institutions, the principal one of which is the hospital. It has been estimated that this structure employs up to approximately 75 percent of these professionals. At the level of the Member State, this institution, in most cases, employs a majority of the nurses (European Observatory on Health Care Systems n.d.; International Council of Nurses Workforce Forum 2013). The hospital in the last few decades has experienced major transformations. Technological advances have been many. Computerized networks have become commonplace. The new economic framework has featured financial efficiency and performance assessment. Patient turnover has increased along with case-mix complexity. Work has intensified and often, working conditions have deteriorated. The changes have been multiple and all have had consequences for the quality of care provided to patients, required skills, and the working lives of nurses at the bedside. These latter elements were to combine via the socio-economic constraints of hospital activity and institutional and work organization (De Troyer 2000).

Health-care reform in the Central and East European Member States was especially extensive. The new political context, born with detachment from the Soviet Union and the transition to democracy, featured a shift from a very centralized approach to a more pluralist model, but still difficulties were encountered in changing the purposes of the hospital structure. As a result, these institutions in the newly acceded Member States perform functions that often differ from those of their European neighbors. There tends to be an overreliance on inpatient treatment inherited from the Soviet health-care system and hospitals are seen primarily as providers of both health and social care. Community care services have been sparse (Index Foundation and Praxis Centre for Policy Studies 2007). For all practical purposes, in this part of the EU, the role of hospitals in the health-care delivery system is more prominent.

Regardless of its functions, the hospital is still the principal setting for nurses' employment and in all Member States, as one might imagine, it is part of the professional scope of practice. Figures for this employment rate are not available for all Member States. According to those reported between 2006 and 2013 (Barros and Simões 2007; International Council of Nurses [ICN] 2007a; International Council of Nurses Workforce Forum 2013; Padaiga, Pukas, and Starkienē 2011; Sicart 2006; World Health Organization: Regional Office for Europe 2013), it appears that Estonia lays claim to the highest hospital employment rate for nurses with 77.3 percent. The percentages then decrease as follows: 74 percent (Portugal), 73.4 percent (Bulgaria), 73 percent (France), 71.1 percent (Lithuania), 66.9 percent (Luxembourg), 64.2 percent (Denmark), 58.8 percent (Hungary), 57.9 percent (Sweden), 57 percent (United Kingdom), 56.2 percent (Ireland), 53.8 percent (Slovenia), 51.6 percent (Romania), 50 percent (Germany), and 46 percent (Finland). Sometimes, figures fail to agree. For example, France is cited as 59 percent by van der Boom (2008) and Germany as 60.6 percent. Such disagreement is illustrative of extensive data problems resulting from the lack of a uniform EU collection system. Most nurses employed in this capacity tend to prefer general hospitals.

As in the United States, throughout the EU, units are distinguished by specialty, type of patient treated, environment, culture, organization, and methods of service provision. Differences pertain to many factors, such as human and other types of resources, planning mechanisms adopted, work patterns, organizational structures, and management styles, to cite a few. Still, in spite of these diversities, resulting from a particular type of health-care delivery system, hospital managers wrestle with many of the same problems.

Staffing Ratios

A major challenge in most Member States relates to the provision of an appropriate institutional staff. In a given hospital or unit, its nature is usually expressed in terms of nursing time per patient per day or a nurse-to-patient ratio. These measures frequently vary depending on the type of facility or unit. Although the notion of staffing includes more than numbers, they are significant. Unfortunately, they often mirror funding contingencies, rather than the needs of personnel or patients. As a result, the need for nurses, their exigencies, and job requirements can lack congruence with existing staff levels. These ratios have generated a great deal of debate with no resulting consensus. There is no universal formula for staffing to guarantee the delivery of safe and high-quality nursing care. Professional associations, relying on the expertise of countries other than their own, have issued staffing guidelines. However, estimates of a specific number or level of nurse staffing for hospitals do not exist (International Centre for Human Resources in Nursing 2009b).

Florence Nightingale in her day enunciated very definite ideas pertaining to nurse densities. At first, she was convinced that the ratio should not exceed one nurse for every twenty-five patients and then she contradicted herself, claiming "twenty five cases are not generally enough" (Nightingale 1954a, p. 72). Being convinced that nurses did not have enough to do, she was of the opinion that "of acute cases, probably, one nurse should take charge of not more than fifty, possibly not more than forty" (Nightingale 1954c, p. 17). Such thoughts are definitely out of tune with those of the contemporary nursing profession.

Staffing ratios have been adopted in some Member States. For example, Belgium and Poland, utilizing a centralized approach have established base staffing levels for all hospital units at twelve nurses for every thirty beds in a twenty-four-hour period and at one nurse per twenty patients, respectively. Lithuania, on the other hand, has assumed a diverse posture by mandating a nurse–patient ratio only for intensive care units in which it has been set at one nurse for every two patients (EFN 2012; Padaiga et al. 2006). Staffing ratios have also been adopted in Greece, Germany, and Italy.

The number of patients for which nurses are responsible, according to the literature, demonstrates variance. In Hungary, each nurse is supposed to have between ten and fifteen patients (*Hungary-Austria: Nursing Emergency* 2006). In Germany, the figure depends on bed capacity or size of the hospital. A higher ratio is found in larger structures. General hospitals with more than five hundred beds have an average of 81.5 nurses per one hundred occupied beds. On the other hand, institutions with less than one hundred beds have an average of 66.4 nurses. At one point in time, Germany utilized nursing time standards, but abolished them because of the unexpected need for many more nurses than envisioned. The nurse–patient ratio in Poland at times has been reported as one to twenty-eight, indicating severe staffing issues. The situation has been even more drastic most recently, in Hungary, where one nurse working a shift has had to care for fifty-one patients (Belcher and Hart 2005; Busse and Blümel 2014; EFN 2012; Weinbrenner and Busse 2006).

In the United Kingdom, the nurse-to-patient ratio has gone from an average of 6.9 patients per registered nurse in the day and 9.1 at night to 7.9 during the day and 10.6 at night. These ratios vary somewhat by specialty (Ball and Pike 2009). Prime Minister Cameron has ordered a review of the nursing situation because of preoccupation with professional standards. A public inquiry is to consider whether rules should be established to guarantee specific staffing levels. The governmental Chief Nursing Officer chose not to introduce mandatory ratios due to the possibility that "instead of becoming the floor they become the ceiling." A recent survey, undertaken in the United Kingdom by *Nursing Times*, indicated that more than 70 percent of the nurse participants favored the introduction of mandatory ratios (Donnelly 2012). These measures are beneficial for patients as well as nurses. A study of the American State of California (McHugh, Kelly, and Aiken 2011), the first State to mandate minimum nurse-to-patient staffing ratios in hospitals, concluded that average skill levels were enhanced and that increased staff levels were identified with better outcomes than those achieved in hospitals located in other States. For medical and surgical units, minimum staffing was established at one nurse for every five patients. Step-down, telemetry, specialty, and other units had diverse ratios. These were not fixed, but must be reevaluated on a regular basis.

Comparative research has also confirmed the link between patient outcomes and nurse staffing. In path-breaking studies, Aiken and colleagues (Aiken 2007; Aiken, Clarke, and Sloane 2002; Aiken et al. 2002) demonstrated that surgical patients in hospitals with high patient-to-nurse ratios faced higher risk-adjusted thirty-day mortality and failure-to-rescue rates. In this setting, consequences for nurses featured a greater likelihood to experience burnout and job dissatisfaction. It is quite clear that inadequate staff levels identify with a galaxy of adverse events, such as patient falls, medication errors, nosocomial infections, and increased readmission rates, all of which have financial connotations. On the other hand, higher densities of nurses correlate with better quality of care, better health outcomes, including reduced patient risk-adjusted mortality and a lower risk of medical complications (Simoens, Villeneuve, and Hurst 2005). Patient outcomes do vary according to the nurse-to-patient ratio.

A recent multination study (Aiken 2011) that included ten Member States revealed that in all of them, a majority of nurses involved reported too few staff members to provide quality care. The percentages ranged from 85 percent in Greece to 63 percent in Sweden. In addition, the adequacy of nursing staff was shown to have significantly deteriorated over a ten-year period. For example, in Germany, it was rated at 37 percent in 1998/99 and in 2009/10 at 18 percent (Zander 2012).

Nurse staffing, as noted, impinges on hospital mortality. In Europe, each additional patient assigned to a nurse accounts for a 10 percent increase in the likelihood of death following a common surgery. On the other hand, the subtraction of a patient from a nurse's workload reduces mortality in hospitals with the best work environments by 9 percent and in those with mixed ones by 4 percent (Aiken 2011). Not only has an enhanced nurse-to-patient ratio improved patient outcomes, it has also contributed quality to the work environment, increased patient satisfaction, and bettered communication structures and nurses' well-being. The associations between the nurse-to-patient ratio, the nursing work environment, nurse evaluations of quality of care, nurse well-being, and patient satisfaction have been found to be significant (Bruyneel 2011). Although perfect nurse–patient ratios have not been identified, the advantages of these ratios have been revealed. It is generally acknowledged that they reap benefits for patients, providers, and health-care costs. As such, they are perceived as a necessary, but not sufficient condition for confronting workplace problems (Gordon, Buchanan, and Bretherton 2008).

Nursing Care Delivery Models

National legislation sets forth the role, duties, and responsibilities of nurses which embrace several categories: prevention, education, care, support, diagnosis, therapy, coordination, reporting, and administration. Most nurses are wed to a holistic philosophy of care, based on the notion that each person is a multifaceted whole, consisting of body, mind, and spirit, and that physical needs cannot be separated from psychosocial ones. Various methods are used to provide services that hopefully represent holistic patient care. There is variance in the delineation of nurses' tasks and responsibilities within the hospital sector and elsewhere, depending on the nursing care delivery model selected.

These frameworks specify the manner in which care is to be delivered by determining the tasks, responsibilities, and authority of the actors involved. They establish the tasks each health-care provider is to perform, who is responsible, and who enjoys the authority to make decisions. Nursing care models are built on the premise that the numbers and types of health-care providers should reflect the needs of the patient in such a manner as to provide services of superior quality in the most cost-effective way possible (Cherry and Jacob 2005). Multiple models of nursing care have been adopted. Basic methods of assignment for providing day-to-day care to hospital patients and others include the case method, total patient care, functional nursing, team nursing, and primary nursing.

The oldest model for nursing care delivery is the case method. It involves one nurse providing care, depending on acuity, to one or more patients. A more modern version of this arrangement is referred to as total patient care or case nursing. According to this framework, in a specific work period, a registered nurse is responsible for planning, organizing, and performing all care required by a group of patients. In carrying out these responsibilities, assistance is provided by other licensed and nonlicensed personnel.

Another early model, dating from the 1940s, labeled functional nursing, organizes patient care in assembly line fashion. Staff members work with groups of patients, rather than providing care for specific ones. Each health-care professional is assigned a precise functional task to be performed under the supervision of a head nurse. For example, one nurse administers medications, another one is responsible for dressings, and so forth. This model proliferates nursing care into a series of tasks carried out by many people. Nursing services tend to be fragmented and impersonal in nature. With patients having to deal with multiple practitioners, often their problems are overlooked because they do not match any defined assignment. Satisfaction on the part of patients and practitioners is not high.

11

Team nursing, developed in the 1950s, followed functional nursing. It was designed to correct the fragmentation of its predecessor and to supply the enhanced demands for professional nurses nurtured by advances in the technological aspects of care. The model features a professional nurse who is responsible for planning, coordinating, and delivering care to a designated group of patients through a team of caregivers that includes auxiliaries with less training. The team leader provides professional direction and distributes work assignments to team members based on their capacities and the acuity level of the group of patients. In essence, it is the team leader's skills that fashion the success of this model which stresses humanistic values and individualized patient care on a personal level, rather than task-oriented care offered on an impersonal plane (Blais et al. 2006; Dison 1992).

Team building is important to this framework. It is an arduous activity. The team chemistry must be fostered and newcomers must be socialized to the unit so collaboration relates to a commonly held philosophy and objective (Estryn-Behar, Le Nézet, and Jasseron 2005). Cross-cultural research on medical errors and injuries in diverse health-care delivery systems has revealed instances in which "rigid hierarchies, fear of vulnerability, and the lack of understanding of the interdependent nature of patient care make effective team work and communication difficult" (Gordon 2005, p. 37). The team chemistry bears implications for the well-being of both nurse and patient.

Advantages of this model are less reliance on registered nurses than found in other frameworks and utilization of less costly personnel who are much easier to recruit. On the negative side, a major flaw of this model has been that often the team concept is diluted. It does not prevail throughout the entire nursing process. Moreover, this arrangement has been criticized because it divides the nurse's role in patient care into segments that can be performed by providers possessing disparate skill capacities. Consequently, it is charged that nursing practice is not perceived as holistic in nature, but merely as a series of tasks to be executed. Moreover, many of them are considered so mundane as not to be worthy of a professional nurse's judgment and expertise (Joel 2011; Weinberg 2003).

Primary nursing, a product of the 1970s, represented an answer to the fragmentation affiliated with team nursing and an attempt to provide comprehensive, individualized, and consistent care. In this framework, the primary nurse is obliged to assess and prioritize the needs of each patient, to identify nursing diagnoses, to develop a plan of care in collaboration with the patient, and to coordinate and evaluate the care provided. These responsibilities embrace all aspects of the professional role including education, advocacy, decision-making, and continuity of care (Blais et al. 2006). In that the primary nurse plans and directs a patient's care over a twenty-four-hour period, this arrangement theoretically eliminates any fragmentation in the provision of nursing services. Accountability and responsibility around the clock are centered in the nurse as the primary care provider.

Primary nursing has been evaluated as being cost effective in terms of decreasing the costs of care and in reducing patient length of stay. Moreover, it helps ensure that competent care is provided throughout hospitalization. In fact, it has improved the quality of care. Patients, their families, physicians, and nurses themselves have assigned this model superior grades. The latter professionals also are pleased with the emphasis on the nurse–patient relationship and the chance to offer more personalized care. They have enjoyed greater autonomy as well. The notion of a single nurse being accountable for holistic care to patients presented a challenge. Often, the result has been greater job satisfaction and the detection of fewer errors and adverse events attributed to nurses. Although primary nursing is often considered the most professional framework, it has its negatives in the form of additional stress, role overload, and role ambiguity (Dison 1992; Joel 2011; Müller-Mundt 1997; Page 2004).

The various nursing care delivery models are not limited to hospitals. They can be used in diverse health-care settings and are of extreme significance. Aiken and Sloane (2002) have indicated that "the organization of nursing care may have an effect on patient outcomes that is independent of, and as important as, staffing and skill levels" (p. 275). These organizational features apparently exert a major influence.

The matter of which nursing care delivery model is the best is open to question. Based on patient and nurse satisfaction, quality of patient care, cost and administrative efficiency, there is little consensus as to which one is best. Moreover, these frameworks know no geographical or care setting boundaries. They have been adopted singly or in multiples in various settings throughout the Member States. Latvia, during the Soviet period, relied on functional nursing. Germany has utilized functional, team, and primary nursing. The latter was developed in the late 1990s in Western Europe, primarily in Great Britain, Belgium, and Denmark. This does not mean that it was automatically accepted in the newer Member States or even in the older ones. In Ireland, hospital nurses, wed to the notion of collective responsibility, had difficulty in embracing primary nursing with its focus on an individual client relationship and the affiliated accountability. Their preference was to work in the traditional task-oriented fashion (McCarthy 2000).

In the newly acceded Member States, especially Poland, primary nursing experienced a slow start, primarily because of the low level of nurse autonomy. Moreover, the matter was not of special significance to the Polish system of nursing (Górajek-Jóźwik 2004; Müller-Mundt 1997; Sandin and Walldal 2002). The level of nurse expertise, support personnel, patient needs and acuity, and the availability of resources vary across settings. In selecting a framework these elements must be given consideration. They are important to the selection of a nursing delivery model. What is suitable to one unit will not necessarily be so to another.

Audit and Feedback

Recently, increased attention has been focused on the quality of services. Across the Member States, there can be a difference in the care patients receive and that they are supposed to receive. Audit and feedback is a mechanism to address this matter. Used to varying degrees in the EU, its purpose is to improve performance of health-care professionals in the interests of quality and safety. It involves a periodic synopsis of clinical health-care performance that is made available to providers of services in such a manner as to permit them to assess and modify their personal practice. This vehicle is not limited to particular health-care settings, individual providers, or combinations of providers. Its universality and flexibility in addressing the wide variation in quality of care witnessed throughout the Member States are noteworthy.

Audit and feedback systems have been utilized in multiple manners, ranging from mandatory arrangements operated by governmental structures to voluntary professional ones. They have represented the internal initiatives of local groups of practitioners, such as nurses, and external ones executed by professional organizations, research groups, or governmental units. Their significance is attributed to their pragmatic approach to relating performance and outcome data to a specific institution or a group of facilities, and to individual health-care providers, or those working in a team.

The mechanism has the potential to influence providers' behavior in a positive manner, but it has not always reaped success in doing so. One would expect that professionals would change their clinical practice, if it was found to be incongruent with accepted guidelines. Such has not regularly occurred. Thus, the effects of this practice, used throughout Europe, have been judged generally small to moderate (Flottorp et al. 2010).

Shift Handover

Regardless of the setting, an important event that occurs regularly in any nursing work routine is the shift handover. Its primary purpose is the transfer of pertinent information from the nursing staff going off duty to the incoming one, so that the latter will be able to assume responsibility for appropriate patient care. More specifically, the report issued during this process serves to provide nurses with information that should aid in making clinical decisions, prioritizing and planning patient care, and maintaining the continuity and quality of care. The methods of transfer vary along with the content of information to be exchanged. The main types of nurse handover are verbal, taped, and nonverbal. The first-mentioned is the most well-known. The impact of these methods on patient outcomes and nursing care is unclear. It is evident that this process is of extreme significance in that erroneous or omitted information can account for undesirable patient outcomes which, in turn, could lead to nurse liability. Financial implications are involved as well. In addition, the shift handover performs other important social, psychological, organizational, and educational functions for nurses. It provides an opportunity for them to evaluate and improve their professional knowledge, nursing decisions, and clinical expertise; to define their role, to mentor newcomers to the profession and/or staff, to deal with job-related stress, to interact with colleagues, and contribute to the team chemistry. In short, its benefits are many. In fact, the Croatian nursing code of ethics recognizes the significance of documentation of planned nursing care, decisions made, outcomes of care and other pertinent information (Croatian Nursing Council n.d.; Hays 2005; Lamond 2000; Martinez and Martinez 2002; Strople and Hani 2006).

In several Member States, nurses have not been happy with the process as executed. In one study of European nurses' perceptions related to it, diversity in the degree of dissatisfaction ranged from 22 percent in England to 61 percent in France. In addition to France, the higher end of the continuum included Germany (55 percent), Italy (53 percent), and Belgium (46 percent). England at the other end was accompanied by Poland (23 percent) and Slovakia (23 percent). The other countries studied featured percentages in the 30s. All considered, the range is great (Meisner et al. 2007). The principal reason for a negative evaluation of shift handover was "too many disturbances." Lack of time was also perceived as an important irritant to a smooth shift changeover, especially in the case of France, which, given the results in the nations surveyed, represents special circumstances. French nurses, since the implementation of a thirty-five-hour work week at the dawn of this century, have severely criticized the reduction of time allotted to the exchange of information and to opportunities for formal and informal exchanges among colleagues (LeLan 2006). Both activities are related to shift handovers. The reduction of work time resulted in a concomitant reduction in staff during peak work periods and often the elimination of overlaps between shifts. The shift changeover procedure was modified as well. Written reports replaced oral ones. Obviously, time for any discussion became a special problem and a high proportion of French nurses expressed concern. Such time constraints are enhanced in other Member States as well by the nurse shortage, increased workload, and financial impact of the shift report. The reduction of time available to relay information decreases organizational knowledge and opportunities for passing on particular skills and knowledge to colleagues. This is reinforced by the increase in work intensity. Shift changeovers are definitely hindered (De Troyer 2001; Strople and Hani 2006).

Other noted causes of dissatisfaction that were assigned lesser weight by respondents included insufficient information exchange, lack of space for the purpose, and poor atmosphere. In large part, these reasons for discontent appear to display an organizational character that reflects poor management. It has been acknowledged that the quality of institutional leadership and collegial support are associated with dissatisfaction with shift changeovers. Furthermore, in most of the European nations studied, discontent was related to professional qualification level and professional seniority, but not to the nursing position held and type of shift worked (Meisner et al. 2007).

Most recently, in the United Kingdom and other nations, including the United States, in an effort to support patient-centered care, experiments with shift handovers at the patient's bedside have taken place. The practice has been adopted as a component of quality improvement programs, in entire hospitals, on selected wards, and sometimes with flexible/integrated approaches appropriate to the individual patient and the specific situation. Staff and patients have had favorable reactions to the practice. However, at this point in time, it is not known if it is a better facilitator for patient care, clinical decision-making, staff support, and education. Further evaluation is required ("What are the Benefits and Challenges" 2012).

It has been suggested that the shift report has the potential to affect not only the quality of patient care, but staff retention as well (Hays 2002). Organizational characteristics are a significant factor in nurse recruitment and retention. Moreover, it is the employees' perceptions of them that are important. A Belgian study revealed that in hospitals nurses considered attractive in terms of their organizational features, various elements, including the handover of shifts, were viewed in a positive vein. Moreover, overall work satisfaction was greater as well (Stordeur, D'Hoore and the NEXT-Study Group 2007).

The role of the shift handover in health-care delivery, its consequences, and its benefits for nurses must be taken seriously and efforts to correct the noted problems and dissatisfactions should be undertaken. A supportive social–organizational environment would enhance its worth. Communication, the basis of the changeover and its raison d'être, should be emphasized. Groups develop their own work and communication patterns and they are capable of modifying an individual's group behavior. However, in nursing, sometimes these can be more arduous. The institutional framework, with its flexible staffing methods and time imperatives, impinge, often negatively, on communication, in general, and especially, during shift handovers. The nature of the group fluctuates constantly. It becomes a collection of nurses who, perhaps, have not established similar goals, specific roles, or even a method of communication (Hays 2005). The social and psychological values of the procedure are lessened and maybe even the professional ones as well. Organizational group management, in some instances, needs to be rethought and paid more attention so as to enhance communication (*Création d'une instance professionnelle infirmière* 2007). Corrective action would benefit a valuable process.

Intentional Rounding

Closely related to nursing service delivery models is an innovative practice concerning provision of care. As part of the British Prime Minister's call for changes in the way nurses deliver care, a new nursing quality improvement initiative, originally developed in the United States as an evidence-based structured process, has recently been introduced in the United Kingdom and elsewhere. Known under various labels, such as care rounds, comfort rounds, or intentional rounding, the practice has been recommended to all National Health Service hospitals as an aid to the consistent delivery of the essential facets of nursing services and to the staff's organization of workload. It involves regular nursing rounds to check on patients in order to ensure their basic care needs are met. Within the framework, there are variations related to the timing of the rounds and the participants. Available evidence indicates improvements in clinical outcomes and patient satisfaction with the practice. However, for a full evaluation more research is required. Effectiveness, cost implications, and impact on staff time are some matters that need to be explored ("Intentional Rounding" 2012).

Hospital Shortages

There is no doubt that there is a shortage of nurses throughout the EU. It is particularly acute in the hospital sector. In fact, in Greece, due to the lack of qualified nurses, patients often hire untrained staff to care for them during the night (Davaki and Mossialos 2005; Papageorgiou et al. 2012). In many Member States, the shortage of specialist nurses is particularly severe, as in England, Slovenia, and Estonia, where it threatens hospital reforms. In spite of the gravity of the situation in reference to specialists, many hospital managers favor a generalized nursing staff, given its flexibility. Nurses can be assigned patients irrespective of their diagnosis, age, placement, or nursing requirements. In other words, they can be used as floaters and assigned to any unit for staff purposes (European Commission 2012b; European Federation of Public Service Unions n.d.). Transfer or rotation of nurses is commonplace in the nursing shortage climate. Routines are destroyed, requiring new ones to be learned. Practicing in a new environment and with new colleagues "means that new alliances must be made, new channels of negotiations found, new conditions of work be handled" (Strauss 2001b, p. 225). The practitioner must learn to manage the new environment. The situation is demanding. Random and frequent transfers often dilute nursing commitments.

Primary Care

European health-care policy in recent years has witnessed a restructuring of the hospital sector which resulted in a decrease in inpatient capacity and shifts from inpatient hospital services to those provided in the community. Greater use of primary care, those services, not requiring advanced medical equipment, and responsible, if necessary, for directing the patient to the appropriate component of the health-care delivery system, has received emphasis as did the construction of a linkage between primary and secondary care and the integration of health and social services. These changes reverberated throughout the nursing profession causing modifications in role and career development.

It is generally acknowledged that "a strong primary care system is the linchpin of effective health-care delivery and that it can help resolve the lack of continuity and responsiveness in health care in general" (Boerma 2006, p. 15). Thus, in many Member States, health-care professionals' roles were redefined with the formation of multidisciplinary primary care teams, consisting of physicians, social workers, nurses, and other personnel, practicing in centers distributed throughout the country and providing an integrated package of care. Denmark, England. France, Germany, Ireland, Italy, Scotland, Sweden, and Wales have been singled out for their integrated service delivery programs (Singh 2008).

In several Member States, these units were to become the base of the health-care delivery system and to serve as gatekeepers to secondary care. Raising the issue of professional work boundaries, the introduction of primary care arrangements bore implications for nurses as well as other professions. These practitioners, depending on the country and its primary care structure, perform diverse roles in the provision of services.

Primary care practices have been distinguished according to the role of physicians. Their attitude concerning delegation of tasks to other providers can create problems. Often, it did, especially in nations, such as Germany, where nurses traditionally have exercised a restricted role in primary care. Moreover, a country's wage system has impacted as well on the assignments distributed by physicians to other professionals. For example, in France, the fee-for-service arrangement hindered collaboration between these practitioners and nurses (Nolte, McKee, and Knai 2008). On the other hand, the general practitioners' contract in the United Kingdom presented no complications. Income was not threatened.

There are those countries, such as France, where general practitioners, for the most part, practice individually or in a group in which all members are in the same field. This has been the case in Germany, the Netherlands, and Italy. In this arrangement, nurses have had a limited role. In Germany and the Netherlands, this role has been attributed to another health-care provider, the medical assistant, who has been

19

preferred by doctors over the nurse for collaborative purposes. In Italy, with minor regional exceptions, the role of nurses has been overpowered by the quantity of physicians.

In the United Kingdom, Sweden, Finland, and other Member States, the situation has differed. Group practices, featuring physicians and other health-care professionals, have been in vogue. In the primary care sector, this model is dominant and multiple positive patterns of interaction and collaboration between physicians and nurses have developed. Initially and often, this was not the case. In the 1950s and 1960s, nurses and physicians in this sector sometimes tended to go their own way. The latter dealt with matters in the office and the former focused on home care. However, with time, things changed. Cooperation developed.

Today, nurses are a significant element in primary care. Prevention, education, health promotion, assessment, and coordination, essential components of primary care and traditional strengths of the profession, are heavily utilized. These elements were incorporated into the project and these practitioners are now in the front line of many centers. In fact, frequently, a patient's initial contact with the health-care delivery system is through a nurse. In Finland, in these health centers, in a given year, patients have experienced fewer contacts with physicians than with other personnel, particularly nurses. This can be attributed to diverse medical traditions, such as the significant role played by nurses, who execute tasks that physicians assume elsewhere (Vuorenkoski, Mladovsky, and Mossialos 2008).

Among the most prominent challenges to health-care delivery in all Member States, are chronic diseases. As populations age, these increase. In fact, most contemporary health care revolves around chronic maladies, such as diabetes, hypertension, arthritis, cardiovascular disease, or mental health conditions. These are diverse from other ailments in that they represent nonreversible long-term illnesses requiring multifaceted services from diverse sources. In the confines of the EU, it has been estimated that at least two-thirds of those persons of pensionable age are afflicted with at least two chronic conditions. Moreover, in England, 80 percent of general practice consultations have focused on chronic diseases. From an economic perspective, they have accounted for up to 7 percent of a nation's Gross National Product (Nolte and McKee 2008a). They certainly take their toll.

In many Member States, nurses have made their mark and have been instrumental in managing these ailments. In those featuring the aforementioned primary health-care multidisciplinary teams, they have often been in the forefront of services to chronics, as in England, Sweden, and the Netherlands. Nurse-led clinics focused on the management of chronic conditions have been an outgrowth of the primary health-care movement. Nurses' role has definitely expanded as they lead these clinics and become involved with discharge planning, case management, and other meaningful responsibilities. As a result, the approach to chronic disease in many Member States has, to a large degree, been led by nurses. This definitely represents a new orientation to the condition. Roles have been redefined in positive fashion.

Similar arrangements have not been adopted in Germany. As noted, in this Member State, the involvement of the nursing profession in the fashioning of the health-care delivery system has historically been minimal. The revamping of Disease Management Programs did not change the situation. They focus on physicians in their role as principal service providers and other professionals are not directly involved. The integration of nonmedical and medical professionals into a care system, such as that for chronics in other Member States, is not even given thought. Such results from the fact that in Germany, nursing is regarded more as an allied profession than an autonomous one with independent responsibilities. It is primarily an extension of medical activities and a complement to medical or hospital care (van der Boom 2008; Siering 2008). As a result, in comparison to those in other Member States, German nursing tasks are more medical and technical in nature.

In addition to economics, a primary reason for the spread of nurse-led clinics was the manufacture of new career opportunities for the profession. The development of a more patient-centered system featuring easy access was of importance as well. This shift in responsibility for chronic care from physicians to nurses has received superior evaluations. It has been demonstrated that the quality of care furnished by nurses is comparable to that provided by physicians. Most important, patients have reaped the benefits of improved health. Moreover, the practice has proven to be more cost effective. Long-term cost savings from complications have been realized and health-care utilization has been reduced (Nolte and McKee 2008b; Suhrcke, Fahey, and McKee 2008). Chronic disease management has improved in nurse-led clinics in multidisciplinary primary care. It is quite evident that the primary health-care sector in many Member States has offered a wealth of opportunities to the nursing profession and, in turn, challenges to the educational institutions responsible for preparing practitioners for the new role. It is recognized that nurses can be trained quicker and at less cost than physicians. Thus, it is logical to expand their practice.

The experience of primary health care in the newer Member States has followed a somewhat different course. In Hungary, at the time other Member States were emphasizing community care, stress was on hospital care. Having the scope of integrating health services, ambulatory care was put under hospital management. Diverse professionals worked from polyclinics that served defined districts or in rural zones from physicians' clinics. Reform realized in 1990, detached primary health care from hospital administration. District physicians became family physicians who served as gatekeepers to the system. This generated the development of a network of mother and child health nursing services to be developed into a wider primary care provider (European Observatory on Health Care Systems 1999).

The Czech Republic also had a later start in the organization of primary care. Even though Czech nurses and other health-care providers were recognized in other Member States as highly qualified, the same did not apply in their home country. Here, they were not perceived as an independent profession autonomous from physicians. It has been difficult to erase this view because physicians were primarily responsible for programs issued by the Ministry of Health and served as faculty and directors of schools of nursing. The same problems have been affiliated with other newly acceded Member States, making it difficult to meet the requirements and spirit of primary care. In Bulgaria, Estonia, and other Member States in the region, there has been an insufficient capacity for long-term chronic care. Slovenia serves as an exception. At the foundation of the national health-care system, there are family medicine–centered primary care units that pepper the country. Nurses have been largely employed in these facilities (Albreht et al. 2009). This represents a departure from the rule of thumb for regional nurses' employment. In spite of the hurdles related to the institutionalization of primary care that had to be conquered in many of the newer Member States, the seeds of this approach were planted. Patients, for the most part and specifically in Croatia, have been more satisfied with nurses' services and behavior than with the organization of practices. Generally, the older and less educated patients have been the most satisfied (Babić-Banaszak et al. 2001).

Closely related to primary care and chronic disease management is the role of the Community Matron in the United Kingdom's National

Health Service. A relatively new title, it was an important part of the government's policy for supporting people with long-term conditions and it offered an additional dimension to career opportunities in nursing. This figure, usually employed in a primary care structure, works as part of multiprofessional and multiagency teams. The Community Matron provides nursing care and also functions as a case manager for patients with complex long-term health needs. A typical caseload consists of approximately fifty very high intensity users of health care or people at high risk of hospitalization. The principal role is to coordinate primary and secondary care and the social services. For the most part, these providers work with all age groups, but some focus on specific client categories, such as the elderly or the very young.

The creation of this position initially caused tension within the nursing profession. Many practitioners already working in the community felt their toes had been stepped on as the newly created role failed to acknowledge their efforts. Initial evaluations of this figure's performance have been mixed. These practitioners have been instrumental in the avoidance of hospital admissions in some localities, but not in others. Emergency admissions to hospitals were not reduced as a result of their services. The area in which they seem to have been most successful is that of chronic disease management where they are involved with other services. Of importance is the fact that consumers have positively evaluated their role (Dubois, Singh, and Jinani 2008; Girot and Rickaby 2008; de Silva and Fahey 2008).

Other Community Nursing Sites

Throughout the EU there are a galaxy of community health-care sites that hire nurses with varied qualifications and skills. These settings include physicians' offices, educational institutions, industry, prisons, rehabilitation centers, ministries, employment and home health agencies, voluntary associations, governments, hospices, and nongovernmental organizations whose mission might not necessarily be to deliver care, but whose activities require the services of care givers. Discussion of all these units is beyond the scope of this work. In the Member States, community nursing features different traditions, development paths, and status. In some, it has been viewed as health care's "poor relative" (Burau 1999). In others, principally Denmark, the United Kingdom, Finland, and the Netherlands, it has been well implanted. However, it seems to be less developed in the Mediterranean countries and the newer Member States. This has

23

occurred because in some nations, such as Hungary, nursing was not appropriately developed for an extended period of time. Distribution of resources and the basic approach to health-care delivery fostered a gulf between medicine and nursing. Only recently, was it accepted that nursing is an organic part of a health-care delivery system and that it is related to the welfare sector and its subsystems. Also, in several Member States, such as Slovakia, Estonia, and Austria, even at the turn of this century, diversified roles for nurses were opposed, principally by physicians, halting the development of community practice (*Nursing in Hungary* n.d.; Pearson and Peels 2001).

Societal changes resulting from the end of Soviet domination in some of the newly acceded Member States took their toll on community nursing. The resulting dislocation impacted both nurses and clients. Caseloads featured a large proportion of troubled families in which the health and safety of children were threatened. In addition, new risk factors made their appearance. The work of nurses was transformed. Their previous well-regulated practice, relatively free of the need to deal with the social needs of poor and poorly functioning families, fell by the wayside. Moreover, given the lack of geographical mobility during the Soviet era, nurses bonded with clients and residents and they were authority figures. The contextual changes, shifting responsibility for health from the collective to the individual, destroyed the traditional role of community nurses as well as that of their clients, suggesting that the former had to develop competences in community assessment, community analysis, and health promotion practice in order to confront the post-Soviet environment (Kalnins 2002).

Community care is provided by nursing staffs with diverse qualifications, ranging from those of a general care nurse to those of an advanced practitioner, depending on their clientele. Specialization is available for nurses desiring to work in the community in Cyprus, England, Portugal, and Sweden, to cite some Member States. The chronic understaffing of nurses in this field has been noted (Buchan and Seccombe 2006) and it continues. Decisions to offer health care in the community created more possibilities for nurses to expand their role in care giving and to increase their autonomy. It seems that gender influences decisions to take advantage of these opportunities and to work in community nursing. The proportion of females engaged in this type of practice has tended to be even higher than that for others (Bessière 2005). In terms of age as well, these professionals have differed from their colleagues practicing in other settings. They have been much older, indicating that nurses' careers, as noted, usually commence in general hospitals which explains the younger age in this sector.

Home Care

Although home care has been provided for over a century in some Member States, the need for it has intensified most recently. A main cause of this phenomenon is the increased longevity of the elderly population, carrying with it, implications for more chronic and mental illness. The highest proportions of senior citizens have been found in Spain (36 percent), Italy (35 percent), Germany, Greece, and Portugal (32 percent each) and the lowest in Luxembourg (22 percent) (World Health Organization: Regional Committee for Europe 2007). It has been generally acknowledged that this population should be able to continue living in their homes or in adopted homes and be supported by ambulant home care facilities complemented by informal care, primarily that furnished by family members. Cost containment, an objective of most, if not all, decision-makers, has also prompted the development of home care along with changing consumer expectations and technological advances that assure quality services apart from the hospital setting. Moreover, nursing at home better supports a patient's well-being and dignity.

In addition, home care in the EU has also been affected by human rights provisions in various legislative measures and treaties. Many make reference to "people's right to proper medical care, protection of their dignity and compliance with their wishes regarding treatment" (Ehrenfeld 1998, p. 62). The 1996 Ljubljana Charter on Reforming Health Care adopted by the European Member States of the World Health Organization (WHO) acknowledged these rights. Also, the Maastricht Treaty makes reference to the improvement of public health and obviating threats to human health. These requirements as they relate to home care have been met in various ways, depending on the Member State involved. Throughout the EU, home care has been assigned diverse meanings and purposes. Given the elasticity of the word "home," there is a pot-pourri of services which are preventive, acute, rehabilitative, or palliative in nature (Boerma and Genet 2012).

Home nursing services have enjoyed a long tradition in Belgium, Denmark, Finland, Ireland, Sweden, the Netherlands, and the United Kingdom. In other Member States, principally the newer ones and those in Southern Europe, including Portugal, Italy, and Greece, they are less developed. Moreover, in these areas, they have encountered financial and legislative hurdles, significant obstacles to meeting changing care priorities and citizens' needs in this sector. These services include rehabilitative, supportive, health promotive or disease preventive, and technical nursing care (Hlavačka, Wágner, and Riesberg 2004; Kerkstra and Hutten 1996). Such activities provide different types of short-and long-term care and support to patients with diverse needs.

To a large extent, the demand related to these services is affected by consumer expectations and views of the role of the family. Throughout the EU, diverse perspectives exist. In the Scandinavian Member States, the culture dictates that aid forthcoming from families is not recognized as an official part of home care, nor is this type of informal care anticipated. Home care is expected from outside sources and it is automatically accepted. On the other hand, in France, Germany, Italy, Spain, Portugal, Austria, Estonia, and other nations, the notion of the extended family has prevailed. The family is considered the first point of care, especially in rural areas. That it looks after its own with the provision of informal care is considered to be a reasonable assumption and normal practice. In Greece, as well, it is believed provision of care is not the state's or its nurse employees' obligation, but the family's. Such a belief mirrors the familial and clientelistic nature of Greek society (Dent 2003a). In these nations, if accepted, the role of services coming from sources, other than the family, is merely to fill in the void when absolutely necessary. There is no tradition of home care. However, social changes have dictated some reductions in the volume of this informal type of caring. The extended family, in many cases, has assumed lesser importance as the significance of the nuclear family has increased. Thus, there are fewer individuals to provide this care. Also, the employment stage for females has drastically enlarged, pulling many more into the labor market.

The home nursing scene in EU nations presents a myriad of organizational patterns and practices. A unique facet of French services, not found in other Member States, is the Hospitalization at Home Program. Its name automatically distinguishes it from other offerings in the sector. It illustrates its orientation toward the medical and the fact that it is organized by hospitals. Its existence attests to the French preference for cure rather than care in matters of health and illness. Moreover, it accounts for the weaker role of home nursing in the French health-care delivery system. In France, even though home care is organized in the community and the private sector, hospitals prefer to organize their own activities, rather than to work with these units. This added feature of home care services has not been available in other Member States (van der Boom 2008).

The division of labor between the different categories of home nursing personnel, other health-care professionals, and informal care givers is often blurred. In part, this results from the fact that in the Member States, boundaries of the social sector are far from homogeneous. Those working in home care undertake diverse responsibilities from country to country and sometimes within countries. Also, they interact with divergent professionals, most of whom have different training. There are also differences in the extent to which services are integrated. In some systems, home care, home help, and social and medical services are represented as a total package and in many others, this is not the case. Complete integration of these elements is a requisite to the delivery of appropriate care. This has been especially difficult in the Central and Eastern European Member States, due to severe shortages of resources and equipment. Lack of such integration makes nurses' communication and collaboration with other actors in the home care delivery system that much more difficult. In most Member States, nurses are at the core of home care. Not only are they responsible for delivering it, but often, they are involved in coordinating it and other supervisory duties. The widest range of home care professionals is found in Belgium, Bulgaria, and Romania. In some Member States, such as Belgium and France, the tasks of these providers partially overlap (Genet et al. 2012).

Even though the autonomy of nurses has been recognized, both professionally and legally, in many Member States, often, it is one thing, in theory and another, in practice. Compared to that of their colleagues working in other sectors, nurses practicing in the home care domain enjoy more autonomy. Working as solo practitioners, and not being under surveillance, for the most part, they have increased opportunities for autonomy in practice. An Italian study of home care nurses (Basso and Salmaso 2004) revealed that 84 percent were satisfied or very satisfied with the freedom of choice they could exercise in their work. In addition, it has been declared that in the Czech Republic, home care represented by far the most successful post-Communist reform and nurses working in this sector were the only ones singled out for treatment as health-care professionals, rather than physicians' handmaidens (Heitlinger 1998). In some Member States, these practitioners do not enjoy this latitude. In France and Germany, for example, home nursing is subservient to the medical profession and in the Netherlands, organizations exercising managerial and bureaucratic monitoring processes restrict practitioners' autonomy. Apparently, Danish home care nurses have enjoyed the most decision-making authority and autonomy (van der Boom 2008).

Home nursing staffs' evaluation of their competence is quite favorable. In a Finnish study (Gronroos and Perala 2008), practitioners attributed it to reading scientific and professional journals, continuing education, decision-making latitude, and work demands. They were confident in helping the elderly meet daily living requirements, answering patients' physical needs, and in collaborating with them and those providing informal care. However, it is most interesting that these practitioners felt deficient in terms of their familiarity with services and benefits available to their clientele, their capacity to adopt evidence-based information in their practice, and their ability to use information technology appliances, such as fax machines and laptop computers. It seems that in their training and orientation, provision of more practical knowledge is necessary.

Shortages afflict the home care sector like many others. The demand for services is not met in many instances. It is generally acknowledged that zones marked by social deprivation undergo greater morbidity and mortality than affluent areas. Often, unfortunately, home care nursing is not reinforced where most needed. At one time, in Estonia, these services were not available in almost one-third of the local authorities (European Commission: Directorate-General for Employment, Social Affairs and Equal Opportunities 2007). France recently adopted a policy to enhance access to home care by improving the regional distribution of nurses working in the field. It regulates nurses' activity in the private sector by limiting practice in areas that are overserved and encouraging it in underserved ones with financial and other material incentives, enhanced functions, and the like (Musques and Naidich 2008).

Shortages of nurses in this sector are high, as in Finland, Germany, and the Netherlands (European Commission 2012b). The situation is particularly acute in rural areas. Frequently, working conditions and remuneration are poorer than in acute care. Absenteeism is also a problem. Often, nurses practicing in home care, not having a solid support system, bear a sense of isolation which reinforces their ambivalence and commitment to their position. In addition, many, having a fear of being reported to authorities, become preoccupied with malpractice. Complaints are also heard about competence development (Josefsson, Sonde, and Wahlin 2008; Josefsson et al. 2007). The percentage of vacancies in the field is elevated. Recruiting presents a challenge, given that many practitioners are deserting the public home care sector in favor of the private or self-employment, as in Germany (www.dbfk.de). Also, the status of this professional arena presents a hurdle because it is rather low compared to other health-care sectors.

Reference has been made to the call for required university preregistration education for all trainees throughout the Member States. This call has been particularly loud in reference to nurses working in home care. This training has been deemed necessary to meet the demands of their supervisory responsibilities and of working independently and with the newly developed advanced procedures used in patients' homes (Ehrenfeld 1998).

Palliative Care

Palliative care, a relatively new and often controversial discipline, was born in the 1970s. An outgrowth of the hospice movement, its early roots were planted in the United Kingdom and the first of these services in mainland Europe was established in Sweden in 1977. From there, over time, the concept spread throughout the continent. It has been described as

> the totality of care provision for patients whose life-threatening disease no longer responds to curative therapies. For the support of these patients at the end of . . . their lives, multidisciplinary care is of the utmost importance on a physical, psychiatric, social and moral level. The major aim of palliative care is to offer the patient and his/her next of kin as much quality of life as possible and maximum autonomy (Corens 2007, p. 120).

Unfortunately, these requisites are not always met in all quarters of the EU.

These services have had different origins throughout the Member States. In Ireland, their foundation was closely connected with religious orders. In many other Member States, they started as a grassroots hospice movement. And, in Spain, they were presented by the national health-care system as an innovation. In some of the newly acceded Member States, they were stimulated by the activities of British foundations. There is no logical sequence to the development of palliative care in the EU (Durán, Lara, and van Waveren 2006).

There has been a rapid and marked increase in the number of countries that provide these services. In terms of quantity and breadth, they are most developed in the West European Member States.

Those in Central and Eastern Europe once again felt the impact of Soviet ideology. Emphasis on physical care and maintenance of the workforce contrasted sharply with the philosophy underlying palliative care. The two had different missions. Not only was the political situation antithetical to the development of such services. Even if there was interest, as in Romania, the lack of economic resources presented a hurdle. Consequently, these services in this part of the world were developed only after the fall of Communism and the independence of Croatia from Yugoslavia and they tended to be created almost without rhyme or reason. Basically, their growth was piecemeal and as in other sectors, stimulated by aid from abroad (Morris 2011; Wright et al. 2003). For example, Croatia took advantage of an educational project in the field with the University of Kent, Canterbury. It featured an interactive approach which was unique for Croatia (Oliver 2005). Also, there is a broad disparity of resources and provision. It appears that Polish services are more plentiful and broader than those in other Central and Eastern European nations. In fact, Polish palliative care nurses have been sought out by other Member States for employment purposes. On the other hand, in Slovenia, palliative care is only in the early stages of development (Albreht et al. 2009; Strózik 2006).

A major challenge faced by supporters of palliative care was a lack of knowledge of the subject, particularly, on the part of the general public and decision-makers. Many, failing to realize its true nature, merely equated it with "tender loving care." In many Member States, major educational campaigns were required. Political opinions on the matter ranged from the majority support of Latvian political parties to the complete opposition of those in Austria (EAPC n.d.).

The culture of a country determines, in part, the reception of palliative care initiatives. Religion, as part of culture, has, to an extent, influenced the manner in which they were received. The Orthodox and Christian traditions have registered hostility. Moreover, in the former, especially as interpreted in Central and Eastern Europe and in urban areas, the matter of death is considered a taboo. It is something not to be openly discussed. In predominantly Catholic countries, much emphasis is assigned to cure over care and hospice, as an institution, frequently bears a negative image. It can represent second-rate medicine. In addition, some aspects of Judaism conflict with the notion of hospice and palliative care (Mosoiu, Andrews, and Perolls 2000; Rocafort and Centeno 2008; www.eapcnet.org).

Lifestyle and the nature of the health-care delivery system have also impacted on the development of palliative care services. These elements account for who will assume responsibility for a terminally ill person. For example, in Greece and Latvia, this obligation is to be assumed by family members and the home is expected to be the accepted site of care. In Estonia, if terminally ill people have close relatives, they have not been able to be admitted to a health-care institution. On the other hand, in Slovakia, families feel no such obligation for care and the burden is cast on health-care facilities (Kalnins 2006; Kiik and Sirotkina 2006). The response has often been similar to that related to home care.

There are significant differences in the modes of palliative care. These relate especially to the number and types of services. Care is furnished in various settings and by diverse providers. Nurses are in the forefront of all. The multiprofessional approach is critical to the service and consumer involvement should be as well. Very often, people wish to conclude their life in surroundings with which they are familiar and to which they are attached—that is, their home. In virtually all of the Member States, with the exception of Latvia (www.éapc-taskforce-development.eu), palliative care is offered in this structure. In Latvia, there has been discussion of initiating these services. There are multiple models of these and the form they assume often depends on the auspices under which a program is organized.

The ideal is to achieve a broad geographic network of mobile care teams so as to allow universal access. Ireland has been singled out for its achievements in this area. In each major geographical subdivision, the county, home palliative care services are available. In some Member States, this care is better developed than in others. For example, in Slovakia and Croatia, lacking quality parameters, it has been deemed inadequate and underdeveloped. In reference to Sweden, the opposite applies. It has been noted that any service in this field that is offered in a hospital can be provided in home care (Džakula et al. 2014; Rocafort and Centeno 2008).

The team of providers can represent various professions depending on the situation. There is no fixed formula. However, teams always include nurses in a prominent role and usually general practitioners as well. Other professionals, such as social workers, psychiatrists or psychologists, and religious leaders are added as needed. These team members have usually taken a special training course. In several Member States, as in the Netherlands, they are backed up by multidisciplinary home care support teams, consisting of three specialist nurses, an internist, a general practitioner, a nursing home doctor, an anesthesiologist, and a pastor. Their role is to inform, support, and advise home palliative care givers in times of need. They are always within reach. In Spain, their distribution is regionalized so as to enlarge availability.

A great many of the Member States, as one might expect, have inpatient palliative care units in hospitals. However, in some instances, as in France, they have not been readily accepted. In Cyprus, the hospital is a principal unit since there are no community nursing services. Home palliative care is offered by two voluntary associations. Hospital treatment requires multidisciplinary specialist care based on team practice. As opposed to those offering palliative care in the home, the hospital teams tend to be more sophisticated. They, too, as well as patients, have access to support teams composed of specially trained physicians, nurses, and paramedics. In the case of Spain, physical and occupational therapists, as well as dieticians, priests, and volunteers are included in the group.

In Belgium and France, these professionals, in addition to acting as consultants in time of need, are to establish a palliative culture, train hospital personnel, and arrange continuity of care for palliative patients on discharge. They are called upon as consultants for a variety of reasons. Technical support or support for families might be required. There might be a need for psychological support for patients as well as health-care providers. In the Netherlands, these teams are responsible for developing curricula for nurses working in this setting. There can be hostility between the hospital support group and its care giving team. The latter has often felt it is in possession of the same level of palliative care capacities as the former. Interaction with it can generate doubt on the part of others as to professional abilities (Rocafort and Centeno 2008).

Other settings for provision of palliative care include the hospice which in some Member States is identified with a negative image. This institution is distributed throughout the EU. Given the pattern of development of palliative care in general and of these structures, many more nurses work in this area in the older Member States than in the newer ones. However, in all cases, it is generally acknowledged that the nurse stands at the core of the hospice staff. Day palliative care is offered in some centers found primarily in Germany, Poland, Spain, Italy, and the United Kingdom. In some places, these centers are undergoing rapid expansion. There is variation in terms of clientele, services provided, and staff (EAPC n.d.; European Parliament: Policy

Department-Economic and Scientific Policy 2008). Nurses are also involved in providing palliative care in nursing homes and residential and long-term care facilities. The development of services in these units has been varied as is their nature. The majority of care in the Member States is delivered in the previously discussed institutions.

Children's palliative care is a recently developed specialty for which opportunities for training and education are few and far between (Downing and Ling 2012). Most palliative care services listed for the various Member States are intended for both adults and children. Many fewer listings are indicated for pediatric patients only. However, most recently, more nations have indicated some palliative care solely for this clientele. These include Latvia, the Czech Republic, Germany, Ireland, Poland, Portugal, Romania, Slovakia, Spain, and the United Kingdom (Centeno et al. 2007; EAPC n.d.). It is noteworthy that the group contains newly acceded and older Member States.

Bereavement support teams provide another palliative care activity with which nurses are involved. Although the list is incomplete, it appears that a majority of the Member States furnish services in this area. Most are available for both adults and children, but almost one-half are limited to adults.

Nurses affiliated with palliative care also provide other types of activities. Macmillan nurses, supported by the Cancer Relief Macmillan Fund and affiliated with the United Kingdom's National Health Service, give supportive care and advice. Their basic purpose is to provide multifaceted information on disease and treatment, as well as that pertaining to financial entitlements and needed equipment for care purposes. They serve as sounding boards for consumers and caregivers. In addition, there are the so-called twilight nurses, some of which are made available by the Irish Cancer Society. These practitioners provide support in the home at night (McDaid et al. 2009; Rocafort and Centeno 2008).

Although palliative care services have made great strides in most Member States, there are still some remaining hurdles that impact on their quality, quantity, and the role of nurses. First and foremost, in several instances, few public resources are committed to them. Furthermore, training in palliative care for EU nurses and other health-care professionals manifests major deficits. Educational programs have been labeled insufficient, primarily because of their lack of volume and failure to adequately integrate the subject matter into preregistration and other offerings. Moreover, many courses have not been accredited by the appropriate authorities. Sweden provides an exception because in this nation an important and prioritized area is nurses' knowledge of palliative care. In addition, in Germany, since 2003, palliative care has been a mandatory component of nurse training (Busse and Blümel 2014; www.cancervard.se).

Although in many Member States, there is a shortage of full-time nurse experts in the field, in general, opportunities for specialization in palliative care are limited. In Hungary, nurses can participate in a program focusing on hospice nursing and coordination of services at the specialist level (www.hospice.hu). Belgian palliative care nurses are accredited and in Poland, this field is a recognized nursing specialty. The examples are few. Efforts have been made to rectify educational deficits. However, many Member States have limited resources. Some in this condition have worked in unison with external units. For example, Slovakia received a grant from the EU designated for the development of palliative care in Eastern Europe. The funds were used for training educators in the field. Lithuania was offered the services of the Polish Society of Palliative Care to train Lithuanian nurses in Poland (Rocafort and Centeno 2008). Education in the area of palliative care is definitely expanding. However, in spite of these efforts, there is no doubt concerning the need to reinforce them.

Palliative care requires multidisciplinary efforts from professionals working in unison. In many settings, the various aspects of it do not receive the appropriate emphasis. In particular, spirituality has often been undervalued, restricting its potential contribution to overall efforts. Arguments have been made as to the importance of this ingredient to palliative care and thus, the need to consider it on an equal footing with the physical, social, and psychological aspects (Amoah 2011).

In some Member States, particularly, the newly acceded ones, the concept of a multidisciplinary team has led to problems. This has been the case in Slovenia, Hungary, Bulgaria, and Estonia. Teamwork was never part of the national tradition in these nations and other factors hindered its development as well. These include the nature of the health-care hierarchy with the physician at the apex, a lack of understanding of the various professional roles encompassed in a palliative care team, and competition between different professions. These factors were so potent that at one time teamwork was not functioning at all in Estonia or Bulgaria. In several instances, its acceptance has been difficult and in Slovenia, nurses have advocated teamwork and multiprofessional cooperation more than physicians (Filej et al. 2009; Kiik and Sirotkina 2006; www.hospice.hu).

To date, palliative care services have not been able to meet the needs of their catchment areas. For example, in Romania, they have covered no more than 5 percent of the country's exigencies and in Cyprus, they are very limited as well. The same is true in Austria where such care is not adjusted to need. The requisites of the individual Member States are met in varying degrees. The aforementioned problems, including others, such as bureaucratic issues, lack of coordination between general and specialist services, and lack of frameworks directed to patients, must be dealt with, if the supply of services is to meet the demand with quality (Hofmarcher and Quentin 2013; Murray, Sallnou, and Aguiar 2012; Theodorou et al. 2012; Vlădescu et al. 2008).

Extended Care

Reference has been made to the increase in life expectancy and chronic illnesses. It is these, in part, which have called forth the need to develop various types of long-term care across the Member States. All were not prepared to do so. For example, in the Czech Republic, development was delayed because of a lack of tradition of such care. Moreover, it costs less to care for this clientele at home, rather than in institutions and like many other governments, the Czech one was under pressure to trim expenses (Schlanger 2003). According to a recent WHO European region survey, extended care was identified as a major need (Büscher, Sivertsen, and White 2010).

Development of this care not only means an increase in nursing services, but also the provision of appropriate education to enable nurses to effectively undertake their important role in this setting which features a work situation diverse from others. The European Council of Nursing Regulators (FEPI) in a response to the European Commission Green Paper on the European Workforce for Health advocated that education related to the elderly and their specific concerns be obligatory for nurses working in extended care. It also argued that specialist training in areas, such as treatment of dementia and chronic diseases, be mandated as well (European Council of Nursing Regulators n.d.).

It is noteworthy that the scope of professional practice encompasses care in nursing homes in all countries except Estonia. This could be because the Nursing Care Master Plan, drawn up in 2001 and to be implemented in 2015, refers to turning small hospitals into nursing care homes by that date (Büscher, Sivertsen, and White 2010; European Federation of Public Service Unions n.d.). Certainly the necessary changes in norms will have to accompany completion of the task.

Evidently, the above-mentioned FEPI proposals were found agreeable to the Swedish nursing profession. In that nation, elderly care consists of two categories: specialization in dementia care with employment in a group residence based on a specific care philosophy and general care of older people with diverse diagnoses. Studies (Josefssen, Sonde, and Wahlin 2007; Josefsson et al. 2007) of practitioners affiliated with these categories revealed basic differences. Greater knowledge and more emotional and conflicting demands were identified with dementia care. Moreover, nurses working in this sector thought they enjoyed greater opportunity to plan and execute daily work routines than to impact the work situation in a wider context. Also, even though support at work on the part of management and colleagues was generally perceived as favorable, it was believed to be higher in dementia care. Although both sets of nurses possessed a broad range of competence, it could have been more developed for some. Competence development was found to be of much greater significance for those employed in dementia care. Nurses working in general elder care displayed other priorities. Their goals were to achieve greater authority in decision-making of importance and to search for another position. There is no doubt that if extended care is to be of superior quality, competence development is a must.

Often identified with poor working conditions, long-term care is a highly labor-intensive domain. The percentage of nurses working in this sector varies greatly across the EU. Thirty percent of German nurses have been employed in this area, along with 24.7 percent of Danish colleagues and 5 percent each of those from Poland and the United Kingdom (ICN 2007a; Widerszal-Bazyl et al. 2003b). The range is great. Very often in this type of work, those providing care have low qualifications. However, in some Member States, such as Hungary and Germany, staff consists of appropriately qualified personnel. In the former nation, 85 percent of all workers in extended care are registered nurses. On the other hand, in many Member States, fewer than half are in the nursing profession (*Help Wanted?* 2011).

The nursing shortage has unraveled in this domain as well. Recruitment and retention present major obstacles, perhaps more so than in other sectors. Continual recruiting, in part, has been attributed to high levels of sick leave among staff employed in this area (Glenngård et al. 2005). Moreover, in general, it does not engender status and prestige and it fails to enjoy popularity. Work organization has been deemed uninviting, the routine monotonous, the challenges few, and organization and leadership of poor quality. Coupled with a lack of resources and quantitative and qualitative staff deficiencies, these perspectives make it difficult to fulfill needs for extended care across the Member States (Albreht et al. 2009; Kloster, Høie, and Skarr 2007).

Turnover rates and shortages of nurses in this domain are impressive. They are high. If younger nurses are not attracted to this type of employment, it seems that sometimes older ones are. As has occurred in the United States, in some Member States, nurses have drifted to the extended care sector in the latter part of their career. Germany, in introducing these services, redesigned nursing processes, making employment prospects more attractive. However, the shortage continued. Member States, requiring further development in this sector, might learn from this experience. The British Prime Minister's commission concerned with the future of nursing called for recognition of the role of this profession in extended care with the development of care pathways ("PM's Commission" 2010). De Raeve (2009) has forcefully asserted:

> Concerning Quality of Long Term Care, we have still a long way to go. Therefore it is of paramount importance we put in place EU standards of care, standards in education and standards in health outcomes, which once in place, should be met at EU level (p. 2).

This task would furnish ideals for the nursing profession and accomplishment would chart the course for quality-extended care.

Advanced Practice Nursing

Advanced practice nursing, a field of employment for some practitioners, is a relatively new development. Initiated in the United States with nurse anesthetists, clinical nurse specialists, nurse midwives, and primary care practitioners, the concept was hailed and imitated by Europeans. This role has been defined in many ways depending on the clinical context and setting and the culture and nation involved. ICN (2010), in an attempt to bring together various efforts, has defined the advanced practice professional as

> a registered nurse who has acquired the expert knowledge base, complex decision-making skills and clinical competencies for expanded practice, the characteristics of which are shaped by the context and/or country in which s/he is credentialed to practice. A Master's degree is recommended for entry level (p. 1).

In terms of knowledge, this role requires new competences in a specific nursing sector that are superior to those obtained at the preregistration level. In practice, the requisites relate to the amalgamation of research, intra- and interdisciplinary collaboration, professional and clinical leadership, autonomy, clinical expertise, and teaching. At this level, the practitioner is assigned more clinical autonomy, accountability, responsibility, and authority (Irish Nurses Organisation 2006).

As any other element, advanced practice nursing is influenced by the environment in which it is introduced. Its development in a country has been impacted by the supply of physicians and nurses. In Europe, this means that it blossomed faster where there was an inadequate number of the former practitioners and a relatively full supply of the latter, leading to a high nurse-to-physician ratio, as in the United Kingdom and the Netherlands. On the other hand, in the Scandinavian nations and France, this supply was sufficient and often, figuring that there was no need to duplicate care, development of advanced practice nursing was at a slower pace (Delamaire and Lafortune 2010; Schober and Affara 2006). Growth in population, decreased access to health-care services, improvements in nursing competence and education, and efforts on the part of individual nurses to challenge professional role boundaries also nurtured advanced practice nursing (National Council for the Professional Development of Nursing and Midwifery 2005). These practitioners use various titles. They include nurse specialist, professional nurse, expert nurse, nurse consultant, advanced nurse in . . . (name of specialty), nurse practitioner, clinical nurse specialist, and so on.

As the role developed in the various Member States, it is evident that currently there is no consensus as to its definition, required education, use of titles, and the regulations that govern it. There are different conceptual frameworks. There are great divergencies in terms of educational preparation and practice. The recommended master's degree is not always achieved. Often, a postbaccalaureate certificate is sufficient. In the United Kingdom, a bachelor's degree, relevant work experience, and on-the-job training is considered adequate (Delamaire and Lafortune 2010). Role functions, scope of practice, and role evaluations are diverse. These differences are not only evident across Member States. Often, there are large ones between subdivisions of a single nation (Björnsdóttir and Thome 2006; Irish Nurses Organisation 2006).

The term advanced practice nursing is really a catch-all or umbrella phrase, indicating nurses practicing at a higher level, but it is not used in consistent fashion. The scope of practice and competences expected are not clear. It is acknowledged that the nursing care provided is expert in nature. Moreover, the professional has expanded competence in a specific field, often including diagnosing, prescribing examinations, tests, and medicines; initiating nursing care and treatment, monitoring patients with chronic illnesses, and coordinating care, to cite some activities. Schober and Affara (2006) have commented:

> What emerges . . . is a pattern of confusion and different interpretations as to what is advanced nursing practice. The large number of titles in use, a lack of agreement over the routes and standards of education and no clear consensus over scope of practice make it difficult to define a clear and distinctive identity for APNs [advanced practice nurses] (p. 13).

This evaluation is still applicable. In each Member State, there are many diverse categories of these practitioners and even more so across the EU.

With the shift from hospital to primary care, it was found necessary to develop community-based nursing. The need was believed to be particularly urgent in the newly acceded Member States. It was in this environment that a new figure on the advanced practice nursing scene, the family health nurse, was born. Launched by WHO in 2000, this role has realized limited acceptance. Only ten of the Member States—Austria, Cyprus, Estonia, Finland, Germany, Greece, Poland, Portugal, Slovenia, and Scotland—have adopted it. Building on the foundation of public health nursing, it was envisioned that health promotion and prevention would be introduced to community settings with the employment of a family systemic approach and a focus on resources and problems in social units. Advanced practice nurses, family health nurses, by visiting, accompanying, advising, supporting, and empowering vulnerable groups would garner their access to a wide variety of social and health services. In this manner, the negative impact of socioeconomic factors on this population would be tempered (Mischke, Schrader, and Schüssler 2006; Thomson et al. 2014). While reinforcing the focus on public health and health promotion, the family health nurse still furnishes curative and palliative services. What was innovative was the manner in which these various aspects of care are combined with stress on the family unit, broadly defined. Also, consumers' participation in the search for responses to their health needs is expected. The various methods related to health promotion and disease prevention used to reach diverse populations were considered novel as well (*Report on the Second WHO Ministerial Conference* 2001).

In some instances, experiences with this advanced practice nurse have been quite successful, as in Estonia. Within primary care teams the role has garnered importance. Moreover, these nurses have assumed some of physicians' responsibilities related to chronic conditions, healthy newborns, pregnancy, etc. Their number of consultations with patients has increased dramatically. In fact, a shortage of these practitioners has been declared (Kopel et al. 2008). Achievements are not as full in some other Member States where prior to the implementation of the family health nurse, roles of nurses already included a family and public health focus. Consequently, tensions arose as professionals already on the scene were uncertain as to how the new arrivals would affect their function. Also, region enters the picture. In urban areas, where a multiplicity of other services is available, for nurses, it is more difficult to implant this role. On the other hand, in rural areas, the task is much easier because access to services is a continuing issue of concern. The function of this figure is congruent with primary health care and community-based health care policy (Büscher, Sivertsen, and White 2010).

Along with a host of other specialties, such as psychiatric, pediatric, and geriatric nursing, advanced practice nursing includes the roles of the clinical nurse specialist and the nurse practitioner, both of which were born in the United States in the 1960s and evolved concurrently. These roles, requiring a setting that appreciates multidisciplinary efforts, resulted from the need to contain costs, enlarge access to healthcare services, reduce waiting time, provide for the underprivileged, and control the health of certain social categories. They too were nurtured by a physician shortage and in the United Kingdom especially, by the Working Time Directive, which regulates working hours throughout the EU. There are clinical specialists in all the principal clinical sectors, and also some who are experts in cancer and perinatal nursing, ostomies, neurological matters, respiratory problems, and other subspecialties. Ongoing experience with patients and their support systems leads to participation in subroles, including direct care research, education, consultation, and management. Much effort is devoted to quality assurance, policy development, and peer review, all activities related to the maintenance of a superior health-care delivery system. The fundamental element in this type of practice is continuous patient involvement with stress on nursing as opposed to a medical care model (Joel 2011).

The nurse practitioner's role is based on knowledge and skills that at one time were viewed as the exclusive province of medicine. For the nurse, this means new areas of service were combined with the nursing role to create a comprehensive practice necessitating collaboration and consultation with physicians and a galaxy of other health-care professionals. The nurse practitioner has the capacity to perform a primary care role and to serve as the first and continuing contact for the consumer within the health-care delivery system. This professional is prepared to undertake a wide variety of activities, including health promotion, disease prevention, diagnoses and treatment of minor acute illnesses, health-care maintenance, and the monitoring and management of stabilized chronic conditions. The nurse practitioners' divisions of practice, including pediatrics, family practice, geriatrics, and adult and women's health, to cite a few, are broader than those of the clinical nurse specialists who often have more circumscribed specialties and subspecialties. These practice areas have featured oncology, geropsychiatry, as well as neurological and medical–surgical nursing. Most recently, the distinction between the clinical nurse specialist and the nurse practitioner has become somewhat blurred.

The nurse practitioner role has a longer history in the United Kingdom than in other Member States. It has been developed in several others, including Ireland, Germany, the Netherlands, France, Belgium, and Sweden, to cite a few. Others, such as Denmark and Finland, have expressed a desire to develop the position. In Germany, after reunification, the role of the nurse practitioner was instituted with aid from the European Social Fund, one of the EU's Structural Funds used to support employment opportunities in the Member States. This professional was utilized in pilot projects, at first, in eastern rural areas to provide primary care with the assistance of eHealth technology and to improve patient access to basic medical services. Primary care physicians were in short supply and distances between care localities and patients were great (Blum 2006). A survey by the Royal College of Nursing (2006) revealed that, according to respondents, core components of the role relate to compiling comprehensive histories, taking autonomous decisions, assessing patients' health needs, doing physical examinations, making new/initial diagnoses and differential ones as well. The main focus of the role, regardless of the site of practice, which includes hospitals, primary care facilities, walk-in centers, telehealth, long-term care institutions, physicians' offices and others, is providing clinical care to patients. The holistic nature of the care offered is of utmost significance.

A major problem has been a lack of awareness and understanding of the nurse practitioner's function. Thus, many of these professionals have felt that their role has not been utilized to its full potential. At the same time, they are of the opinion that their efforts have been limited by restrictions on nurses' prescribing privileges and the issuance of requests for imaging (National Council for the Professional Development of Nursing and Midwifery 2005; Royal College of Nursing 2006). As for all types of nurses, for nurse practitioners, time pressures are weighty. Implementation of the role requires the cooperation of physicians and employers. In many instances, as in the United States, the former were not always supportive of the concept. This was the case in the Netherlands where payers also joined the opposition. Other stakeholders, such as the media, consumers, civil society, and governmental institutions, have held more positive attitudes (van Dijk 2003). Often, it is general practitioners who feel threatened with the implementation of the nurse practitioner figure. In general, many have preferred to work with a nurse having only basic preregistration education. Hostility was also engendered from the nursing profession itself. With the assumption of some medical tasks, it was charged that these advanced practitioners were selling out and trying to become junior physicians (Schober and Affara 2006). Moreover, they were accused of stressing cure rather than the care traditionally identified with the profession.

On the positive side, evaluations have indicated that this advanced clinician has reaped success in terms of significant contributions to patient care. Services provided have been judged timely, holistic, superior in quality, cost effective, and comprehensive in nature. Moreover, nurse practitioners have become important members of multidisciplinary teams and have been widely applauded by patients (National Council for the Professional Development of Nursing and Midwifery 2005, 2007). In terms of quality of service, it has been found that they allow for longer consultations and greater continuity of care. For physicians, the existence of this figure reduces the workload and furnishes time for activities they had difficulty accomplishing previously. In terms of costs, there are financial benefits as well. Task delegation from physicians to these specialists has maintained or increased the quality of care. In addition, the continuity of care has been enhanced and the substitution of physician care by nursing care has not resulted. It has been affirmed that if work relates to specialized nursing duties, it is most likely an addition to the duties of physicians, rather than a substitution. When a medical task is carried out, substitution might be greater (Groenewegen 2008). It has been demonstrated that role substitution has had a positive influence on patient outcomes and experiences. Nurse practitioners enhance the accessibility and availability of primary care. In addition, they are important contributors to its quality. Moreover, research has indicated that these professionals and general practitioners provide comparable care (Dierick-van Daele et al. 2009, 2010). In short, the benefits of utilizing nurse practitioners are several and they have been recognized.

The clinical nurse specialist role has been created in Ireland, Malta, and the United Kingdom and is in the process of being developed in Belgium and Germany. These professionals, primarily based in hospitals, offer support to staff nurses, patients, project leaders, and quality control managers. They contribute specialist knowledge and skills to the workplace in terms of the assessment, planning, provision, and evaluation of care. They are involved in patient and staff education, the development of care protocols and standards, the improvement of the quality of care through support of evidence-based practice, and the facilitation of system change. Their role necessitates that they relate to both medical and paramedical professionals. In addition, they are expected to undertake research and audit activities and to act as consultants to their colleagues and multidisciplinary teams for educational and clinical practice matters. The role is based on a direct and indirect clinical focus, patient advocacy, education and training, audit and research activities, and inter- and intradisciplinary consultation. Leadership pervades all facets of their duties and responsibilities are broad in nature. These professionals have experienced difficulty in allotting time to all these activities, due to the pressures of meeting clinical demands. Time for research has been especially scarce. Research undertaken, for the most part, focuses on patients, but much also relates to the specific role in question. Research and audit activities have been the least well-developed aspects of the role (Delamaire and Lafortune 2010; National Council for the Professional Development of Nursing and Midwifery 2007).

As in the case of nurse practitioners, initially, there was a lack of understanding of this function which led to little cooperation from relevant stakeholders. In addition, being new, it was not universally defined and thus, much ambiguity resulted. Moreover, this new professional at the workplace raised suspicion and skepticism. These barriers to role development, among others, had to be overcome. Networking on a local, regional, and national basis was of great utility, along with the construction of strong interdisciplinary working relationships, both formal and informal, internal and external to the workplace. Networking was particularly important because the risk of remaining isolated at the workplace was great. The motto in Ireland was: "Our job is to empower, not to take away from other staff" (National Council for the Professional Development of Nursing and Midwifery 2004). In spite of the initial hurdles encountered, clinical nurse specialists have realized success. Their role and performance have received accolades from many quarters. Directors of nursing, staff nurses, other health-care providers, patients, and clients have unanimously recognized their merits. It appears that these professionals have responded to service demands in a flexible and innovative manner.

The practice of prescribing and administering medicinal products has often accompanied the development of advanced practice nursing, as in the United Kingdom, Spain, Ireland, and Sweden. However, it is not operative in all Member States. For example, Danish nurses are not allowed to independently prescribe medicines. The development of prescriptive authority is related to an increase in professional spe-cialization, lack of access to appropriate health care in underserved and rural areas, a decrease in the supply of physicians, and an increase in the quantity of advanced practice nurses (An Bord Altranais and National Council for the Professional Development of Nursing and Midwifery 2005; Irish Nurses and Midwives Organisation 2013).

Limits to this prescriptive authority are fashioned by the model uti-lized and the legislative and professional norms of a nation. Prescribing models include independent prescribing, collaborative or multidisci-plinary prescribing, group protocols, involving written guidelines for the supply and administration of medications to distinct groups of patients, and time and dose prescribing. All require professional and legal responsibility on the part of the nurse performing the adopted model's requirements. The requisites for nurse prescribing qualifica-tions vary from nation to nation and, as in other cases, there can be diversity within a country. In general, some type of postregistration education is required. There is no fixed standard. Evaluations of this practice have been most positive. It has proven to be cost effective. Consumers have reacted enthusiastically because of the approachability of the practitioners, the nature of encounters with them, and the con-venience and saving of time offered by this practice. Moreover, it was found that patients' medication management showed improvement (An Bord Altranais and National Council for the Professional Development of Nursing and Midwifery 2005).

Advanced practice nurses represent a small proportion of all practi-tioners. Working in numerous settings, they provide important services to disparate populations. Regardless of their title or site of employment, they have definitely proven their worth from a variety of perspectives and, at the same time, have enhanced their influence on the health-care delivery system. However, given the lack of consensus pertaining to definition of role, educational preparation and qualification, use of titles, and regulation, cacophony, not symphonies, pervade their stage throughout the Member States. The EU's focus on the development of the internal market dictates that the nursing profession, in collaboration with it, rectifies this deficiency related to advanced practice.

Walk-In Centers and Telehealth Nursing

Updating of health-care delivery systems in some Member States, such as Sweden, Ireland, and the United Kingdom, included the introduction of telehealth nursing and walk-in centers. These resulted from concern with out-of-hours services and general access to health care, caused partially by an increased number of females in the medical profession which influenced working hours, enhanced consumer expectations, and remote areas' lack of attractiveness as a site for health-care providers' practices, among other factors (Hartmann, Ulmann, and Rochai 2006). These innovative and important methods of providing care are usually carried out by nurses working in advanced and specialized roles.

Walk-in centers in the United Kingdom were launched in 2000. Enlarging access channels to care, they are located in supermarkets, shopping malls, subway stations, and other sites which attract large numbers of people on a daily basis. In these settings, nurses undertake health promotion activities, treatment of minor health problems, and provision of information and advice on illnesses and various local services. Walk-in centers have been found to be particularly useful to the elderly and for palliative and end-of-life care (Bourgueil, Marek, and Mousques 2005; Johnson 2011).

Equally as innovative as walk-in centers are the nurse-led telephone triage services, originally established in England in 1998. In this Member State, they are known as NHS Direct (National Health Service Direct). In Scotland, they were born as NHS24 and in Wales as NHS Direct Wales. These units offer consultation on line and by telephone around the clock. Nurses direct patients toward the appropriate health-care structure or, if necessary, they aid in solving the problem (Bourgueil, Marek, and Mousques 2005; Longley et al. 2012). In Sweden, there are similar arrangements. Nurses employed in these sites undertake triage as well. Performing this function, these professionals join physicians as gatekeepers to the health-care delivery system. In fact, it offers the nursing profession a new power base.

Employment in telehealth has presented its challenge to nurses. Swedish practitioners have often been perturbed by "second-hand consultations," meaning they are unable to speak directly with the person seeking aid. Instead, they are forced to communicate via a third person. Such a process makes decision-making that much more difficult. Not seeing the patient and perceiving the unspoken, frequently create uneasiness. Appropriate decisions must be made from the caller's description of symptoms. Remedies include training in active listening for decision-making purposes and training to understand callers from different cultures in order to avoid social conflict (Wahlberg, Cederound, and Wredling 2003).

These units have been successful primarily because of the staffs' high degree of specialization in certain chronic pathologies, such as diabetes, asthma, and hypertension. In the United Kingdom, nursing advisors are equipped with at least five years' experience making clinical assessments and offering advice. In addition, they have been prepared for this type of employment by participation in an intensive training course (Hartmann, Ulmann, and Rochai 2006). These programs have led to more appropriate use of health-care services. Furthermore, they have received accolades from trade unions, governmental authorities, and most important, from their users (Buchan and Calman 2005; Com-Ruelle, Midy, and Ulmann 2000).

Independent Practice: The Self-Employed

Another employment option for nurses is self-employment or independent practice. This opportunity is not available in all Member States. However, it is permitted in some, such as France, Poland, Belgium, Estonia, Romania, Austria, the Czech Republic, Portugal, Germany, Bulgaria, Croatia, Hungary, the United Kingdom, and Slovakia. Even though Maltese licensed paramedical professionals are not permitted to practice independently, some, including nurses, informally do. Sometimes, before undertaking employment in this capacity, certain requisites have to be met. For example, in the Czech Republic, a nurse needs ten years of training prior to being able to practice independently. There has been discussion to shorten this period to seven years. Demands are less in France, where the professional experience requirement is a minimum of twenty-four months. For the most part, self-employment is not especially prevalent throughout the Member

States ("Czech Hospital Nurses" 2009; European Working Conditions Observatory 2014; Muscat and Grech 2006; www.infirmiers.com).

Nurses working in this sector practice their profession in a variety of ways. First of all, they can create their own firms. In Poland, the government, in an attempt to limit the consequences of the serious employment repercussions resulting from modifications in the health sector, initiated a retrenchment support program, a phase of which offered credit to nurses for the purpose of establishing private practices (Domagala et al. 1999). There are also opportunities to provide services based on individual contract. These can be negotiated with physicians' offices, insurance companies, sickness funds, health authorities, and other institutions in the public and private sectors. It is quite common for physicians to sign contracts with nursing practices or to collaborate with them in the delivery of services. In Poland, when the self-employed sign contracts with health insurance funds, they are granted certain privileges awarded to private health-care providers. These include permission to prescribe pharmaceuticals at reduced prices. Freelance nurses also act as entrepreneurs in areas such as spas, travel health, and cosmetic treatments. In Estonia, self-employed nurses have faced restrictions. School health services, which have not been clearly defined or adequately funded, have represented the one area in which they have been able to operate their practice, provided they are specially qualified, even though they are marginalized (Jesse et al. 2004; Strózik 2006).

Increasingly, self-employed nurses fulfill a substantial part of rehabilitation and home care needs. This seems to be the case in Belgium, France, and Germany. As part of a relatively recent reform in France, the role of these practitioners in the management and coordination of care for dependent patients has been reinforced. They became responsible for the development of nursing care plans that integrate health and social care for this population. Improvement in care was to result from enhanced coordination between various professions. In addition, the independent practitioners' role was further strengthened with the transfer of greater responsibility to them related to the management and coordination of care for the elderly. These professionals were also assigned new limited prescribing privileges and authority to perform a number of tasks previously reserved to physicians (van der Boom 2008; Midy 2003a; Naiditch 2007). The role and position of French self-employed nurses has definitely expanded in regard to health care and social services.

Independent practice seems to be gaining in popularity, especially in France and Germany. In the latter Member State, since the introduction of long-term nursing care insurance, the number of self-employed nurses has steadily increased. In France, as soon as they have met the requirements for this type of employment, 4 percent of recent graduates usually leave their position in favor of independent practice. The self-employed have accounted for 14.6 percent of French nurses (Chevreul et al. 2010; Marquier 2005; Sicart 2006). On the other hand, in Hungary and Poland, the rate has been much less, ranging between .54 percent and 1 percent. Interestingly enough, nurse practitioners, for the most part, tend to prefer community-based clinical settings over private practice. The quantity of independent practice nurses varies greatly from one Member State to another. The proportion working in entrepreneurial roles is far from large. Not very many are involved in large-scale developments, such as heading new provider organizations or becoming full partners in general practice arrangements (Currie, Chiarella, and Buckley 2013; *Front Line Care* 2010; Ordem dos Enfermeiros 2011; www.eski.hu). As opposed to their colleagues working in other situations, independent practitioners, to a large extent, work on a fee-for-service basis. Financial reimbursement and the nature of existing legislation represent significant challenges for nurse practitioners. To maintain the attractiveness of this employment site, a recent Belgian contract specified that discrimination must be avoided between independent and salaried nurses since they perform the same tasks.

It is generally acknowledged that nurses working in this capacity enjoy job satisfaction. However, some negative aspects, similar to those of their colleagues employed in other sectors, have been identified. These include heavy workloads, especially the administrative facets, and difficulty in finding substitutes when needed. Moreover, dealing with a patient in this setting differs from the same in another. For example, in the hospital, activity is team-oriented, well-codified, and ordered according to a system, whereas for the self-employed this does not hold true (Midy 2003b).

Agency and Bank Nursing

Given the magnitude of recruitment and retention problems for nurses and the use of recruitment moratoria from time to time, health-care institutions have had to increasingly rely on a specific facet of the internal labor market in the form of bank nurses as well as the external labor supply industry and its agency nurses. Staffing agencies are entities that provide a wide variety of health-care facilities with nursing staff for temporary or supplemental assignments. On the other hand, the bank, having the same scope, is operated by the health-care institution itself and consists of an internal temporary register of nurses containing the names of practitioners known to it, often former staff members or even professionals from its own permanently employed nursing workforce, who also provide their services on an on-call basis (Hardill and MacDonald 2000; Purcell, Purcell, and Tailby 2004). A large part of the literature pertaining to these units refers to the situation in the United Kingdom. There seems to be a paucity of case studies or comparative research in this area focusing on EU Member States.

Both bank and agency nursing are important to meeting staffing needs. For some nurses, they are the equivalent of a second job and for others, their main employment. Nurses selecting this type of undertaking do so for several reasons. Primarily, they are interested in a flexible work schedule and being able to control their working hours. They want to be able to choose when to work and have a choice in work assignment, even if they have to sacrifice a higher stipend. Then, there are those practitioners who want to supplement their salary and thus, work independently. Sometimes, the choice is made on the basis of a desire to avoid institutional politics or even to make certain that a main work unit, often one's own, has adequate staff. In addition, practitioners without a permanent post often desire to maintain their professional skills (Ball and Pike 2006b; Cowart and Speake 1992; Review Body for Nursing and Other Health Professions 2007).

This type of nursing has definitely increased in significance for health-care institutions. Even though it represents a solution to nagging and continuous problems, there are issues of concern for nursing practice and nursing personnel. Managers often find it more arduous to control and monitor nursing practice with part of the staff exempt from institutional sanctions and rewards. Members of the permanent workforce often have to assume additional responsibilities related to the orientation of supplemental colleagues, the care of more complex patients and the execution of organizational administrative routines concerned with forms, requisitions, reporting, and the like. These burdens potentially can lower morale and generate resentment. Both managers and nurses on staff seem to agree that a prime concern relates to quality control (Purcell, Purcell, and Tailby 2004). Supplemental nurses, like any others, vary in quality, experience, and personal competence. Sometimes, doubts have been raised about their qualifications.

Nursing practice issues involve inexperience, medication errors, and lack of continuity in patient care, all matters that carry implications for the quality of services.

Nurses providing supplemental staffing frequently experience lack of support from other personnel and exclusion from a health-care team. They are often perceived as outsiders and relationships with permanent staff members can be strained. This creates difficulties for managers. Shifts in assignments provide diverse experiences for the practitioner working in this capacity, but they can have negative implications for the patient who, receiving services from different nurses, might have to bear the brunt of a lack of continuity in staffing and nursing care. Furthermore, shifts in assignments can make supplemental nurses more vulnerable to committing errors. Studies have revealed that reliance on these practitioners has led to higher workplace accident rates attributed to a lack of familiarity with on-site personnel and equipment that impacts negatively on teamwork and communication, reducing the quality of care (Bourbonniere et al. 2006; Institute of Medicine of the National Academies 2004). The cost to an institution of reliance on this type of personnel is debatable. There is a lack of consensus as to whether the saving costs of longevity related to vacations, pensions, raises in salary etc., fringe benefits, and related administrative costs offset the expenses of orientation, possible low productivity, required extra supervision and coordination, and decreased morale of regular staff.

The accountability of agency nurses has raised concerns. The question is to whom do they feel more accountable—the institution where they are working or the agency that placed them there? Lack of support on the part of other staff members can be interpreted as lack of institutional support. This reaps implications for supplemental nurses, particularly inexperienced ones, who may seek support elsewhere. An obvious point would be the staffing agency. If they manifest more accountability to the agency, relationships with the health-care institution can be damaged and if allegiance to the latter is dominant, they can antagonize the agency and possibly risk being released by it (Hood and Leddy 2006). There is the potential for the development of a catch-22. A balancing act is required.

From the nurses' perspective, those employed in this type of work have expressed positives and negatives. Like their colleagues in other sectors, stress is a part of their working life. However, its magnitude is said to be greater because of a lack of familiarity with the workplace and the possibility of being the only qualified nurse in an unfamiliar unit. Another ingredient of stress is the resentment exhibited by regular staff members. The lack of opportunities for professional development and promotion has also been cited along with job insecurity and not being part of a team. In addition, there is a preoccupation that this type of work might have a negative impact on one's career, in general, and specifically, on possibilities for permanent employment. Evaluations from nurses in advanced practice are more positive. With the demand for their services being so great, they have been, so to speak, in the driver's seat, being able to dictate a wide range of stipulations concerning their employment, including such things as schedules and assignments. They claim a relatively stress-free environment in comparison to that of their regular employment (Arnold et al. 2003; Ball and Pike 2006b; Purcell, Purcell, and Tailby 2004).

Nurses working as agency or bank nurses are involved in a sphere with employment conditions that differ significantly from those of their colleagues hired on a regular basis in various types of health-care facilities. The European Commission was of the opinion that the working conditions of persons employed in this capacity should be "at least those that would apply if they had been recruited directly by [the] enterprise to occupy the same job" (Forde and Slater 2005, p. 250). The result of this concern was Directive 2008/104/EC which underscored the principle of equal treatment for these employees.

Other Employment Choices

A frequent practice in some Member States, is to work in a couple at the same time. For example, many Polish nurses live and work in Poland and also commute to posts in Germany. Their Estonian colleagues have engaged in the same practice. They work certain days of the week in Estonia, according to a shift system, and then also offer their services in Finland, Sweden, or Norway. Also, as noted, there is the same mobility between Luxembourg and neighboring countries and also between Spain and Portugal (Kautoch and Czabanowska 2011; Lai et al. 2013; López-Valcárcel, Pérez, and Quintana 2011; Saar and Habicht 2011). Then, throughout the EU, it is known that nurses often hold second jobs. Many public service employees hold second jobs in the private sector or work in a self-employed capacity.

In a few Member States, numerous nurses have assumed positions on the very periphery of the health sector, primarily for financial reasons. As of 2009, in Estonia, this constituency represented 25 percent of the nursing workforce which was employed in health spas, beauty salons, and other facets of the service sector. Such a practice bears more consequences for the sustainability of the health-care system than migration. The same relates to Hungarian nurses who participate in cosmetic and fitness endeavors in Austria. They provide massage, chiropody and manicuring services, among others. Hungarian hospital managers are aware of this activity and in order to keep these nurses as employees, they provide flexible work schedules. Somewhat different is the Croatian situation. Nurses are employed in spas and medicinal mud baths. Using natural mineral springs, they provide preventive, curative, and rehabilitation services (*Human Resources* 2008; *Hungary-Austria: Nursing Emergency* 2006; Saar and Habicht 2011; Vŏncina et al. 2006).

Skill Mix

The number of nurses in an area is important, but the key is to have the appropriate number of these professionals employed in various capacities, some of which have been discussed here, in the right place at the right time and in possession of the right skills. In any health-care setting, to deliver quality services, it is of utmost significance to have the proper mix of skills for the job that has to be completed. Moreover, those practicing their profession should ideally be well-educated and trained, highly motivated, and adequately distributed and supervised. Geographical deployment and skill mix furnish the foundation for nursing services of superior quality.

Defined as "the combination or grouping of different categories of workers, that is employed for the provision of care to patients" (McGillis-Hall 1997, p. 31), skill mix relates to the competences of an individual practitioner, the ratio of senior to junior grade staff in a single profession, and the combination of different professions within a multiprofessional team. The term may also refer to personnel from either a national or subnational perspective. Furthermore, it may imply the combination of activities or capacities necessary for each position within an organization (Buchan and Dal Poz 2002). Currently, skill mix is on the center stage of most Member States' health-care delivery system. Its importance has been underscored by modifications in the ways used and structures in which services are provided. As noted, primary and other care in the community has experienced rapid development as have complex medical and surgical procedures performed in hospitals, necessitating a larger and more sophisticated workforce. Reference must also be made to the restrictions of the Working Time

Directive, budget constraints, cost efficiency, shortages of certain provider groups, their incorrect deployment, underqualified or misqualified staff, the need for quality improvement, and changes in other health-care professions. These elements have been some of the drivers necessitating an enhanced focus on skill mix and work redesign. The nursing profession, as a result, presents a new face.

Decisions concerning skill mix must be viewed in light of the framework in which they are taken. Even though workforce planning has been labeled "at best an inexact science" (Buchan 2007), there are several contextual elements which influence its course. Thus, human resource planning requires dealing with a wide array of issues, including the broader political, regulatory, professional, and work environment; resource availability, culture, custom, practice, power of the various health-care professionals, current configuration of the health-care delivery system and the demographic characteristics of its workforce, and service delivery needs. The pieces to the puzzle are many and the elements are complex. Any of them can either facilitate or hinder change in the skill mix. In short, skill mix is determined by the organizational and systemic context, but, at the same time, it is a determinant of this framework. Influence is reciprocal (Buchan and Dal Poz 2002).

These contextual factors assume an importance at three different levels: the macrolevel, the mesolevel, and the microlevel, all of which are used to make skill mix decisions. At the macrolevel, the influence of regulations related to scope of practice and economic factors assume importance. The mesolevel is of significance when a skill mix program is being established and it relates to the setting and its impact on desired objectives. Last, the microlevel concerns the day-to-day staffing of a profession involved in the skill mix project, including its interprofessional relations with colleagues. Factors at all three levels are involved in the outcome of skill mix decisions.

As it happens, at times these three levels are not always synchronized, as in Spain, where it is difficult to coordinate the centralized regulation of professional education, training, and working conditions with the decentralized system of health-care delivery. Practices governing wages, industrial relations, and the negotiation of working conditions are affiliated with the civil service system as established by the central government. As a result, health-care managers at the meso- and microlevels have practically no flexibility in experimenting with diverse staffing models, tailoring incentives, and developing professional commitment to a skill mix formula. Germany finds itself in similar circumstances (Bourgeault et al. 2008). Center–periphery relations are critical to the outcome of skill mix practices.

Recognizing the significance of context to skill mix decision-making, global associations of diverse health-care professionals, representing over 25 million of these providers, including midwives, nurses, pharmacists, physical therapists, dentists, and physicians, have issued a joint statement on the subject. According to these professionals, such policies should be country-specific and should be made giving consideration to the above-mentioned factors. In other words, there is no "one-size-fits-all" model.

There are a variety of approaches used in skill mix decision-making, ranging from task-based analysis that focuses on the transfer of tasks between professionals and conditions necessary to assure quality to the role-based approach, concerned with the total number of nursing hours required per patient day and the proportion of registered nurses to total nursing staff. The latter is more widely used (International Centre for Human Resources in Nursing 2009b). Most often, a variety of methods is adopted and it is assumed that quality, safety, and cost effectiveness are in the equation.

Rather than creating a comprehensive strategy concerned with wages, working conditions, and recruitment and retention issues, most skill mix efforts are centered on established training numbers and related costs. In fact, most Member States, instead of assuming a proactive stance, are reactive in that they respond to skill mix problems in their acute and politically sensitive stage (Dussault et al. 2010). Moreover, it has been noted that few efforts include a strong economic facet. As a consequence, the economic rationale for decisions taken, especially in the context of this global economic downturn, is less weighty than it might be. Economic modeling, evaluations, and randomized controlled trials would aid in making cost/quality tradeoffs and titrations of staff members and staff qualifications (Rafferty and Clarke 2009).

Work redesign, as part of skill mix, has become a sign of the times. Nursing in a variety of settings, having become a prime target for such efforts, has undergone a recent transformation in roles. Trends in the Member States have changed the way in which nurses, in particular, and all health-care professionals, in general, work. There are several techniques to redesign the professional role. In that the boundaries between nursing and medical care have always been fluid, these mechanisms have, to a large extent, focused on the relationship between these two professions, often giving rise to professional disputes. One method to change roles is enhancement, meaning an increase in the depth of a position via an extension of the role or the skills of a particular category of provider. For the most part, enhancement efforts have focused mostly on nurses. Substitution is another mechanism that is often utilized. It involves an expansion in the breadth of a position, especially by working across professional boundaries or by exchanging one category of worker for another. Delegation comes about when a task is moved either up or down a traditional unidisciplinary scale to arrive in the purview of another provider. Innovation is a vehicle that brings about new positions, via the creation of a new type of provider, for example, the health-care assistant. These mechanisms have been used to directly transform roles. Indirectly, they have been modified with changes in the interface between services, that is, where they are furnished (Bourgeault et al. 2008; Buchan and Calman 2005; McKee, Dubois, and Sibbald 2006).

Task shifting has taken place primarily between nurses and physicians, but also between nurses and nursing auxiliaries and others. As noted, nurses have assumed responsibility for some tasks previously located solely in the medical domain. This has raised questions about the separation of nursing from caring, and thus, detraction from professional advancement. In addition, enhanced technical competence affiliated with professional growth may distance practitioners from those for whom they care (Bach n.d.-a; Kirpal 2003; McDonald, Campbell, and Lester 2009). When a task has been transferred from one professional domain to another, both undergo change as does their power on the health-care delivery stage. Professions are constantly undergoing change and practices at the workplace do not fail to create new relationships for them. New roles can be perceived as a threat and thus, it is important that all professions affected by skill mix decision-making be included in the process. This could make acceptance of an outcome, even if it is a bitter pill to swallow, that much easier. Also, this practice is useful in building good will. Trade unions form another sector to be involved. In the Member States, skill mix changes, spurred by economic and qualitative incentives, have relied on diverse mixtures of the aforementioned mechanisms in a variety of settings with different outcomes.

Once a skill mix has been decided upon, the job is not finished. Very often, role conflict and ambiguity arise in settings that have experienced work redesign. This situation has been known to contribute to error production circumstances, the reason being departures from established routines (Page 2004). Health-care providers have to be adequately oriented to the new environment so as to avoid such situations.

In addition, legislation and regulatory provisions must be made congruent with the agreed upon skill mix. Professional education and training qualifications, roles and responsibilities, working conditions, remuneration, career opportunities, available support, and codes of ethics are some elements that need to be addressed. Concern has also been evidenced about scope of practice as it relates to transfer of tasks. Debates on the subject usually focus on specific duties, such as prescribing, and thus, do not value to the fullest professional judgment and competence. On the other hand, the United Kingdom's approach to the matter is rather unique. The regulatory framework allows for enlarged practice following exhaustive and professional reflection and decision-making. The framework recognizes the elevated competence of nurses and their obligation to take decisions in the best interest of patients (Büscher, Sivertsen, and White 2010). This approach is slowly being regarded as worthy of consideration elsewhere. Malta's scope of professional practice (Malta: Council for Nurses and Midwives 2002) is of the same spirit. It allows individual practitioners to formulate their specific roles in accordance with their personal perceived knowledge and experience. The practice in both the United Kingdom and Malta recognizes the professionalism of nursing and allows for the increased flexibility in exercising the nursing profession that is necessary in the contemporary health-care environment. The planning of nursing human resources, like that in other professions, is complex. However, if done appropriately, the benefits are many for service providers, employers, patients, and society as a whole.

The Public and Private Sectors

Nurses have a galaxy of opportunities for employment, only some of which have been presented here. However, those mentioned provide the reader a notion of the employment scene which in all Member States is divided between the public and private sectors. Although complete and detailed data on the subject referring to the Member States is not available, it is quite evident that nurses have a clear preference for work in the public sector. In Ireland 95 percent of these professionals are identified with this line of work and in Sweden 92 percent, in Denmark 87 percent, in Finland 86 percent, in the United Kingdom, Slovenia, and Cyprus 80 percent, in France 78 percent, in Poland 72 percent, and in

Germany 60 percent (Albreht 2011; ICN 2007a; International Council of Nurses Workforce Forum 2013; LeLan 2004; Pike and Williams 2008; Sagan et al. 2011; Theodorou et al. 2012). The pattern has been established. Sometimes, as in Portugal, where only a few professionals work exclusively in the private sector, health-care providers, including nurses, work in both sectors simultaneously.

Public sector nurses in some Member States are automatically a part of the civil service system. This happens in Cyprus, Portugal, Greece, Malta, and, as noted, Spain. It means that recruitment and job placement contrast with practices familiar to many American nurses. Health-care professionals in Cyprus are allocated to employment sites via a centralized system. They are only allowed to move if a vacancy exists. However, the picture of the relationship between a facility's need and the alleged lobbying related to the distribution of health-care providers has been somewhat hazy or blurred (Golna et al. 2004). The Greek civil service also embraces employees of the National Health Service. It has been contended that it "lacks the tradition, organizational coherence, status, class assets and expertise commonly associated with West European civil services" (Davaki and Mossialos 2005, p. 146).

The case of Spain is unique. Nurses are in possession of rights similar to those of civil servants. They garner access to public sector employment on the basis of their results on a mandatory examination. Once they secure entrance, they are granted a permanent position. One of the labor rights they enjoy is ownership of one's position, a regulation originating in the Franco era. In Malta, as well, nurses in the public sector are subject to the Public Service Management Code, meaning that all employment conditions, including promotions are in the domain of a central unit, the Public Service Commission. Portuguese nurses working for the National Health Service have civil servant status as well and thus, the standard civil servants' career path (Barros, Machado, and Simões 2011; López-Valcárcel, Quintana, and Socorro 2006; Muscat et al. 2014; Muscat and Grech 2006).

In some Member States, the employment of nurses in the private sector has blossomed. For example, Cyprus underwent this experience and it was interpreted as a manifestation of greater utilization of richer nursing staffs in this setting. The same occurred in Greece and was attributed to the deficiencies and lack of competitiveness of public health services, due to extreme underfunding (Golna et al. 2004; Tountas et al. 2005). In several Member States, such as France and Spain, nurses employed in the private sector frequently wend their way, as soon as they are able, to employment in public institutions. The path traveled usually leads from the private to the public arena, but not necessarily in all instances. In Sweden, many nurses working in public elder care services deserted them and sought employment in the private sector. In fact, the traffic on this road tripled ("Editorial" 2008; Josefsson et al. 2007; Marquier 2005). However, as noted, often, geriatric care is perceived as not the most appealing place to work from a variety of perspectives. Also, of note, is the fact that frequently, as in Spain, the public and private sectors compete for practitioners with various incentives, such as job security, higher wages, enlarged clinical freedom, and the like (López-Valcárcel, Pérez, and Quintana 2011).

Professional Practice: Work Styles

Nursing, being a social institution, cannot be abstracted from the society in which it operates. There is variance from country to country in the manner in which roles are interpreted and executed. Culture definitely impacts nursing practice and, in part, accounts for diversity in diagnosis, assessment, and intervention strategies as well as the methods nurses invoke to mediate conflict, communicate, or interpret different behaviors. Throughout the Member States, nurses, educated in the same manner, bearing the same titles, and working in the same field, but affiliated with varied cultures, will practice diversely. Even though there is a general consensus as to the notion of caring in nursing, differences between the perspectives of nurses, hailing from varied Member States, have been detected. These originate in the assignment of disparate levels of importance to individual aspects of the caring concept. These similarities and divergencies may be attributed to cultural differences related to dominant social values, facets of nursing education and training, as well as the institutions in which nurses are employed (Watson et al. 2003).

Work styles are often differentiated by national boundaries. A study (Martinez and Martinez 2002) of the practices of nurses employed in intensive care units in Spain and the United Kingdom demonstrated diverse paths. Even though nurses of both nationalities performed many of the same activities, based on the concept of nursing care, those in the United Kingdom were said to have more leeway in terms of decision-making related to treatment. In addition, Spanish nurses were found to undertake more technical procedures. Differences in attitude toward patients and relatives were also identified. All is not "sweetness and light" and if, in Spain, a nurse finds the behavior of a patient or a family member or members irritating, it is permissible to make this known to the party or parties concerned. Sincerity is underscored. Other variations between the two systems related to organizational procedures. It has also been affirmed that in Member States, such as the United Kingdom, Denmark, and the Netherlands, nursing tasks are specifically nursing in nature, whereas those in Germany are perceived as derived from medical responsibilities (van der Boom 2008). Health and health care are embedded in value systems which dictate, in part, why and how health-care problems are confronted in specific cultures.

Studies of foreign nurses practicing in a nation have also highlighted the different scenarios. A majority of these professionals working in Portugal have revealed significant contrasts between their home countries and the host nation. These related primarily to diversity in methods, functions, competences, autonomy, interprofessional relations, and work conditions. Spanish nurses remained the most impressed with differences. They reported that auxiliaries in Spain execute many of the tasks performed by their Portuguese colleagues. Also, they affirmed that in Spain, nursing professionals enjoy more autonomy and perform more technical procedures (da Silva and Fernandes 2008). Professional practices do not necessarily cross borders, but instead reflect cultural differences.

Cultural diversity may also be viewed from another perspective, that of age divisions within a nursing workforce. These, being more heterogeneous than previously, divide an institution's nursing staff into diverse groups based on year of birth. Each one features a distinct set of characteristics, values, beliefs, and preferences. In reality, the individual group has its own culture which dictates its members' distinctive wants, needs, and behavior, including work style. Each cohort also brings diverse assets and liabilities to its site of employment. These generational identities can provide onerous assignments for managerial personnel (Manion 2009).

Professional Practice and the New Social Scene

The Tallinn Charter of 2008 called on the WHO Member States in the European region to reinforce their health-care delivery systems in light of the social, cultural, and economic diversity pervading the area. This initiative has significance for the EU Member States and it was welcomed by the EFN. Given globalization, Europeanization, and the growth of the internal market that stimulated demographic transformations, the existence of the multicultural societies patterning the

59

Member States, with few exceptions, can no longer be overlooked. A consequence of this phenomenon is the placement of new claims on the nursing profession. It has been demonstrated that nurses are not always in possession of the necessary capacities to respond to these demands due to organizational, professional, and personal limitations. This has been shown for professionals working in institutional frameworks and in the community (Hultsjö and Hjelm 2005; Peckover and Chidlaw 2007).

The needs of the new clientele in terms of its migrational and cultural background have not received adequate responses on the part of health-care providers. There have also been failures in meeting its language and communications exigencies. In short, more equitable care for culturally diverse communities must be forthcoming. This requires that nurses, regardless of their work setting, have the requisite skills for culturally competent practice. As has been underscored, they must be able to supply appropriate services to culturally diverse clients.

Problems with cultural education have been identified (Peckover and Chidlaw 2007). This is a serious matter because culture has a major impact on health beliefs and health-care behavior. Health culture orients the thoughts and feelings of group members, how they think and feel, and the direction of their actions and their outlook (Stevens and Diederiks 1995). It fashions how they view illness, health and health care, how they experience them emotionally, and how they behave in reference to others and their environment. It is a potent mechanism. Nurses must be familiar with the norms, values, ideas, habits, and customs in reference to health and illness of the diverse groups in a society. That is asking a great deal, but it is requisite to the provision of adequate care. Diversity issues are of prime importance in contemporary times. Congruence between nurses' education and social needs must be assured. Transcultural, multicultural, and intercultural nursing have all acquired a new significance.

The Maltese government has recognized this fact with its creation of the Migrant Health Unit within the Department of Primary Health Care. This organ resulted from the large influx of irregular immigrants. It offers them community-based health education and aids them with access to health-care services. Other activities include on-site cultural mediators' assistance to practitioners and their patients in order to temper language and cultural barriers. Moreover, the structure is also responsible for training health-care professionals and students on cultural diversity issues as they relate to health care (Muscat et al. 2014).

If nurses are to provide services to people from diverse cultures who hold varying values, beliefs, and perceptions of health and illness, ideally, a workforce should mirror its clientele. To do so, most contemporary ones must lose more of their homogeneity and become more multicultural in composition. Attracting the appropriate newcomers to their ranks is a major challenge. Further attempts must be undertaken to achieve racial, gender, and ethnic diversity throughout the profession in all Member States. Increases in the cultural and ethnic diversity of client populations will undoubtedly continue. Hopefully, throughout the Member States, the same will take place at an appropriate pace in the nursing profession and its student bodies. Regardless of their site of employment, nurses must be prepared to practice in this new climate that has transformed the social fabric of the Member States. They must be transethnic, transcultural, and transracial in order to adapt their services to changing societies.

Turnover

Turnover has been defined as the "number of people changing jobs within an organization or leaving an organization within a given year" (Baumann 2010, p. 7). It refers to both internal and external movement in workplace settings and it varies from country to country. Very few make known their turnover rates. Also, comparisons are most difficult, as in other instances, because not all nations use a common definition and a uniform methodology for computation (Gillies 1994). Nurse turnover varies throughout the Member States. In Lithuania, it has been labeled minimal (Padaiga et al. 2006). This is understandable in light of the prominent job insecurity and the high unemployment rates that are found in many of the newly acceded Member States. On the other hand, in Malta, it is high and directed toward the private sector, in part, because of the differences in working conditions (www.sahha.gov.mt).

Discussions of the phenomenon in the United Kingdom illustrate the data problem and the issuance of different figures. The specific rates are discordant, even though they refer to the same time frame. The rate has been cited as between 20 percent and 30 percent (Bridges and Hyde 2007). Ball and Pike (2009) report that it has increased to 16 percent and another study (Review Body for Nursing and Other Health Professions 2007) indicates a figure near the 10 percent range, as does the ICN (2007a). A more recent source (International Council of Nurses Workforce Forum 2013) reports the rate as 8.2 percent. In the past, the chances of turnover have been greater in the private sector

(Ball and Pike 2003). Sweden's turnover rate reflects stability which is better than great variations. It has involved, for the most part, transit between employment settings and not exit from the profession. It has been recorded at around 7 percent (Hasselhorn, Müller, and Tackenberg 2005; ICN 2007b; Josephson et al. 2003). On this, diverse sources agree. Turnover rates reflect recruitment and retention problems. This is evident in the Danish and Irish cases. In Denmark, the rate is cited as 32 percent and in Ireland, as 11 percent, but in some large facilities, it rises and ranges between 15 percent and 17 percent ("INO-PNA Submission" 2007; ICN 2007a; International Council of Nurses Workforce Forum 2013). It is generally acknowledged that these rates, to a large extent, are affiliated with the behavior of the newer entrants to the profession. As mentioned, there is a tendency for turnover to be elevated in the first year of service. Usually, it remains high within a group and might even augment during the following year before decreasing. Patients in facilities with turnover values higher than 22 percent have a greater possibility of dying and a longer length of stay (Gordon 2005).

Predictors of turnover are multitudinous. A list of these variables includes age, tenure, job satisfaction, organizational commitment, views concerning employment opportunities elsewhere, and supervisor's behavior. Also listed are various environmental elements, such as management style, level of stress, relations with supervisors, opportunities for career development, and inflexible administrative policies. In short, organizational, demographic, and environmental elements plus personal factors have an impact on nurses' turnover intentions (Hayes et al. 2006). High turnover rates indicate that work conditions are not as expected.

In health care, turnover, as an issue, has been assigned top priority because of its wide-ranging consequences. Financial and other costs are involved. In practical terms, it is a costly activity causing additional expenses for recruitment, hiring, orientation, added supervision, and the new employee's development to full productivity, as well as other matters. Furthermore, it carries implications for a health-care delivery team's satisfaction and that of patients, safety, perceptions of the quality of care, greater pressure on nurses to practice in an increasingly fragmented and unsatisfactory atmosphere, and the nurse–patient relationship. Regardless of the health-care setting, high turnover rates negatively reflect on the experience level of nursing staff and its productivity. Not only is organizational continuity threatened, but the overall ability to care for patients and the quality of care provided are brought into question (Institute of Medicine of the National Academies 2004; Lum et al. 1998).

In spite of all the negatives, turnover does have some positives. The introduction of new faces into any organization is always welcome. It brings with it possible benefits. Often, it permits elimination of dead wood and career progression. Furthermore, it creates the chance for new ideas and new skills to be incorporated into the institutional framework (Baumann 2010; Hutt and Buchan 2005). In a sense, it can be equated with fresh air. Even though there are advantages to turnover in organizations, a happy medium as to its appropriate amount must be found. Stability is the objective.

Nurse Employment and the Financial Crisis

Reports (Adams 2011; International Labour Office 2010) have indicated that health care, experiencing an increase in employment, was more fortunate than other sectors in weathering the global economic crisis. This might be the case in general. However, it certainly does not hold in reference to the EU's nursing profession. Aggregate figures do not reveal that, in many Member States, contracts with temporary or nonunion workers were canceled and staffing levels were frozen, leaving posts vacant.

A common response throughout the EU to the crisis was a reduction of health-care budgets. Such took place in several Member States, including Bulgaria, Ireland, Hungary, Estonia, and Latvia. In the latter case, the budget cut, totaling 40 percent, was most significant. In several instances, the health-care facility scene was redesigned with the closure of smaller structures, amalgamation or downsizing of others, along with similar procedures, frequently meaning lay off for many nurses. In addition, the number of nursing posts was often reduced, as in Lithuania, Greece, Portugal, Denmark, Italy, Romania, Germany, and elsewhere. Other reactions resulted in a freeze on hiring and a moratorium on replacements, as in Cyprus and the Netherlands, or authorization for only partial replacement, as in Finland and Greece, and the encouragement of early retirement. Conditions of employment in many Member States underwent change. Wages for many practitioners were cut, especially in the public sector. Some nurses realized reductions of up to 40 percent, as in Greece. Often, employees' pension contributions were enlarged and benefits and promotions underwent a freeze along with an increase in taxes. In Ireland, change included, in addition to cuts in salary for those with stipends over a certain figure, an increase in working hours, reduction in overtime, increment delays, and abolition of twilight payments for services provided between 6 PM and 8 PM This scenario has caused many practitioners in the Member States to emigrate in search of more fruitful employment or to accept opportunities outside of nursing. For example, in Hungary, nurses have been attracted to supermarkets and shopping centers for employment purposes (Buchan, O'May, and Dussault 2013; Dussault, Buchan, and Wismar 2013; Eke, Girasek, and Szócska 2011; EFN 2012; Irish Nurses and Midwives Organisation 2013; "New Report" 2012).

With the crisis, health-care employment might have continued to gain as generally asserted, but certainly not for all nurses (International Labour Office 2010). Unemployment rates for these professionals have grown and continue to grow. In Denmark, the rate has increased to 1 percent, in Finland to 1.6 percent, and in Latvia to between 5 percent and 6 percent. In Germany the rate registers at <1 percent and in Sweden at 0.5 percent. On the other hand, Cyprus, Croatia, and Bulgaria report high nurse unemployment. The impact of the crisis on the latter Member State was particularly severe. With restructuring, nurses lost jobs. Ten thousand abandoned the profession and two thousand five hundred left the country to seek more positive employment conditions. In several Member States, such as Luxembourg and Italy, nurses were often substituted with nonqualified staff. Also, in some instances, they were downgraded in the staff hierarchy, even though they continued to execute many of the same professional responsibilities affiliated with a higher classification (Džakula et al. 2014; EFN 2012; International Council of Nurses Workforce Forum 2013; "New Report" 2012).

Another situation that is prevalent among nurses and that has raised its head higher during the financial crisis is underemployment. This state refers to those practitioners who are employed in the field, but not in work that takes full advantage of their knowledge, skills, and capacities. With mass layoffs and the reduction in nursing posts, in several Member States, many of these professionals have been forced to take positions that are inferior to their abilities and potentially threaten patient outcomes. Due to the scarcity and inadequacies of available data in many Member States, nurse unemployment and underemployment have been referred to as "a hidden problem" (Spetz 2011). Both circumstances should be fully exposed. They merit the utmost attention of decision-makers. EFN has vehemently urged the EU to take notice of the situation. Moreover, it is noteworthy that to date, a systematic comparative analysis of the Member States' responses to the financial crisis has not been undertaken. Efforts have concentrated on overviews (Mladovsky et al. 2012).

Given the impact of the financial crisis on the EU nursing profession, in 2013, a new international association, Global Nurses United, was born. Its principal objectives are to make known the negative effects of austerity measures, privatization, and decreases in health-care services and to increase protest against them.

It is noteworthy that the crisis, in some cases, had a positive side. Appropriate reactions were able to generate improved productivity and the elimination of unnecessary and unproductive expenditures. In addition, in some instances, the allocation of resources became more efficient and primary care and ambulatory services were expanded as greater cohesion developed among the various levels of care (Dussault, Buchan, and Wismar 2013). In spite of these positive happenings, the financial crisis has taken its toll on the nursing profession.

The European Union and Health-Care Human Resources Management

The importance of skill mix and other good human resource management practices has been recognized in research that has validated better patient outcomes affiliated with more favorable nurse staffing (Aiken 2007; Needleman et al. 2011). The European Commission has acknowledged this significance in its Action Plan for the EU Health Workforce. Its goals are to enhance health workforce forecasting and planning, to achieve a better understanding of skill needs, to encourage exchange concerned with recruitment and retention and to underscore ethical recruitment. Moreover, this significance is also recognized in its program related to sector councils on employment and skills at the EU level. These units are "platforms at sector level where stakeholders seek to gain insight into the likely developments in employment and skill needs with the aim of assisting policy making within or for this sector" (European Commission: Directorate-General Employment, Social Affairs and Inclusion 2010, p. 1). Similar to these entities are the transversal councils which focus on trends and developments in two or more sectors of the labor market.

Sector councils have been established in fourteen of the Member States and transversal units in sixteen. In Belgium and Spain, given their division of authority, the structures are regional and not national in nature. Sweden has a program for the establishment of these units and Austria, Bulgaria, Latvia, and Lithuania are noted for their absence.

The track records of these last-mentioned nations are quite different. The system for forecasting human resources needs in Austria is said to be of excellent caliber, whereas in the other nations, experiences have been cited as poor and problematic (ECORYS Research and Consulting 2010).

In many Member States, these units are of recent origin and thus, in their early stages of development. Also, some structures have the same purpose, but under another name. Moreover, it happens that employment issues are sometimes determined in national transversal councils, but from a sector perspective. These structures have been found to have a positive effect on the sectors concerned and their enterprises, employers, and employees (European Commission: Directorate-General Employment, Social Affairs and Inclusion 2010). Cross-national collaboration between these councils has been rare. However, it is expected that this will change with actions to be undertaken by the European Union Sector Councils. Such cooperation could be valuable to all stakeholders.

The interest of the EU in human resources planning is evident in other activities as well. Funded by the Seventh Framework Programme of the European Commission, the Registered Nurse Forecasting Study (RN4CAST), a major analysis of human resources management for nursing in Europe, focuses on the injection of new factors concerned with the workplace environment and qualifications of the nursing workforce into traditional forecasting methodologies, so as to be able to relate them to the quality of patient care and safety (Sermeus et al. 2011). In that there has been a dearth of research focusing on skill mix decision-making, this effort is most welcome. It is claimed to be one of the largest nursing workforce projects ever undertaken in the EU (www.rn4cast.eu). Results provide many instruments to overcome the deficiencies identified with the comprehensiveness and accuracy of the traditional models used for forecasting staff requirements. Furthermore, by addressing both the volume and quality of nursing staff and the quality of patient care, the project contributes significantly to EU policy making concerned with nurse workforce planning (Sermeus 2012; Sermeus et al. 2011).

Exhibiting a different focus is an EU joint action program concerned with forecasting the needs of a health-care workforce. The purpose is to engage the Member States and professional associations in a partnership so as to improve the personnel situation throughout the EU. Dialogue and exchange of experience form a central thrust of the effort

(European Commission 2012b). Most Member States favor consistent collaboration at the EU level so as to be able to exchange best practice. Support for such international cooperation is considerable.

It is hoped that such initiatives will result in the production of an overview of evolving skill needs in the health-care sector until 2020. This picture with the common multilingual classification of occupations, qualifications, and skills is to serve as a resource for nurse educators and those in the general health-care sector. In addition, in an effort to close the gap between the world of work and education, the construction of a skills alliance in the health-care arena is on the EU's agenda. It will investigate opportunities for establishing new sector-specific curricula along with innovative methods of teaching and training.

Admittedly, health care, in terms of state expenditures, symbolizes an economic burden. However, concurrently, in terms of employment and economic regeneration, it represents an asset. The key objective of realizing economic growth partially from the contribution of innovative and sustainable health systems is articulated in the EU's proposed Health for Growth Programme (2014–20). Efforts are to aid Member States in the development of common instruments at the level of the EU for the purpose of confronting a lack of resources and facilitating innovations in health-care delivery (European Commission 2012b). This program will complement earlier initiatives, such as the Commission's measures for EU job-rich recovery which included health services and other fields. It must be remembered that health-care provides an important link to other industries, such as business and pharmaceuticals. It is for this reason that health-care delivery has been and is a significant actor in European integration (Goodwin 2006). This is the rationale for the general recognition of the health workforce crisis and its European dimension. EU action certainly adds value to the efforts of the individual Member States. Policy initiatives at both levels should be aligned.

Over the years in the Member States, there has been a shift, as noted, in nurses' sites of employment which obviously influences their scope of practice. On the one hand, they have shifted toward more fundamental forms of nursing care, such as that found in residential services for the elderly or in the community. On the other hand, they have also followed a diverse direction, inspired by the development of highly specialized and technical forms of care, leading to a broader and more sophisticated scope of professional practice. Changes in the patterns of care and the institutions in which it is given are always on the horizon and it appears that they will remain. This means that the Member States will continue to be challenged by the need to refashion the size and scope of the nursing workforce so that it is congruent with changing needs and transformations in care giving at the local, national, and international levels. How this challenge is met depends, in part, on practitioners' output. It is the workplace as an institution that, in part, fashions and develops roles.

> Work situation and institution must be regarded in the light of the particular professional segments represented there: where the segments are moving and what effect these arenas have on their development. Since professions are in movement, work situations and institutions inevitably throw people into new relationships (Strauss 2001a, p. 22).

It is these contacts that assign a changed posture to a profession.

Nurses are usually perceived as a homogeneous, single professional group. However, their institutions of employment, some of which have been referenced in this chapter, and their workplace lives are highly differentiated. They are part of a segmented profession with wide variations, deriving, to a large extent, from their workplace institutions. Thus, the following chapters focus on various aspects of the employment scene which impinge either directly or indirectly on nurses' output and professional development.

2

Industrial Relations and Payment Mechanisms

Introduction

Industrial relations, a significant component of civil society, weigh heavily on the settlement of social conflict, the achievement of consensus, economic modernization, and the legitimacy and stability of democracy. They color the various aspects of daily life for the employed and have implications for society as a whole. In the EU, the diverse facets of these relations are integrated under the rubric of social dialogue and the European social model. The latter features the parallel and complementary character of economic development and social progress and economic dynamism and social equality. Organized diversity, extensive social integration, and the institutionalization of social equality, via social security and an appropriate income distribution, and regulation of the labor market through the adoption of appropriate strategies by the state or other entities are critical to this model (Kohl and Platzer 2003).

Industrial relations represent the framework within which conditions of employment are developed and they are a determinant of the manner in which social dialogue, focusing on social and economic strategies, is carried out. They involve the coming together of employers' and employees' representatives for the purpose of determining the nature of their relationship. These relations concern the rules, processes, and mechanisms that regulate the connection between the two constituencies and also that between them and the state and its agencies. It is to be underscored that industrial relations are nationally embedded. Their essence in any nation is closely linked to the formal and informal aspects of the environment. It is the specific political, social, economic, and cultural forces that fashion a system, its operation, its outputs, and its effect. These elements account for the usual consensual environment in which Danish industrial relations take place and the opposite atmosphere that characterizes Estonian circumstances. More specifically, diversity in industrial relations focuses on the relationship between collective bargaining and legislation, the levels at which collective bargaining occurs, trade union density, membership in employers' associations, and social dialogue mechanisms, to cite a few elements.

Industrial relations policies in general, and, in particular, those related to wages, employment, and social protection are largely within the realm of national responsibilities. They are not considered major competences of the EU. Thus, EU regulations pertaining to these areas, for the most part, are restricted compared to those of the Member States and fragmented and complementary (Keune 2008). Consequently, the social models of the Member States display much diversity. This cross-national divergence characterizes most institutions and procedures related to industrial relations as well.

The original Treaties of Rome, which founded the European Economic Community, subsequently to be called the European Union, contained little law on employment and labor relations. Most legal statements on these subjects are lodged in other EU materials, primarily directives. Amendments to these treaties, found in the Single European Act, the Maastricht Treaty, the Treaty of Amsterdam, the Treaty of Nice, and the Lisbon Treaty have given more form to these matters. Thus, the EU's competences in these areas are now more developed and may be exercised via legislation, European social dialogue, or the open method of coordination. More specifically, the Nice Treaty provides for the institutionalization of collaboration among social parties via a social dialogue procedure that could lead to the creation of community agreements (Articles 138, 139). Furthermore, the document obliges the social parties to participate in a balanced and sustained social process through collective bargaining and consultation (Article 2).

Other pertinent references to the Europeanization of social rights include the 1961 European Social Charter, the 1989 Community Charter of the Fundamental Social Rights of Workers and the 2000 Charter of Fundamental Rights of the European Union. The last-mentioned document provides for the right to collective bargaining, the backbone of social dialogue in the Member States. It affirms: "Workers and employers or their respective organizations, have in accordance with Community law and national laws and practices the right to negotiate and conclude collective agreements" (Article 28). Collective bargaining, the voluntary negotiation between organizations representing employers and employees for the purpose of regulating terms and conditions of employment by collective agreement, has definitely been sanctioned by the EU along with the rights to establish and join trade unions. These have been presented as fundamental social rights.

European industrial relations activities were nurtured by three specific historically related phenomena: (1) the creation of organized interests in the form of trade unions and employer associations at the sectoral, national, and supranational levels; (2) the recognition of the potential contribution of these groups and their role as participants in industrial relations; (3) the enhanced interest of governments and decision-makers in industrial relations (Vandenbrande et al. 2007; Weiler, Newell, and Carley 2007). Each of these factors was impacted by the social, political, and economic circumstances of the day and of the nation concerned, accounting for diversity in the organization of industrial relations systems throughout Europe.

Trade Unions

The European Convention for Protection of Human Rights and Fundamental Freedoms (1950) protects the right to freedom of assembly and association, including the right to establish trade unions (Article 11). Freedom of association and the right to form organizations, such as trade unions, are recognized throughout the Member States as well. Although these rights are guaranteed, the sources that sanction them differ. For example, in some instances, it is the constitution of a nation that delivers these rights, such as in Germany, Malta, and Romania. Or, it might be a combination of the constitution and other legal measures, as in Greece, Finland, and Estonia. Other instruments that perform this function are the Labour Code in Hungary or solely the law, as in Spain (Federation of European Employers 2004). Several means have been utilized throughout the Member States.

Trade unions in the EU tend to be organized on a sectoral or occupational basis, according to a confederate structure. Some Member States have more confederations than others. A single confederation unites the individual trade unions in Austria, Germany, Ireland, Latvia, Slovakia, and the United Kingdom. At the other extreme are the cases of Hungary and France where six and seven confederations, respectively, perform the same task. In several nations, divisions between the confederations are based on politico-ideological or religious considerations, although ideological differences have tempered in recent times. Political divisions color relations between confederations in Belgium, Cyprus, the Czech

Republic, Spain, France, Italy, and Portugal, to cite a few illustrations. However, most recently, confederations are distancing themselves from political parties. In other Member States, such as Greece, Estonia, Slovenia, and Malta, the factor dividing confederations is sectoral—the public versus the private sector.

Also, autonomous unions, not affiliated with any confederations, exist in some countries, such as in Italy, Lithuania, and Luxembourg. Many of these associations represent professional and managerial employees, the service sector, and, in some instances, specifically nurses. Nursing Up and Nursind in Italy are prime examples. Sometimes, as in the United States, a professional nursing organization serves as a trade union as well. Trade unions, regardless of their structure, are established to defend the interests of workers at the work site and in the larger social, economic, and political realms. Their impact is multifaceted and broad in scope. In addition to their workforce effects, from the institutional and societal perspective, they also exert an economic impact. Furthermore, they influence the administration and quality of patient care. Their activities also impinge on unions themselves (Friss 1989).

Many discussions of trade unions make reference to density, the share of employees who are members of a union or the ratio of actual to potential membership. Accurate comparisons of trade union membership between Member States are difficult, due to variations in calculation methods, the nature of data sources, and their quality. Still, the density rate has been labeled an important indicator of the level of trade union participation. Moreover, it has been identified as the most significant external determinant of the workplace psychosocial safety climate, health, and Gross Domestic Product (Dollard and Neser 2013; European Commission: Directorate-General for Employment, Social Affairs and Equal Opportunities—Unit F-1 2006). Unfortunately, data related to EU nurses' membership is not abundant and what exists is highly fragmented and incomplete. Thus, discussion must be at a somewhat more general level.

Throughout the EU, there is a divergence in unionization trends on a geographical basis and also between the private and public spheres. In general, unionization rates are higher in Europe than most other parts of the globe, including the United States. It is noteworthy that health-care workers and specifically, EU nurses, have been unionized for a longer period of time than their American counterparts. Moreover, unionization for these professionals did not generate such heated and charged debates as it did in the United States. Membership registers enormous differences throughout the Member States, where density has ranged from 80 percent in Denmark, at the top of the scale, to 8 percent in Germany and France, at the bottom (Vandenbrande et al. 2007; Weiler, Newell, and Carley 2007). In general, the Nordic Member States along with the Mediterranean islands of Cyprus and Malta feature the highest density rates and Germany, France, and most of the newly acceded Member States, the lowest. However, unionization has been relatively high for French public sector nurses (Kirpal 2003). Also, it is noteworthy that the website (www.mumn.org) of the Malta Union of Nursing and Midwives reports that 98.4 percent of the nursing population is included in its ranks. Midwives in that nation score even higher.

Over time there has been a continuing decline in unionization in a number of European countries, the most dramatic of which took place in many of the newer Member States, specifically, Cyprus, Hungary, Croatia, Slovenia, Latvia, and Greece. An increase in density rates has most recently been witnessed in Belgium, France, Malta, and Germany (Curtarelli et al. 2013; Eurofound 2012; Waddington 2005). In most countries, trade union membership is either static or continues to decline. Of significance is the fact that health-care workers have traditionally experienced a high degree of unionization and that the greatest trade union density is found in the health and social services and public administration. In the new EU Member States, the strongest unions in the public sector in terms of membership are those that include nurses (Kauppinen n.d.). Seago and Ash (2002) in an American study, concluded that trade union membership is affiliated with better patient outcomes and more spirited debate about patients' needs and concerns.

The low unionization rate in the Central and East European Member States has been attributed to several factors. With the change in regimes the unitary system of social partners was replaced with pluralism. With the recognition of freedom of association, membership shifted from an obligatory to a voluntary basis. Many people perceived trade unions as structures to be rejected because of their affiliation with the past. There was a legacy of distrust some unions carried over from the pre-transition period in which they were viewed as too close to the central government and the Communist Party. Negative attitudes and lack of trust were manifested by management, government, and employees. In addition, economic restructuring and the privatization process, both of which transformed institutional structures and distribution of employees, took their toll as well. Most recently, the financial crisis has added its weight. A decrease in trade union membership as a result of mass dismissals has been attributed to it (Alford 2003; Cziria 2013; Lado and Vaughan-Whitehead 2003).

The role of trade unions was modified with the transition to a democratic regime. Their automatic economic and political incorporation into the state was terminated. Also, membership, in part, suffered because these bodies were often overlooked by government and decentralized layers of health services management. Many workers came to believe that trade unions were not capable of fully protecting them, leading to apathy and resignation on their part. This combined with the negative attitude of employers generated by privatization created difficulties for trade unions (Korkut 2006; Philips 2006; Rosskam and Leather 2006; Tomev, Michailova, and Daskalova 2003). Decreased membership means decreased resources, financial and otherwise; decreased authority, and challenges to unions' legitimacy and their claim to be the collective voice of a group of workers. However, it is noteworthy that union membership had a better survival rate in the health arena than in other facets of the public and private sectors.

Employer Organizations

In the world of the labor market, counterparts to the trade unions are the employers' associations who defend the interests of this constituency in industrial relations and the political arena. All Member States have established employer federations organized on a general or sectoral basis. As in the case of trade union confederations, they vary in number. They range from one in Austria, Estonia, Denmark, Spain, Luxembourg, Latvia, and the United Kingdom to the twelve in Italy that reflect the highly fragmented political culture. Their main purpose is to organize the nation's entire private sector. This is not always accomplished. Usually the state sector and public interest enterprises are excluded from these groups. These entities participate in collective bargaining on a separate basis.

The presence of a single or prominent employer association does not always ensure a key role in collective bargaining. This has better chances of happening in the smaller economies. Thus, in some Member States, such as Germany, Cyprus, and Denmark, these organizations are structured on a sectoral basis. It is this type of association that tends to be more important in large economies (European Commission: Directorate-General for Employment, Social Affairs and Equal

Opportunities--Unit F-1 2006). The power and structure of employers' organizations are not uniform. They vary throughout the Member States. In some, the confederations are more significant and in others, the sectoral associations triumph. Both trade unions and employers' organizations may be labeled intermediate structures, due to their role as a liaison between the state, their counterparts, and their memberships. Both entities are propelled by membership and authority. Furthermore, they blend the interests of their diverse constituencies and represent them in various arenas. These are the major industrial relations actors.

Collective Bargaining

The right to bargain collectively is most significant in that this process is considered to represent the best method for enhancing the terms and conditions of health-care workers in both the private and public sectors (ILO Sectoral Activities Program n.d.). As in many other areas, there is also variation in the legal status of collective bargaining throughout the Member States. In most of them (15), the process is established by law. In some (11), it is sanctioned by the constitution and in a few (2), it is a voluntary system in that there is no mention in the fundamental law or in statutory regulations.

Traditionally, throughout a large part of Europe, collective bargaining has been autonomous allowing wage decisions and working conditions to be reached freely. This autonomy was promoted by certain legal principles that included "freedom of association, presence of collective parties, generalized enforceability of agreements through legislation or other administrative measures and the procedural function of collective agreements which may predetermine the contents of collective agreements at a lower level" (European Commission: Directorate-General for Employment, Social Affairs and Equal Opportunities--Unit F-1 2006, p. 10). The relationship between collective bargaining and the law in Member States generates much debate focusing on the issue of autonomy. EU law, such as the Working Time Directive, which assigned employees rights related to the workplace, and the frequency of derogations from the law and collective agreements lead to questions concerning the proper relationship between autonomous industrial negotiations and legal mandates.

The major output of negotiations is the collective agreement, a contract describing the terms and conditions of employment. This document focuses on the rights and privileges and obligations of both the employer and employees. A contract negotiated by a trade union and the employer in some circumstances can be made compulsory by binding arbitration or by legislation. Most recently, during negotiations, principal stakeholders—governments, employers' organizations, and trade unions—have frequently adopted a partnership approach to address key issues and achieve consensus.

The conditions and influence of collective bargaining, its scope, and the way in which it is operationalized differ significantly throughout the Member States. There is much variation, determined primarily by institutional diversity and disparate roles assigned to the actors. Collective bargaining remains the dominant method for concluding a contract, but the level at which bargaining is conducted varies among nations. One of the major systemic differences relates to the level at which negotiations take place. Industrial relations operate at different levels: the national level, the industrial or sectoral level, and that of the workplace. In the first instance, industrial relations determine a framework policy. This is often developed by representatives of government, employers, and employees. At the industrial level activities focus on a specific sector of the economy, such as health care. Usually the principal participants at this level are the employers' organizations and the trade unions. At the workplace or enterprise level the key players are the employer and trade union representatives. Collective bargaining does not usually take place solely at the sectoral or enterprise level, as in Slovakia. For example, in Latvia, health-care negotiations occur at the national and enterprise levels (Cziria 2012; Lai et al. 2013). Every system has a mix that involves, directly or indirectly, various elements, but not in equal measure.

A majority of the Member States are accustomed to an organized multilevel system of collective bargaining on a centralized level (cross-sectoral or sectoral) and at the workplace level. Most of them rely on the sector as the main bargaining unit. Sometimes, as in Belgium, Finland, Greece, and Slovenia, agreements concluded at this level elaborate on and implement general intersectoral agreements taken earlier at the national level. The latter provide guidelines for all lower-level negotiations and thus, offer a framework for sectoral activities. In the newly acceded Member States, sectoral labor relations are weaker and much less importance has been assigned to collective agreements reached at this level. Although sectoral negotiations take place in these nations, the individual enterprise has remained a most important bargaining level, particularly in Latvia, especially in the public and ex-public sectors; Lithuania, and the Czech Republic (European Commission: Directorate-General for Employment, Social Affairs and Equal Opportunities--Unit F-1 2006; Leisink, Steijn, and Veersma 2007a, 2007b; López-Valcárcel, Quintana, and Socorro 2006; Peña-Casas and Pochet 2009; Vandenbrande et al. 2007; Weiler, Newell, and Carley 2007; Wiskow, Albreht, and de Pietro 2010). Sectoral level bargaining usually takes place at the national level. However, in some countries, such as Germany and Spain, this type of negotiation is carried out at the regional level, illustrative of division of power in the nation and a general trend toward decentralization in labor relations. In a nation, the level selected for negotiation activities is not always the same in the public and private sectors. For example, in Malta, the enterprise level is predominant in the private sector and sectoral agreements prevail in the public arena. On the other hand, in Denmark, the sectoral level is utilized in both instances.

In most European countries, employment relations in the public sector differ from those in the private sector. In the former, for the most part, labor relations tend to be strongly collectivized with a rather centralized bargaining structure and trade unions enjoy a more authoritative position than their private sector colleagues. In addition, public sector organizations display certain characteristics that distinguish them from their private sector counterparts. Assigning much importance and attention to health, safety, and welfare issues, they are associated with a paternalistic notion of government and having become accustomed to adopting standardized employment practices, public sector workers have come to expect job security and lifelong employment, as in the case of French public sector nurses. Collectivized labor relations in the public sector provide a significant role for trade unions. Furthermore, the public organizations involved strive to be ideal employers serving as the model for private entities to emulate. These traits are peculiar to most EU Member States, excluding the newly acceded ones (Leisink, Steijn, and Veersma 2007a, 2007b). As an aside, it is interesting that in Lithuania, health-care agreements are concluded by the usual partners as in other Member States, but the National Association of Patients must give its approval as well. This atypical practice certainly manifests the significant consideration given to the consumer, as it should be. Of importance, is the fact that all stakeholders are included.

In the United Kingdom, the National Health Service opted for alternatives to traditional collective bargaining. Whitley Councils named after their founder, J. H. Whitley, and originally established to temper industrial unrest, developed into public sector wage negotiation bodies. Representing employees and management, the Whitley system was adopted by the National Health Service on its birth in 1948. Functional groups within the system determined the salaries and work conditions of specific occupational categories and a general Whitley Council established the conditions of service common to all National Health Service personnel, subject to ministerial approval. A pay dispute occurred in 1982 that led to the creation of an independent pay review body for nurses and midwives, removing them from the Whitley system of bargaining. It was called the Review Body for Nurses and Allied Health Professionals. The expectation was that these groups in the future would not ally with other health-care workers in a sector-wide salary campaign (Bach 1999). This new independent unit, composed of people from professional, business, and academic backgrounds, was to advise the government on the pay of these National Health Service employees.

Following the 2004 introduction of the Agenda for Change, an extraordinary attempt to revamp the National Health Service pay system, the scope of the review body, having been extended over time, was further enlarged to include others involved in the delivery of health care. Thus, it eventually became the National Health Service Pay Review Body. It reviews materials on pay and related issues from government, staff, and management organizations and its recommendations apply to all National Health Service staff with the exception of physicians, dentists, and the most elite managers.

Mention must also be made of the role of the state in terms of intervention in collective bargaining. Depending on national legal arrangements, it can attempt to influence negotiations in many ways, including by providing the institutional structure for dialogue, furnishing the norms or ceilings for wage bargaining, imposing settlements in the private sector, or suspending negotiations. Influence can also be exerted by establishing minimum wages, tax-based income policies, or threats of sanctions. Furthermore, government may utilize its role as an employer in the public arena to influence negotiations in the private sector. The role of the state is important in some countries and in others, such as Sweden, the lack of state involvement in the bargaining process is notable. In the newly acceded nations, there has been a pronounced emphasis on the state, given the underdevelopment and weakness of the intermediate collective bargaining structures, leading to their inability to meaningfully negotiate independently (Kauppinen n.d.; Kohl and Platzer 2003). Perhaps, this strong role has actually contributed to their particular weakness. One must also remember the importance of the state in the Central and Eastern European Member States prior to their transition to democratic regimes.

Recently, reports concerned with the involvement of government in collective bargaining have indicated that intervention has been great in Belgium, Finland, Hungary, Ireland, Luxembourg, the Netherlands, Portugal, and Slovenia, meaning that government directly participates by furnishing norms or ceilings. On the other hand, the least amount of government intervention, signifying government is only involved in the setting of a minimum wage, has been affiliated with Austria, Cyprus, Denmark, and the United Kingdom (European Commission: Directorate-General for Employment and Social Affairs 2004; Jacobs 2005; Vandenbrande et al. 2007; Weiler, Newell, and Carley 2007). Still, Bach (1999) has adamantly criticized the role of the state and its relationship to National Health Service collective bargaining prior to the adoption of the Agenda for Change, the present pay structure. He posits:

> Limits imposed on free collective bargaining in the National Health Service demonstrate that the state has always strictly controlled public expenditure to the detriment of nurses' pay, undermining its claim to be 'model employer'. . . . For nurses the state as a model employer always lacked substance (p. 114).

The time frame assigned to collective agreements in the various Member States differs as well. In some nations, such as Austria, France, Italy, the Netherlands, Portugal, and Slovenia, an annual or uncoordinated sectoral bargaining cycle exists, whereas in other nations, a more formalized multiyear cycle ranging from two to four years is adopted. Most of the newly acceded nations seem to fall into the variable category. For example, in Croatia, in terms of duration, collective agreements may be applicable for an indefinite or definite period. The latter lasts for three years, but may be prolonged with clearly specified reasons. (Carley et al. 2010; Croatia: Ministry of Economy, Labour and Entrepreneurship 2011, Article 10; Curtarelli et al. 2013; European Commission: Directorate-General for Employment and Social Affairs 2004; European Foundation for the Improvement of Living and Working Conditions 2007a, 2009a; Weiler, Newell, and Carley 2007).

Extension of the provisions of collective agreements to entities and workers not party to the document is possible in most Member States. In

79

fact, it has been a common practice for employers to extend agreements to both unionized and nonunionized employees. Exceptions to this practice are provided by Cyprus, the United Kingdom, Denmark, and Malta. In three nations there are no regulations governing the procedure. Contracts are usually extended by legislation or action on the part of a member of the government, such as the Minister of Labor, as in Croatia. Austria is unique in that permission comes from a diverse source, the Federal Arbitration Office. In many instances, certain requirements must be met before extension is granted and very often, it is automatic, as in Spain and Belgium. It so happens that the practice has been utilized more in some countries than in others. For example, it is adopted frequently in Estonia and the Netherlands, but rarely in Hungary and Germany (European Commission: Directorate-General for Employment and Social Affairs 2004; European Commission: Directorate-General for Employment, Social Affairs and Equal Opportunities--Unit F-1 2006; European Foundation for the Improvement of Living and Working Conditions 2007a; Köhler and Begega 2007; Vigneau and Sobczak 2005; Weiler, Newell, and Carley 2007).

Adoption of this procedure serves as a shield against declining trade union membership. In spite of the decreasing level of trade union density, the coverage rate of collective agreements increases via the extension of accords. This is the situation in France where the state actively intervenes in favor of collective bargaining by imposing almost complete collective agreement coverage through application of the extension procedure. The same has held for the Netherlands where low trade union membership has contrasted with a high rate of collective agreements, due to the state's extensive use of a statutory extension process (Rose 2005).

The principal subjects around which collective bargaining revolves are pay and working time. However, an economic crisis can shift the focus of negotiations from pay raises to job security. In addition, many other matters are often discussed. These include workers' social guarantees, work conditions, benefits, various types of leaves, allowances for specific purposes, health and safety at work, the work environment, work-related stress and other occupational ailments, promotion, work–life balance, educational opportunities, procedural issues related to grievances, dismissal, and the power and status of trade union groups at the workplace, among other items. The list is incomplete and long. A comparison of collective agreements in the various Member States reveals variance in their basic nature. In terms of their scope, some are broader than others. There is no fixed formula. However, in Spain, the law (Spain 2003) details the numerous subjects to be covered in negotiations (Article 79). On the other hand, in the new Member States, the content of accords has been termed "limited" and "weak" (Lado and Vaughan-Whitehead 2003; Vaughan-Whitehead 2007) because the range of issues covered is narrow. In general, reference is made to pay and bonuses and infrequently to working time. Tending to regurgitate mandates of other legal documents and establish measures in the most general terms, sectoral agreements, in particular, in these nations, have been cited for their poor contents and thus, their frequent ineffectiveness as regulatory instruments.

Basic Wages

Health care is a labor-intensive industry in which a significant portion of the expenditure is devoted to workers' salaries. In fact, according to the WHO European Region, nurses and midwives account for approximately 60 percent of most health-care budgets in the area (www.euro.who.int/nursingmidwifery). One of the most important activities of the Member States' industrial relations systems is wage bargaining. The collective bargaining process has an important role in determining employees' salaries. Pay and other aspects of remuneration lie at the core of collective negotiations throughout the EU and in some Member States, particularly, the newest ones, they can be the only matters on the bargaining agenda.

Representing a major expenditure in any health-care system, not only do stipends in the broadest sense have an immediate impact on the cost of its operation, but they are significant components of any health-care human resource strategy. They partially determine how an institution relates to external labor markets through staff recruitment and retention. Thus, they are of fundamental importance to an understanding of health-care worker and, in this case, specifically, nurse shortages. In addition, pay systems, depending on their nature, contribute to the culture of an institution and impinge on staff behavior, motivation, and performance. Given that pay has been found to be a most important dimension of nurses' job satisfaction, this limits institutional efforts to enhance gratification. Furthermore, wage levels and benefits symbolize the attractiveness of the profession and explain much of its collective action. Also, they influence the degree of interest in part-time employment and appropriate ones are important to positive practice environments. Socioeconomic security is closely related to efficiency, effectiveness, and the quality of care and, in turn, to the health of any community (Buchan and Evans 2008; International Council of Nurses et al. 2008b; Lane, Antunes, and Kingma 2009; OECD 2009; Willem, Buelens, and De Jonghe 2007; World Health Organization: Europe 2006). Given the significance of pay systems, it is not surprising that they furnish a popular subject for public debate and throughout the Member States have occupied a prominent place on the nursing profession's agenda.

The European Social Charter (1961) affirms the right to fair remuneration (Part I (4)) and "the right of men and women workers to equal pay for work of equal value" (Part II, Article 4(3)). The notion of fair remuneration can be interpreted in two different ways. From one perspective, it could mean that it is not appropriate to pay an employee below a certain limit or it could also signify that in terms of wage structures, they must be related to factors that establish who is to be paid more and who less. A notion of what is fair and just is set forth by collective agreements in that they define elements to be considered when individual stipends are set. All in all, this means that differences in wages must be objectively justified, if they are to be viewed as just (Ahlberg and Bruun 2005). Moreover, the International Labor Organization's (ILO's) Nursing Personnel Convention (1977b) endorses remuneration of nursing personnel fixed at levels that are commensurate with their socioeconomic needs, qualifications, and responsibilities, and that are likely to draw people to the profession and retain them. In addition, in an instrument of wider scope issued over three decades earlier (Medical Care Recommendation 1944, No. 69), the ILO refers to adequate income for health-care professionals so as not to distract their attention from the maintenance and improvement of their patients' health.

Many Member States in the health-care sector utilize formal career and pay structures. These are found where there is a differentiated system for nurses with positions at different levels of a scale and payment is related to the position and often to performance and qualifications as well. Frequently, education and professional experience in terms of the number of working years are linked to wage levels. There are various possible combinations. For example, Portuguese nurses employed in the public sector receive a salary in conformity with a civil service pay scale. It rewards workers according to a matrix that relates professional category and length of service, but performance is given no consideration. In Malta, nurses as part of the civil service, as opposed to the practice for other health-care professionals, can only enter the service at the lowest possible salary level, irrespective of their qualifications and experience. These employees are paid according to a scale system. Croatian nurses' salaries are classified according to a job complexity index (Barros and Simões 2007; Muscat et al. 2014; Muscat and Grech 2006).

Illustrative of a formal career and pay structure is the aforementioned Agenda for Change, the system designed and adopted by the National Health Service in the United Kingdom. Having as an objective the enhancement of staff recruitment, retention, and motivation, it introduced new pay arrangements in the interests of modernization. The remuneration system of the National Health Service now features a series of pay spines, one of which is for staff that was in the purview of the aforementioned Pay Review Body for Nurses and Allied Health Professionals. In turn, these spines are divided into nine pay bands. Individual nurses are assigned to one of these bands on the basis of job weight as measured by an evaluation scheme. They then progress annually from one band to the other provided their performance is satisfactory and they can demonstrate possession of the appropriate capacities for their classification. The latter are evaluated yearly according to the Knowledge and Skills Framework, a critical component of the pay structure. It defines and describes the level of knowledge and skills staff need to perform effectively in a specific position and to deliver health-care services of superior quality. It is relied on to determine the wages and career progression of each individual employee (Agenda for Change Project Team 2004). It is expected that staff will normally progress from one pay point to another on an annual basis until the top of the pay spine is reached.

The system is constructed on the value of work, not job title. To make certain that the principle of equal pay for work of equal value is implemented, the scheme was reinforced by the job evaluation, based on various elements or factors, each of which has identified levels, and a point score is obtained for each position. Development of these factors and the weighting and scoring systems were deemed innovative. For the first time, with the implementation of the Agenda for Change, all positions could be evaluated. In addition, the plan also harmonized the terms and conditions of employment. Managers have positively evaluated the system, pointing to its fairness, provision of harmonized conditions for various types of staff, equal pay claim protection, and opportunities to introduce new positions (Buchan and Evans 2008).

At the other extreme, lie the decentralized pay arrangements where wage structures are determined locally. Salaries at this level may also be based on performance and contributions to activities at hand. Such a system is congruent with the Ljubljana Charter signed in 1996 by the Member States of the WHO European Region. The document defines the values and principles that should govern health-care reform in Europe. Decentralization was favored, sanctioning devolution of decision-making, and enhancement of local management so services would match local needs. Illustrative of this practice is the Polish situation. Here the minimum level of pay is set in negotiations involving trade unions and employers at the national level. Then, at the work site, there is more collective bargaining in which the employer and employees' trade union representatives participate. These discussions focus on employment conditions, such as wages and working time. It seems that, in the case of Poland, such an arrangement has allowed for "passing the buck." Polish nurses' wages have been a source of collective action. The Ministry of Health insists that any decision on nurses' pay arrangements is the responsibility of the individual hospital director. Yet, those occupying this position claim that wages, leaving to be desired, are the fault of local authorities and the Ministry (Holt 2010). Accountability is lacking.

Payment mechanisms are somewhat different for the self-employed nurse. In France, these practitioners are paid directly by the client on a fee-for-service basis. Questions concerned with incentives involved in this method of payment have been raised. The health insurance system then partially reimburses the patient. These professionals cannot determine their own fees. They practice according to agreements that detail their relations with insured clients and the health insurance funds. Thus, their rates must reflect those of these official accords which are specific to each profession and usually have a duration of four to five years. Agreements with nurses include an annual target for expenditure. If the target has been met, rate increases are sanctioned. Moreover, nurses are required to respect an individual annual ceiling related to earnings. If they fail to do so, they must reimburse the health insurance funds part of the fees collected (Breuil-Genier 2003; Sandier, Paris, and Polton 2004).

Self-employed nurses in Ireland follow a fee structure posted by the Irish Nurses Organisation. Rates are established according to the day of the week, time of day, calendar date (holiday or not), time spent on service, and type of shift, if applicable. Moreover, escort rates have been established along with on-call fees, in addition to charges for other services. Payment of these rates by the patient are due to the nurse involved within one calendar month (Irish Nurses Organisation 2005). Self-employment has also attracted many Polish nurses as well. However, the payment process is somewhat different. In this case, practitioners are paid directly by the health insurance funds who are allowed to determine the manner and type of payment. Strózik (2006) has asserted that these "payment mechanisms have not been adequately regulated" (p. 94). The Dutch Healthcare Authority in the Netherlands determines the rates for independent professionals who must not charge more. They may also charge less and as individuals, they may agree with local health insurance companies to a lower rate than the maximum one. Self-employment has been an attractive option for some EU nurses. As these few examples demonstrate, the economic facet of practice of the profession in this manner is not uniform. It has been operationalized in diverse ways.

Comparison of nurses' actual salaries is a difficult task once again because of the nature of the available data which is drawn from diverse sources using different definitions, work sites, categories of nurses, and types of employment, to cite a few elements (OECD 2009). However, in spite of this, some generalizations may be made. In many nations, health-care workers, in general, and, especially, nurses, have received lower wages than employees in most other sectors of the economy. It might be that, in part, these low salaries result from the dominance of females in the profession. The situation is particularly dire in most of the newly acceded Member States. With the transition in regime, many health-care providers realized a decline in wages and job security, resulting from harsh economic times and restructuring of the health-care delivery system. Even with some substantial increases in pay over time, they remain in an inferior position. Throughout this region, the wage levels in health care are lower and often, significantly lower than the workforce average. Moreover, salaries are lower than those in the older Member States. For example, Polish nurses earn four to six times less. Also, the difference in the remuneration of different professions is less pronounced.

In general, health-care wages in the Central and East European Member States have been labeled shockingly low. Nurses' salaries in Hungary, Slovakia, the Czech Republic, and other nations are lower than the average wage and colleagues in Luxembourg earn four to six times more (OECD 2009). Again, illustrative of this state is the Polish situation. Nurses earn less than one-half of the average remuneration of an employee in the national economy. Of all specialized professions, they earn the lowest wages. Thus, they have had one of the most substandard salary levels in Polish society. In Slovakia, circumstances are somewhat brighter, but still a matter for concern. Health-care workers earn significantly less than the average monthly wage in the general economy. The general wage gap is at 30 percent. In spite of wage changes, the average earnings of professionals in this sector are below those of persons in other fields. Nurses' wages represent approximately 85 percent of the national average. Very often, hospital executives, here and elsewhere in the region, in order to achieve a balanced budget and avoid debt, single-handedly decrease salaries. In Bulgaria, salary reductions have ranged from 10 percent to 50 percent. Labor has requested a pay structure that would guarantee minimum wages in the individual health professions and also allow for more differentiation of salaries based on performance and quality of work (Büscher, Sivertsen, and White 2010; Gajdzica 2007; *Health Care in Central and Eastern Europe* 2001; OECD 2009; "Polish Nurses" 2007; Strózik 2006).

The picture has been of the same type in other newly acceded Member States. In Hungary, health-care workers have been the fifth lowest paid full-time employees in the economy's fourteen main sectors (Gaal 2004). In Latvia, the average salary level for health-care professionals has been 9 percent lower than the overall average in the public sector, in general, and, in particular, 25 percent less than in public administration. More specifically, it should be noted that on average, nurses, due to a shortage of personnel, work the equivalent of 1.4 full-time jobs for their basic salary of one full-time job. In Lithuania, health-care professionals in the public sector have earned 83 percent of the national average wage. In Estonia, the figure registers at 81 percent. In an optimistic vein, it is to be noted that between 2006 and 2012, Estonian nurses' salaries increased by 57 percent (Karnite 2007; Lai et al. 2013; Padaiga et al. 2006).

It is evident that, in this group of Member States, pay levels for health-care providers in comparison to those in other sectors of the national economy leave to be desired. In this region, health-care stipends have traditionally been low. This type of work has been perceived as being unproductive. Thus, the pay level was always less than that affiliated with the so-called productive employment found, for example, in the manufacturing and trade sectors. Also, the health sector's bargaining power has been weak in comparison to that of other sectors that can easily prove their importance to economic growth. Such a perspective is erroneous. A healthy population is most important to a healthy economy. Further complicating the situation is the fact that the majority of health-care providers are female (Alford 2003; Rosskam and Leather 2006). It is noteworthy that with the advent of the most recent economic crisis, in many of these nations, public sector wages, being already low, were frozen or decreased. Cuts were realized in Latvia, Greece, and Lithuania and freezes took place in Bulgaria, Estonia, Hungary, and Slovenia. Often, in response to the loss of public revenues, as in Latvia, the clinical nursing staff's working hours were increased (Carley et al. 2010; International Labour Office 2010; "Public Sector Spending" 2011).

Soon after the transition, general economic difficulties in many Central and East European nations led to the nonpayment of wages to health-care providers for periods of up to six months. In essence, they were paid late, if they were paid at all. Obviously, such a situation has serious consequences not only for the workers and their families, but also for the quality of services delivered by the individual health-care systems involved. In-kind benefits vanished and staff became more vulnerable to inflation. Workers' mobility was severely limited because people could not leave employers who owed them back-pay. Survival was, and often, still is, a challenge as any notion of economic and/or job security vanished. In many instances, a sizeable army of working poor was groomed (*ILO/PSI Workshop* n.d.; Rosskam and Leather 2006; Tomev, Daskalova, and Mihailova 2005).

In an attempt to rectify this situation, the Hungarian government introduced a minimum wage for certain health-care professions. This was the inspiration and rationale for Slovakian and Estonian requests to do the same. The Estonian Nurses Union in negotiations with the Estonian Hospital Association fixes minimum hourly pay for the profession. One can appreciate the following statement contained in *Slovakia: The Manifesto of the Government of the Slovak Republic* (2006): "It will be an important task for the Government to restore the citizens' trust toward health care providers, to humanize the health care staff's attitude to patients, which, however, is conditional upon adequate improvement of health care staff remuneration." This affirmation has a more general application than just to Slovakia. Unfortunately, according to Rosskam and Leather (2006), in this geographical area, "nurses . . . can continue to labour for sub-standard public sector salaries with little prospect of any significant improvement" (p. 42). This statement is still valid.

In the older Member States, the same types of pay differentials are evident. For example, in Finland, the salaries of nurses have been lower than the average wage (OECD 2009). In the United Kingdom nurses' salaries do not compare favorably with those of teachers. These professionals earn 19 percent less than primary school teachers and 25 percent less than those at the secondary level. This difference increases with age. Older primary and secondary teachers, those in their forties, get 30 percent and 34 percent, respectively, more than nurses. A similar difference is evident for all age groups. In terms of responsibility, nurses with management duties earn 23 percent, 29 percent, and 13 percent, respectively, less than primary and secondary teachers and police officers with supervisory obligations. At the same time, these professionals earn less than primary and secondary teachers with no managerial responsibilities and only slightly more than a junior police officer without supervisory tasks to perform. Public sector spending cuts as a reaction to the economic crisis, as in other instances, took a toll on nurses' earnings. All National Health Service employees with salaries over a certain amount had their wages frozen and pension entitlements reduced. The situation is somewhat different in Germany where nurses' stipends are on a par with those of policemen and primary school teachers. In fact, their wages are above the OECD average (Busse and Blümel 2014; German Nurses Association n.d.; Pike and Williams 2006, 2008; "Public Sector Spending" 2011). Traditionally, in most European nations, teachers have been likely to earn more than nurses. More specifically, with the exception of Italy and Austria, nurses' wages have been less than those of primary school teachers. Again, except for Austria, teachers at the secondary level in all countries have had higher salaries than nurses. In Cyprus, a teacher at any level has been paid more than a nurse (*Informe* 1999; International Labour Organization Sectoral Activities Program 1998). This trend is still evident.

In Austria, those employed in health care have hourly wages that are 12 percent below those in the economy as a whole. Nurses in France on their first job are better paid than their cohorts with equal qualifications. However, over a five-year period their increases in salary are significantly less. Thus, they do not maintain their position (Hofmarcher and Quentin 2013; Marquier 2005). Irish nurses are paid less than compatriots in either the public or private sector with similar qualifications. In fact, in terms of public servant salary scales, Irish staff nurses find themselves at the bottom of the ladder and they continue to fall. Wage cuts, due to the economic crisis, have not been limited to the newly acceded states. As noted, Irish nurses' salaries have been reduced as well. Moreover, higher pay for agency specialist nurses has been eliminated along with that for the so-called twilight shifts. The overall reduction has been estimated to be 14 percent for low and middle-income nurses. Sweden is atypical in that the salary level of nurses with a university education is above the national average ("Agency Nurse Plans" 2011; Büscher, Sivertsen, and White 2010; Hofmarcher and Rack 2006; "INO-PNA Submission" 2007; International Labour Office 2010). These comparisons afford an idea as to the relative financial attractiveness of nursing compared to other occupations in the Member States. Even though many of the pay gaps in the older ones are significant, they are less critical and of lesser weight and dimension, given the overall economic situation. Still, they merit serious attention.

With few exceptions, there is a general tendency throughout the Member States for wages to be higher in the public sector than in the private. Sometimes a different salary structure is used for nurses employed in the private sector. For example, in the United Kingdom, most private sector nurses are not paid according to the provisions of the aforementioned Agenda for Change. The majority receive salaries based on other scales. Nurses employed in the public sector in Bulgaria, the Czech Republic, Lithuania, Latvia, Slovenia, France, Ireland, the United Kingdom, and Spain, to cite a few examples, have earned more than their counterparts in the private sector. The same does not hold for Denmark. The extent of the gap between the two sectors varies. The differential has been as low as 3 percent in France for starting nurses, but across all hospital professionals, it has ranged from 7 percent to 15 percent ("European Nurses" 2008; Marquier and Idmachiche 2006; Wait 2006). For this reason, French hospitals in the private sector have found it difficult to recruit personnel. In other nations, the difference has been greater. In the United Kingdom, it has registered at 21 percent, in Bulgaria, at 33 percent, and in Spain, at 50 percent (Daskalova et al. 2005; Frijters, Shields, and Price 2007; Gancedo 2006; Pike and Williams 2006). Interestingly enough, in Latvia, Austria, and Finland, the wage level in both sectors for nurses is about the same—low. The challenge for the Dutch has been to maintain an equilibrium between the two sectors (Hofmarcher and Quentin 2013; Jacobs 2005; Karnite 2007; Vuorenkoski, Mladovsky, and Mossialos 2008).

In Bulgaria, Estonia, Poland, and Hungary, in the private sector, there is a difference between the declared wage and the real one. An established practice is to conceal the real value of wages so as to reduce labor costs. Often, employers declare a wage that is much less than the one actually paid to the employee. Making a declaration of this type, employers decrease their taxes and social insurance contributions. Transparency is lacking. Such a practice, obviously, generates superficial and artificial pay data. In addition, the state budget and the social security purse are negatively affected because of the lower contributions. Workers suffer as well. Their future pension entitlements are automatically reduced (Daskalova et al. 2005; Tomev, Daskalova, and Mihailova 2005; Vaughan-Whitehead 2007).

In spite of various pronouncements issued by EU institutions over the years, parity of stipends between males and females has not been realized. Discrimination to the detriment of the latter is quite evident in several Member States. The EU average gender pay gap stands at 16.2 percent to the advantage of men. This figure varies greatly throughout the Member States. The continuum ranges from 0.9 percent in Slovenia to the Estonian 27.7 percent. Other nations on the positive side include Poland (4.5 percent), Italy (5.3 percent), Luxembourg (8.7 percent), Romania (8.8 percent), Belgium (10.2 percent), Croatia (10.6 percent), Portugal (12.8 percent), Malta (13.4 percent), Bulgaria (13 percent), Ireland (13.9 percent), Lithuania (14.6 percent), Sweden (15.4 percent), Latvia (15.5 percent), France (15.6 percent), and Denmark (16 percent). The remaining Member States are in negative territory, having exceeded the average. Spain is exactly even with it. In some cases, even though the difference between male and female stipends might be small, it has been found to be statistically significant (Christensen 2009; D'Árgenio 2007; Eurofound 2012; European Commission 2013; Marquier 2005). Much conflict within the profession has been sparked by this inequality, especially in Denmark and other Nordic nations.

Sweden has managed to reduce its gender pay differential via provisions of the Equal Opportunities Act. It requires all employers with a certain number of employees to determine on an annual basis if unwarranted pay differences between the sexes exist. As a result of this type of scrutiny over an extended period, gender pay divergences within the same profession have greatly decreased. The Netherlands has faced the matter in a somewhat different manner. Not having legislation that focuses on equal pay for men and women, it relies on the aforementioned principle of equal pay for equal work by both sexes as found in the Act on Equal Treatment of Men and Women. Moreover, it has extended this concept by applying it to part-time and full-time workers (Ahlberg and Bruun 2005; Jacobs 2005). In March 2011, the

EU Social Affairs Ministers adopted A New Europe Pact for Equality between Women and Men: 2011-2020. Its purpose is to ensure equal pay for equal work of equal value and more. It also promotes women's empowerment in decision-making in the political and economic realms. Hopefully, this instrument will enjoy more success than its predecessors.

Other factors account for various types of pay gaps. Decentralization, for example, as permitted by the aforementioned Ljubljana Charter, allowed devolution of decision-making, local management, and combinations of ownership and organization. This arrangement has raised problems concerned with equity. In fact, employment became fragmented and much inequity resulted. Pay disparities between regions, between staff, and within professions were magnified, rather than resolved. For example, in Poland, nurses in the same hospital, performing the same jobs, have received different salaries because they were employed on different contracts by different levels of government. Attempts to decentralize pay decisions to afford greater flexibility are very complex (Alford 2003; Bach n.d.-b). Also, the work site accounts for differences. For example, French nurses working in hospitals have higher pay than their colleagues practicing elsewhere. The opposite has occurred in the United Kingdom, where nonhospital nurses have enjoyed a greater reward than their hospital colleagues (Pike and Williams 2006). Within the hospital sector, the type of facility involved has generated pay inequities, as in Slovakia, where wages are higher in teaching hospitals than in general hospitals. Institutional inequities also exist in Bulgaria. They are caused by agreements that provide for the distribution among staff of 40 percent of the revenues derived from clinical care paths. The problem is that they are distributed disproportionately and have created big differences within and between different professions in hospitals and between these facilities as well (Daskalova et al. 2005).

Wage differentials are also based on geography, regions, institutions, specialties, type of worker, or nature of employment. For example, in France, salary has been linked to type of contract and region. Nurses, practicing in rural areas, have earned less than those working in major urban centers (Marquier 2005; Marquier and Idmachiche 2006). This is true in many nations. In the United Kingdom, practitioners affiliated with an agency used to resolve nursing personnel shortages have commanded higher salaries than those holding an institutional contract. Thus, many National Health Service nurses have used their annual leave and spare time to moonlight. This is not always the case. In Ireland, trade unions advised agency nurses not to work for the lower wages established in the 2011 cost-cutting initiative. This move brought their pay below that of the permanent nursing staff ("Agency Nurse Plans" 2011). In the various Member States, there are considerable differences in the use of agency personnel and their working conditions. The aforementioned Directive 2008/104/EC accorded these workers the right to equal treatment that includes equality in terms of pay, leave and maternity leave, as well as equal access to collective facilities, such as childcare units. Moreover, agencies are obliged to improve access to training and childcare in between jobs, so employability will be enhanced. Field of practice has also led to pay gaps. Certain specialties generate a salary differential. In Sweden, geriatric nurses have earned more than cohorts in other nursing sectors (Hasselhorn, Müller, and Tackenberg 2005). Often, differences become enlarged, if the specialty is experiencing a shortage. Wage gaps are a fact of life in the nursing world throughout the Member States. They can vary according to gender, position, power, practice, the setting, geography, and a galaxy of other factors, but they still are present.

Supplements to Basic Wages

As in the United States, most nurses in Member States are paid according to a salary-based approach and within this framework various practices are adopted. Sometimes, there are automatic increases in stipends, especially in nations, such as Portugal and Belgium, where earnings are linked to the cost of living. Of note is the Swedish situation. In many new health-care endeavors, workers are awarded short fixed-term contracts. Thus, management is not bound to engage in collective bargaining or to give obligatory wage increases (ICN 2007b). Very often, there are certain allowances, some of which qualify for additions to nurses' basic pay in specific Member States. These include rewards for working unsocial hours, overtime, and certain shifts, as well as stand-by or on-call duty. Location allowances are also used in various Member States, such as the United Kingdom and Ireland. Location may be viewed from two different perspectives. From one, it has a geographical significance, referring to a specific type of region. For example, nurses in the United Kingdom are eligible for high cost area supplements, if they practice in inner London, outer London, or on the fringe. According to the Agenda for Change pay scale, they are privileged to receive extra payments equal to 20 percent, 15 percent, and 5 percent, respectively, of their basic salary. From another viewpoint, location refers to the structure or unit where nurses perform their duties. For example, Irish nurses working in Units for Severe and Profoundly Handicapped in Mental Handicap Services, in Care of the Elderly and Alzheimer Units, or in Acute Admission Units in Mental Health Services are eligible for a location allowance (Irish Nurses Organisation 2005). Qualification allowances in specialist areas have been used as well, but not in Finland, where there is no wage difference between primary and specialized nursing (Vuorenkoski, Mladovsky, and Mossialos 2008). Language proficiency is a qualification that garners extra rewards for nurses in Estonia.

Bonuses may also be performance-related and linked to either individuals or teams. In the case of Spain, by law, these rewards apply to part-time employees as well (Spain 2003). Due to the general lack of objective and measurable indicators of outputs and the cost of implementing a merit-based program, the effectiveness of performance-related pay as a motivator has been questioned (Bach n.d.-b). Another type of bonus is found in some of the new Member States. The widespread payment of bonuses is a practice used in exchange for the acceptance of poor working conditions. Workers are content with these as they inflate their income (Vaughan-Whitehead 2007). A practice not widespread in the United States, but in existence in Italy, Greece, and other Member States, is the so-called thirteenth month. All employees, regardless of the nature of their employment, at the end of the year, based on collective agreement or law, automatically receive an extra month's pay that is not dependent on performance. In addition, years of service also provide a rationale for augments to a pay check. In France, nurses annually receive a 1 percent bonus for each year of service up to a maximum of 30 percent (www.infirmiers.com).

Recruitment and retention premiums are often used in areas where management is not able to construct and retain an adequate nursing staff. These imply a targeted approach in that rewards are aimed at certain professionals in short supply. Those targeted have usually included senior nurses and those in fields experiencing severe supply problems. Sometimes, in the same vein, supplements have been offered to professionals who left the profession or a country to work abroad with the hope that they will return to the national ranks of their profession. Finland has had major campaigns, especially in London, to recruit Finnish nurses back to their homeland. The Pay Review Body for Nurses and Allied Health Professionals in the United Kingdom was skeptical of these supplements, claiming they would only rotate shortages, rather than compensate for more general supply side deficiencies (Bach n.d.-b).

Incentives have been linked to nurses' basic remuneration in many Member States. A persistent problem in the health-care world, as noted, has been the gap between the supply of and demand for service providers, especially nurses. In an attempt to reduce the severity of this difficulty, many nations have taken to using various incentives, if they have not developed a full-fledged reward scheme. A focus of such efforts has been enhancement of recruitment, retention, and performance of staff (Global Health Workforce Alliance 2008). Purposes have also included the achievement of a particular objective in a service unit or a change in staff behavior. In some instances, the scope of such rewards is formally specified along with criteria for their distribution. This is the case in Spain. Law 55/2003 (Spain 2003) details these matters. Also, facilities in some Member States enjoy fewer opportunities to develop their own incentive programs and to use a reward strategy as a lever for change. It is noteworthy that Lithuania is a nation in which the stipends of health-care providers have not been linked to any incentives that would increase their productivity, the quality of their work, or their retention. Austria adopts these additional rewards. However, in part, they depend on the subnational unit in which the person is employed. Thus, income comparisons between different groups of employees and regions prove most difficult. These rewards may be distributed to professionals, as individuals or as members of a team. They may be formal or informal, direct or indirect, and monetary or nonmonetary in nature (Hofmarcher and Quentin 2013; Padaiga et al. 2006).

Monetary incentives include a wide variety of direct and indirect payments, such as salary bonuses, pensions, insurance policies, allowances for transportation, parking, childcare, housing, uniforms, and other items; as well as various kinds of financial support related to fellowships, scholarships, tuition reimbursement, and loans. Very often, bonuses are dependent on performance or they are linked to length of service, as in Hungary. The Hungarian human resources development program provides for a "loyalty bonus" to an annual stipend for nurses with at least four years of service (*Health Chapters* n.d.). In the public sector, Germany has introduced yearly payments related to individual performance (Beese 2006). In the United Kingdom, new entrants to nursing have received additions to their pay checks.

Perhaps the most unique incentives have been offered to Czech nurses. In exchange for renewal of contracts, a private clinic has offered complimentary German lessons, five weeks of vacation, free liposuction, and silicone breast implants. Nurses were allowed to choose their one-time reward from a list that included these and other procedures. Also, they were offered lunch vouchers and day care. Management claimed these incentives were less expensive than increases in wages. Such a program did not escape criticism. Critics asserted it demeaned the profession and reinforced a cultural view of those in its ranks as sex objects and play things. On the other hand, these procedures were justified by the fact that nurses claim they are under pressure to have a captivating and pleasing appearance and that attractiveness is as important as their clinical skills. Social values as manifested in the print and electronic worlds have underscored these standards. As a chief of plastic surgery affirmed: "If you want to have good employees, you have to have good incentives, and we are offering free breasts. Others could offer free Mercedes" (Bilefsky 2009).

Not all economic incentives have met with success. In fact, in Spain, in spite of the aforementioned legal mandate, these measures, rather than improving performance, "created conflicts between colleagues, a bad working atmosphere and suspicions of arbitrariness" (López-Valcárcel, Quintana and Socorro 2006, p. 125). The scheme backfired. It is generally acknowledged that monetary incentives do not solve supply-side problems, nor do they necessarily serve as motivators. An empirical European comparative study of community nurses (Kingma 2003) confirmed the attitude that nursing as a profession is not likely to be influenced by or interested in this type of financial gain and thus, it expresses a lack of interest in monetary rewards. Moreover, it was reiterated that these strategies fail to impinge on nurses' professional conduct. Economic benefits related to educational endeavors were given a positive grade. However, they were not perceived as having financial connotations. Instead, they were viewed in terms of professional development. In addition, performance-related incentives were labeled inappropriate for the profession, primarily because of the whole question of evaluation criteria. In regard to available economic incentives, many nurses, assigning importance to the relative salary and its relation to social status, favored a salary increase instead.

In terms of incentives, nonmonetary rewards are important. They include the provision of a positive work environment, flexibility in employment arrangements, support for career and professional development, including effective clinical and personal supervision; coaching and mentoring structures, access to services, and intrinsic rewards related to job satisfaction, personal achievement, commitment to shared values, respect for colleagues and community, and membership in a team (ICN et al. 2008a). These rewards, providing important motivating forces, such as recognition, appreciation, and opportunities for career progression, are highly prized by nursing professionals. People want to feel part of an organization. They want to feel valued for their contribution to it as members of a team which means recognition and respect from colleagues and managers. Nonmonetary rewards allow for this. A study of Belgian nurses (De Gieter et al. 2006) reported that these nonfinancial and psychological rewards were assigned great value. In fact, they have been found to contribute to motivation more than financial incentives (Monecchi and Peroni 2007; Shaw 2006). Recognizing this, Kingma (2003) has suggested that the language used in connection with reward schemes should manifest the idea of appreciation for a job well done, rather than incentive or bonus implying extra work and effort are required.

Reward systems mean different things to different people, but exactly what they mean and to whom, and why they are perceived in a certain manner, and what are the outcomes of diverse programs are some questions that have not been fully explored. There is a dearth of research on these matters. Programs must be tailored to the nature of their audience. They must mesh with its preferences and characteristics in order to be effective. Many factors impinge. Age, gender, stage of career, professional background, general economic conditions, and the nature of the labor market are some elements that influence the structure of a reward program and the reception it might receive. Constructed in an appropriate manner, these schemes could be an important instrument in the grooming of a superior nursing staff. The alternative points to a three-tier shortage: a lack of nurses willing to accept current wages and work conditions, a scarcity of these professionals as the demand for their services increases, and a deficiency in the nursing care patients are provided (Gordon 2005; ICN et al. 2008a).

Overtime may be compensated with premium pay rates or time off in lieu. It also may be unpaid in any form—no extra pay and no time off. Compensation, whether in the form of premium wages and/or time off, is determined in most Member States by legislation and/or collective agreements. There are many different schemes. Illustrative of their diversity are the following examples. Latvian labor law requires that excess hours be rewarded by a pay rate of 100 percent extra over and above the standard rate. In Romania, the practice is the same, but there is also another option, time off in lieu within the subsequent thirty days. The Bulgarian Labour Code sets parameters. It provides that the premium rate for excess hours must be established in an accord between employees and the employer and must not be less than 50 percent extra for work on normal working days, 75 percent extra for the effort on weekends, and 100 percent extra for the same on public holidays. Some Member States, such as Finland, specify compensation based on the sequence of excess hours. The Finnish Working Hours Act states that the first two hours of overtime are to be rewarded with regular pay plus 50 percent extra. Additional hours require regular pay plus 100 percent more. Weekly excess hours receive regular pay in addition to a 50 percent increment, regardless of the number of hours worked. Portuguese legislation establishes that overtime is to be compensated with a pay rate of 50 percent extra for the first hour and 75 percent extra for subsequent hours, or in lieu time off at a rate of the time worked plus 25 percent (Carley 2007).

Once again, it must be noted that data related to nurses' overtime, how it is compensated in practice, and whether it is rewarded, is sketchy. Sometimes, compensation is one thing, in theory and another, in actuality. For example, in the United Kingdom, the Agenda for Change Agreement provides for a pay rate of time-and-a-half for overtime. Yet, it has been noted that in spite of the number of hours worked overtime, very few nursing professionals are likely to be paid at the requisite rate. Nurses working in the independent sector are usually paid for excess hours at the normal rate and those affiliated with the National Health Service are more likely to be offered time off. Moreover, senior nurses tend to be unpaid. It turns out that in the United Kingdom, nurses have been less likely than other health-care personnel to get the premium pay rate in overtime situations (Ball and Pike 2005, 2007; Pike and Williams 2006). Perhaps, this practice is related to their status. Also, in a neighboring nation, Ireland, 73 percent of nurses, who have had to work hours over and above their contracted time, have reported they were unpaid for their efforts (Adams and Kennedy 2006).

Similar occurrences have been identified in the newly acceded Member States. In one study, 90.8 percent of Lithuanian respondents noted they never or rarely received overtime pay. The percentages for Romanian and Czech Republic participants were 53.1 and 37.2, respectively (*Health Care in Central and Eastern Europe* 2001). Although these professionals did not always receive their overtime stipends, their capacity to generate extra funds was increased. By working extended hours their contact with patients was extended as well. This means that they were well-placed to garner additional informal payments. So, in one way or another, their pay was enhanced. Overtime has been of major concern to these nurses.

In a discussion of nurses' remuneration in the EU, mention must be made of these informal payments which have remained an unsolved problem. There appears to be little agreement on a definition of the practice. However, one offered by Gaal et al. (2006) seems appropriate in that its scope is inclusive. They refer to the informal payment as "a direct contribution which is made in addition to any contribution determined by the terms of entitlement, in cash or in-kind, by patients or others acting on their behalf, to health-care providers for services that the patients are entitled to" (p. 276). The important feature of this definition is that the payment is over and above the terms of entitlement. Various labels have been attached to this transaction. It has been referred to as a gratitude payment, a gratuity, an under-the-counter payment, an unofficial payment and an envelope payment, to cite a few. The labels are many.

For the most part, the practice of making unofficial payments to health-care providers has been and is common, especially in the newly acceded Member States of Central and Eastern Europe, with the present exception of the Czech Republic and Slovenia. In the latter two nations, health-care salaries have been relatively high compared to those in other transitional societies and they have kept pace with inflation (Afford and Lessof 2006; Stanojovic and Vehovar 2007). In Greece, the practice has been referred to as an "ingrained social institution" (Liaropoulos et al. 2008). Obviously, the phenomenon is more widespread in some countries than others. For example, it is quite common in Poland, Hungary, and Croatia. In the latter Member State, the practice is well-known, even though Article 7 of the Nursing Code of Ethics (www.hums.hr) states that practitioners "shall not accept any gifts . . . which could be interpreted as an attempt of gaining personal benefits or privileges." On the other hand, the phenomenon is now relatively rare in Estonia (Kopel et al. 2008; Võncina et al. 2006). The players in this game include individuals, institutions, patients, relatives, and most health-care providers. Those on the health-care team score by receiving various types of informal payments.

Certain distinctions as to their nature may be made. A basic difference concerns payments made to facilities and those to individual practitioners. In-kind payments are distinguished from monetary ones.

Then, at the individual level, there is a difference between transactions that contribute to the basic costs of care, those that provide the costs of care, those that afford patients superior services, and those that offer patients no particular benefit and that result from the fact that a health-care provider has exerted power (Ensor 2000). For the most part, these payments are offered in the hope of obtaining access to services, a higher quality of treatment, quicker services, scarce high quality goods, or out of fear of getting no treatment at all (Legido-Quigley et al. 2008; Liaropoulos et al. 2008; Thompson and Witter 2000). In fact, in Slovakia, it has been reported that 71 percent of the public believe that in order to receive reputable and reliable health-care services, one must offer an informal payment.

Many of these transactions involve money, ranging from small to huge sums, but offerings may be nonmonetary, involving goods and services. Gifts may include home-made food which is common in rural areas, as well as sweets, flowers, alcohol, coffee, or a combination of these and food products of various types, ranging from meats to fruits. Invitations to dinner, trips, and luxury items, such as perfumes, works of art, and jewelry, have been used as well. Other offerings include services provided by patients or their families or political and social favors (Balabanova and McKee 2002; Gaal et al. 2006). These categories feature items to suit all income levels. Obviously, some people give more and some less, depending on their personal circumstances.

As noted, there are several players in this game, ranging from individuals to institutions. The latter no longer score in this informal payment game as they did in the past. These payments are, for the most part, unequally distributed among health-care personnel. The physicians, especially specialists, are the important scorers, reaping the largest portion of the prize as the captain of the team. Other health-care providers score in lesser fashion. Those professions with lower wages, such as nursing, tend to receive smaller monetary payments, for example, as in Poland (Strózik 2006), and sometimes, instead, they are awarded nonmonetary gifts. This has been used to explain why nurses value contact with patients' relatives, who are the ones that often make the monetary offerings, and why they take advantage of every opportunity to be in service.

The setting in which these payments are made is important as well. They are more common in some than in others. It is generally acknowledged that they are more prevalent in the inpatient sector than in outpatient services. More specifically, they are more widespread in hospitals and specialized facilities as opposed to primary care structures. In fact, in Hungary, the frequency of these payments was found to be the highest for hospital care and the lowest for outpatient care (Gaal 2004; Szende and Culyer 2006). Then, specific units of the setting manifest diverse tendencies. Staff working in surgery, urology, ophthalmology, and obstetrics-gynecology are likely to receive more of these rewards than personnel in other areas.

Economic, cultural, legal, and ethical reasons are set forth as explanations for this phenomenon. From the economic perspective, it is generally acknowledged that it represents a legacy carried over from pretransition Communist regimes in which it was commonplace to find an informal economy side-by-side the formal one. Part of the former included gratitude payments in the health-care sector, resulting from a system that featured shortages necessitating these informal transactions. Thus, they were common before the transition and after it took place, they persisted. It has been suggested that the lack of financial resources is closely related to the extent and types of informal payments (Gaal et al. 2006). The size of this informal economy is not really known because the boundary between the formal and informal is not clear. There seems to be a sizeable gray area. All is not black or white. Estimates as to its financial worth in various countries reveal no real consensus.

The practice has also been related to a nation's culture and tradition. In this sense, the informal payment represents gratitude, gratitude in the form of a gift to show appreciation for being cured (Gaal, Evetovits, and McKee 2006). The legal perspective demonstrates that the practice was aided by the nature of the norms and controls internal and external to a profession. Being defective, they failed to function appropriately. Regulations lacking specifics were applied haphazardly. Thus, the phenomenon flourished. The ethical interpretation refers to physicians' greed and abuse of power to extract payments from patients, resulting from their market position and control of resources (Ensor and Witter 2001; Gaal and McKee 2004).

The practice of informal payments is not without its consequences, some of which have been referred to as positive (Liaropoulos et al. 2008). Helping to inflate the recognized low salaries of nurses, these transfers not only enrich their pay envelopes, but they raise morale as well. This is important to performance. In addition, they serve as an aid in retention, tempering the outflow of personnel from the health-care sector. Also, they benefit patients because they provide them an opportunity to show appreciation and respect to providers who meet their expectations. Yet, on the other hand, there are serious implications for staff security from several perspectives. Even if staff profits, in the short run, from these transactions, benefit and pension programs do not because they do not take them into consideration. Thus, a nurse who retires would most likely realize a bigger decrease in income than is officially the case, simply because the pension would be calculated on the basis of formal wages (Alford 2003). From this perspective, informal payments could be a cause of insecurity. Furthermore, professionals, having direct contact with patients, are automatically at an advantage in terms of receiving gratitude payments. Obviously, physicians are in pole position to control the whole system and thus, their pockets.

In some cases, income from these payments is considerable. This fact could make recipients adverse to innovations in the health-care delivery system. Barriers to reform could be constructed (Gaal et al. 2006). Moreover, moral issues must be given consideration. These transactions inject the potential for corruption into health care. In Latvia, results of a survey of the populace indicated that 51 percent of the respondents were of the opinion that unofficial payments to health-care professionals constituted corruption and 49 percent believed they did not. The latter viewed them as acts of gratitude (Tragakes 2008). Trade unions have claimed these payments can only be curbed by increasing salaries in the health-care sector. It would seem that to arrest the practice's damaging effects, such action only represents part of the picture. Low salaries are a problem and they are related to informal payments, but given their multiple origins, much more is needed. Florence Nightingale, even before these transactions gained prominence in the newly acceded nations and elsewhere, commented on the subject and offered her solution. In her words:

> Any nurse asking or accepting a present, whether in money or in kind, from any patient, or friend of any patient, whether during his illness or after his death, recovery, or departure, must be at once suspended from duty, her pay immediately cease, and the Superintendent-General be appraised of it, who, if satisfied of the truth of the charge, should immediately dismiss her (Nightingale 1954a, p. 54).

Wage Evaluation

Problems specific to the nursing profession include wages. Dissatisfaction on the part of these professionals is great and the matter has generated much conflict. Also, often, throughout the Member

101

States, they have served as the cause of various types of collective action. In fact, there is not a single one in which this theme has not raised difficulties at one time or another. The vast majority of nurses express considerable dissatisfaction with their stipends. This creates concern because in a study of Belgian nurses (Willem, Buelens, and De Jonghe 2007) pay was found to be the most important facet of job satisfaction. Moreover, it has been included among the many factors that stimulate nurses' departure from the profession and, in Sweden, it has been found to be the most important factor (Hasselhorn, Müller, and Tackenberg 2005).

Research focusing on European nurses' evaluation of their wages (Hasselhorn, Müller, and Tackenberg 2005) reported that in all countries, a majority was dissatisfied. To be more specific, dissatisfaction among these professionals in various nations ranged from 58 percent to 90 percent. These figures are significant. Negative reactions have been particularly pronounced in Finland (Flinkman et al. 2008), Italy (Hasselhorn, Müller, and Tackenberg 2005), and a bulk of the Central and Eastern European Member States. Not only are nurses highly critical of their salary levels, but they are especially perturbed by the gap between their wages and those of other comparable professions. This feeling is particularly evident among younger practitioners. Expression of this dissatisfaction is found in the Spanish nurses' basic guidelines which declare that these professionals should have a salary not less than 80 percent of that of physicians. Dissatisfaction also relates to the lack of equilibrium between salary, responsibilities, work demands, and conditions and effort required. Economic harsh times have been reported by nurses in the older Member States, such as the United Kingdom, Ireland, Germany, and Finland, but, particularly, by those in the newer ones, such as Poland, Slovakia, Bulgaria, Romania, and Estonia, where income insecurity is prevalent (Hasselhorn, Müller, and Tackenberg 2005; Rosskam and Leather 2006). This absolute lack of security and general dissatisfaction nurture transactions in the informal economy.

In a more optimistic vein, reference must be made to France and the Netherlands where nurses were found to be more satisfied with their pay than colleagues in other Member States. Among younger French nurses, those having worked in the field for only five years, 56 percent of male participants in a survey thought they were well paid or very well paid. The figure for female respondents was 66 percent (Marquier 2005). However, as noted, these positive evaluations do not always endure. In a survey of the Netherlands (Hasselhorn, Müller, and

Tackenberg 2005), 67 percent of all nurse respondents indicated good or very good economic circumstances.

The low level of salaries in many of the newly acceded Member States, as noted, has nurtured nurse migration. Illustrative of this fact are several examples. In the recent past, approximately one thousand two hundred Czech nurses have headed abroad, principally to Germany and England. In addition, a galaxy has flocked to Austria where a large number work, many illegally, in the private sector in a facility or for elderly individuals. Evidently, authorities have been somewhat lenient in administering the law, not wanting to alienate the elderly who are dependent on these service providers (Alda 2006). Numerous Latvian nurses are eager to be recruited for work in Norway and Germany. Their Polish colleagues travel in the same direction. Their most popular destination has been Italy with Scandinavia, the United Kingdom, Ireland, and the United States being attractive as well (Kalnins 2006; Krajewski-Siuda and Romaniuk 2006; "Polish Nurses" 2007). Romania and Slovakia have experienced the same phenomenon. Now that Croatia is a Member State, authorities there are worried about losing hundreds of nurses in the first years of membership.

Primarily, nurses' adventures to other countries have been undertaken in search of better wages and job security. For example, Estonian nurses desiring to work abroad have high expectations. Some of them hope for salaries three to four times higher than their present earnings and others think in terms of at least six times more. Evidently, Slovakian practitioners, who work in Austria, the United Kingdom, the Czech Republic, or in Scandinavia, receive three to four times more than they do at home. Polish nurses report they can earn at least four times their Polish stipend doing the same work in the United Kingdom, Ireland, and Italy (Dragu 2006; Holt 2010; Vörk, Priinits, and Kallaste 2004). Needless to say, the outflow creates problems for many facilities and programs. For example, the Czech Republic already has a significant nurse shortage and Estonia is in need of nurses with specializations. It is the most qualified that are leaving their native countries. Obviously, these exoduses, primarily from East to West, and partly organized through bilateral accords, such as the one between Poland and the Netherlands, influence the quality of health services delivered and often, in negative fashion. Many health-care executives in these newly acceded Member States are concerned, even though the outflow of nurses has been less than originally expected. With the hope of decreasing this outward flow and ideally of stopping it, they have offered nursing personnel incentives, some of which are innovative and imaginative. Income security is a sensitive matter that merits attention because of its far-reaching consequences, only one of which is the emigration of these professionals.

Social Security and Pensions

As part of their resources that allow for adequate household consumption needs, social security is important to all citizens and it can be considered a facet of personal income. The European Union Charter of Fundamental Rights (2000) acknowledges entitlement to social security benefits. Providing that they recognize the basic principles of equality of treatment and nondiscrimination, each Member State is to determine the details of its own social security system, including the nature of the benefits to be provided, their value, and the conditions of eligibility (ETUI-REHS Research Department 2005). The EU has also acted on this subject, particularly as it relates to employed persons and their families moving from one Member State to another. Once again, focus is on free movement. With all due respect to the mosaic of existing national social security systems in existence, the EU has assumed the role of coordinator of these schemes (Council Regulation 1408/71, 118/97) so as to facilitate workers' freedom of movement.

These mobile people and their dependents are assured that these benefits will not be forfeited when they change residence within the EU. They are guaranteed equality of treatment with nationals of the host Member State. More recently, Regulation (EC) No. 883/2004 firmly acclaimed that linking social security rights to place of residence cannot be justified. Furthermore, the regulation applies to a broad list of benefits related to the multiple facets of social security. Coordination of the various national social security systems and not the creation of a single European arrangement was selected as the best policy, given the diversity in schemes and varying standards and cost of living across the Member States.

Pension benefits are also a significant part of anyone's remuneration package. The nursing profession, consisting, for the most part, of females with variations, deviations, and divisions in career paths, presents a challenge to pension funds. In the EU, there are three different models or pillars of national pension systems. There are statutory retirement pensions provided by the state. Occupational pension plans are those developed in the framework of a professional activity and provided by employers for their workers in connection with their employment. These may replace state pensions or serve as a supplement. Last, there are personal pension plans not related to employment that represent individual savings for retirement.

For the most part, in the EU Member States, public programs serve as the main source of pensions for nurses and others. However, the employer privately managed schemes are growing in significance. These second pillar arrangements are important in the Netherlands and Ireland and of lesser importance in Denmark, Belgium, Germany, Sweden, and the United Kingdom (Sarfati 2010). The newly acceded nations, in particular, feature a state retirement scheme and a private one built as a funded tier of statutory arrangements, which are mandatory for people below a certain age and voluntarily accessible to older folks. In fact, in Estonia, Latvia, Poland, Hungary, and Slovakia, the private schemes are obligatory for new entrants to the labor force; in Bulgaria, for those born after 1959, and in Croatia for those under forty. In Lithuania, on the other hand, they are purely voluntary (Asenova and McKinnon 2007; European Commission: Directorate-General for Employment, Social Affairs and Equal Opportunities 2006; www.regos.hr). Within this framework, there are variations in terms of funding, accessibility, and types of benefits. The pension landscape, like many others in the EU, is quite heterogeneous, even though all systems are dedicated to common objectives. All are aimed at providing sufficient and sustainable pensions by guaranteeing adequate retirement incomes, the financial sustainability of pension programs, and schemes that are transparent and congruent with the needs of their clientele and the requirements of modern society (European Commission: Directorate-General for Employment, Social Affairs and Equal Opportunities 2007).

One of the major differences between and within these models relates to funding. Public state pension plans are based on contributions made throughout one's working life by employee and employer and/or taxes. In most cases, both employer and employee contribute to the public pension scheme. The contribution rate represents a percentage of one's wages. The employers' responsibility ranges from a low of 6.3 percent in Cyprus to a high of 24.87 percent in Belgium. On the employee side, these percentages vary from a low of 2.5 percent in Lithuania to a high of 20 percent in Croatia. The funds receive an injection of state contributions from tax revenues in some nations, such as Germany, Greece, Luxembourg, and Austria. Moreover, in Denmark, public pensions are financed solely by taxes. Both employees and employers contribute in equal fashion in Germany, Cyprus, Luxembourg, Malta, and Poland.

Slovenia represents an outlier because it is the only nation in which employers pay much less than the workers (European Commission: Directorate-General for Employment, Social Affairs and Equal Opportunities 2006; www.regos.hr). As far as occupational pension plans are concerned, some are financed only by the employer and others require employee contributions as well. Personal pension arrangements rely on individual payments, but sometimes the employer or government also contribute, as in the Czech Republic, Hungary, and Slovakia. It is clear that the pension funding scene contains much diversity, given the nature of participation assumed by employees and employers.

In terms of who gets what as far as pensions are concerned, again there is a great deal of variety. Payments are calculated in a different manner from country to country. The relative income of retirees in several Member States is close to 75 percent of their previous earnings and in some, it reaches 90 percent. However, there is the other side of the coin, where it is particularly low. A European Commission report (European Commission: Directorate-General for Employment, Social Affairs and Equal Opportunities 2007) indicates pension entitlements, especially in statutory pension arrangements and in well-structured private ones, such as those based on collective agreements, provide approximately 70 percent of retirement income. It concludes that pensions, in general, guarantee adequate income in most Member States. However, it is noteworthy that Lithuania and Ireland have extremely low pensions in comparison with other Member States. Moreover, most recently, Greece and Ireland have reduced pension benefits.

Studies (International Centre for Human Resources in Nursing 2009a; Sarfati 2010) have indicated some skepticism in reference to the adequacy of nurses' pensions. More specifically, their benefits in Bulgaria, Lithuania, and Latvia are below the poverty line. In the Czech Republic, they amount to approximately 40 percent of previous earnings and in Sweden, the first and second pillar benefits combined equal 65 percent of one's last salary. Often, benefits are not calculated according to actual take-home pay that includes the extra remuneration for extraordinary work (night shifts, on call, overtime etc.). Base pay is used for the calculation, so the nurse is penalized. In Member States, there are significant gaps in the sufficiency of the income of important segments of the nursing profession. This is especially true of those who have worked in long-term care and community care services. Furthermore, gender imbalances are identifiable as well. It is noteworthy that in Malta, pension benefits are the same for a male and a single female nurse. However, if a nurse is married, her pension is calculated on the basis of her husband's. This practice, which seems quite atypical, applies to all females, not just nurses (Sarfati 2010). Still, in spite of these problems, it is claimed that public plans provide a better guarantee of pension rights for nurses, given their employment behavior characterized by career breaks, transfers among sectors, and part-time work.

Sarfati (2010) has singled out Finnish pension arrangements for special attention and as being advantageous for nurses. According to the plan, all gainfully employed people in Finland, regardless of the nature of their work, accrue earnings-related pensions, provided their wage reaches an established minimum per month of 47 euro (approximately $51.23). Even when workers are not paid, for example, during various types of leaves, pension rights continue to accrue. The same applies to those employees receiving unemployment, workers' compensation, or other payments. The same accrual rates apply to all economic sectors and occupational groups. However, the rate depends incrementally on age category. This system seems to accommodate nurses' career patterns.

The statutory retirement age in most Member States is sixty-five and in the Czech Republic for women it depends on the number of their children. In some nations, women have an earlier retirement age than men. For example, in Lithuania, females may retire at sixty and males at 62.5 and in Romania, the age for females is sixty and sixty-five for males (Galan, Olsavszky, and Vladescu 2011; Padaiga, Pukas, and Starkienē 2011). Even though there is a legal retirement age in a nation, this is not necessarily the average age at which people retire. The statutory retirement age and the effective average age of retirement rarely coincide. Many European nations, such as Belgium, Germany, Italy, Denmark, Ireland, Sweden, the United Kingdom, and Finland, have general early retirement options, often subject to age and/or number of insured years which generally apply to all public sector employees. Finland has such an option specific to nurses. Also, in Belgium, most nurses are entitled to retire early from age fifty-eight on because nursing is considered a profession involving arduous activity. In most Member States, workers retire well before reaching the official retirement age. For example, the average age of Irish nurses who depart the workforce is sixty, in Denmark, it is sixty-one, and in the United Kingdom, between fifty and sixty, well below the statutory retirement requirement. These examples are not atypical. In some nations, it is possible to retire at age fifty, as in the

United Kingdom, or age fifty-five, as in Denmark. Since the early 1990s, many nurses have taken advantage of such options, creating a deficit in the workforce of these professionals over age fifty-five. In France, the majority of hospital nurses retire at age fifty-five. However, 17 percent of their male colleagues and 20 percent of the female ones have already departed the profession (Dubois, McKee, and Nolte 2006; *Formation et trajectoires* 2011; International Centre for Human Resources in Nursing 2009a, 2010; Manion 2009). In some Member States, there are strong incentives for persons of a certain age to retire. Also, often an existing retirement culture or mind-set can dictate that workers leave their employment as early as possible. In addition, mandatory retirement ages in some nations, are stringently applied. A wealth of experience has been lost. On the other hand, in Romania, nurses over the age of sixty-five are allowed to continue practicing, but only in the private sector and with proper annual authorization (Galan, Olsavszky, and Vladescu 2011).

Many nations authorized a decrease in the effective retirement age during the 1970s and 1980s which ran counter to the significant augment in life expectancy in these decades. This raised some issues. The number of contribution years to pension funds decreased, while the number of years' benefits was due to individuals increased. The sustainability of pension systems became a challenge. Moreover, as noted, some countries have diverse retirement ages for men and women. This practice creates inequity of benefits. In Italy, Austria, Belgium, Poland, and Portugal, female public employees, can retire at age sixty, whereas their male colleagues must wait until they reach age sixty-five. In Slovakia, the age for females is fifty-five. According to the EU, such a practice violates Article 141 of the Treaty of Maastricht on European Union (1992) concerned with equal treatment of men and women in working life (Bonanni 2010; D'Árgenio 2008). In the eyes of the Court of Justice of the European Union (CJEU), the prohibition on age discrimination is merely a particular expression of the general principle of equal treatment. It is also noteworthy that in its decision in Case C-262/88 (1990), *Barber v. Guardian Royal Exchange Assurance Group*, it reaffirmed the principle of equality between the sexes as it relates to pension systems. It ruled that pension benefits are considered to be wages and thus, must comply with the notion of equal pay for men and women (ETUI-REHS Research Department 2005).

Many Member States have or are taking steps to meet these problems. They are attempting to make their programs congruent with the realities of the modern world, that is, the increase in life expectancy and the need for a new and appropriate relationship between contributions and benefits. A prime objective is to limit expenditures and guarantee sustainability of statutory programs. The challenge is to provide sufficient resources for adequate pensions. Another prime issue being addressed is how to assure adequate pension benefits for nurses in light of their new flexible career structures. On the one hand, along with options for early retirement, disincentives to work longer are being tailored and, on the other, incentives to remain part of the workforce are being strengthened. For example, in the United Kingdom, a flexible retirement initiative that allows one to delay withdrawal from the workforce and to work in another manner is available to nurses. They may select the Wind Down option that permits them to work part-time or the Step Down alternative, according to which, they move to a more junior position. Neither of these options reduces pension benefits and, in fact, in the long run, retirement income may increase. Legislation has been enacted in France to maintain the workforce. Its scope is to prevent discrimination against older folks who want to remain in the world of work (Bennett, Davey, and Harris 2007; Camerino et al. 2006). These efforts and similar ones are especially important as far as nurses are concerned, given the widespread shortage. These professionals may be compared to wine. Often, in terms of vintage year, older is better from a variety of perspectives. The same may be said of nurses. Also, many pension funds are recalculating benefits in terms of increased life expectancy and, in addition, most countries, in order to meet EU requirements, are phasing out differences in the legal retirement age based on gender.

For the most part, national nurses associations have not been especially vocal or active in the realm of pensions. They have not asserted themselves in the various facets of the policy process related to these arrangements, much less in the administration of programs. Exceptions to this trend are provided by the United Kingdom, Denmark, and Finland. Especially in the latter two nations, nurses' organizations are actively involved in many aspects of pension programs. The International Centre for Human Resources in Nursing has issued a call for more meaningful participation on the part of nurses in pension matters. This is sage advice, in particular, in light of the challenge to balance the supply of these professionals with the demand for their services. Failure to seriously enter the pension arena means nurses are only penalizing themselves in many ways. They should respond in the affirmative to this call. It is in their interest.

Europeanization and trade liberalization have created many changes in the health-care sector, including those related to nurses' mobility. One of the basic rights enshrined in multiple EU materials, as noted, is workers' freedom of movement. However, many pension schemes and especially, provisions related to portability of pension rights presented a barrier to this principle. Pension rights, like social security, had to be protected, if nurses and other workers were to become part of the mobile society and move within the confines of the EU. Coordination of social security pension schemes allows mobile workers to maintain their accrued statutory pension benefits. However, supplementary or occupational arrangements of the second pillar posed a portability problem and still do. Failure to solve this problem reduces the flexibility and effectiveness of the labor market. The Council adopted Directive 98/49/EC concerned with the safeguarding of these pension rights for those persons moving across borders within the EU. Guarantees against the loss of all or some of these benefits were detailed. More precisely, equality of treatment concerning preservation of pension rights and cross-border payments were assured. However, the document did not concern conditions of acquisition of supplementary pension rights, their transferability, or portability.

The Commission has demonstrated an intense interest in pension issues, relying, to a large extent, on the open method of coordination because it permits "mutual learning, benchmarking, best practice and peer pressure to achieve objectives" (ETUI-REHS Research Department 2005, p. 11). It has been particularly interested in an EU harmonized funding regime. In the interests of examining retirement more intensely and from a broader perspective, in 2000, it established a Pensions Forum in which representatives of government, employers, employees, and pension programs discuss issues concerned with occupational pensions and cross-border mobility, such as tax obstacles, vesting periods, and waiting periods. It has put forward several proposals, none of which have been approved. It is still in search of a directive to reduce barriers to mobility without creating major difficulties for pension programs. In a positive vein, the so-called Pension Fund Directive, Directive 2003/41/EC of the Parliament and the Council, established a general framework for pan-European pension arrangements covering the institutions for occupational retirement provision. Also, in 2010, it was agreed that retirees were to get a single pension check from the Member State in which they are resident. Each nation in which they worked is to contribute to the amount based on the percentage of their working life spent in that country. Progress has been made as far as pension benefits and mobility are concerned. However, it is slow, given the complex nature of the matter and the fact that pension systems are, in the eyes of many, a national issue. More remains to be accomplished.

Conclusion

Materials presented in this chapter highlight the diversity in industrial relations throughout the confines of the EU. Not very much in this area has been Europeanized and, for the most part, these relations are practiced in a national framework. There has been discussion of possibly building European wage formation structures through collective bargaining and collective agreements. The establishment of an industrial relations system at the European level has been proposed as a means to counter the internationalization of capital, to create greater worker participation in European economic development, and to avoid a downward spiral in employees' social guarantees. It has been argued that such a harmonization would be congruent with the free movement of labor. Optimism prevailed for some supporters of such a project, due to the strong commitment of the European Commission and advances in the structures of social dialogue. However, wage determination, a prime element in industrial relations, was not included in the realm of harmonization (Blanke 2005a).

To realize this objective certain obstacles related to other institutions and the regulation of labor relations must be overcome. Harmonization is hindered by the great variety of national arrangements and practices in industrial relations and the diverse bargaining cultures. The legal binding effect of collective agreements is regulated in a different manner throughout the Member States. Moreover, at the EU level, there is no legal basis for such transnational collective agreements. Employer and employee structures are organized in European networks, but they do not enjoy "a mandate for wage bargaining which directly binds trade union membership in all countries" (Blanke 2005b, p. 160). Extreme diversity characterizes interests and institutional commitments of individual trade unions. Even though national industrial relations systems face similar economic and social challenges, they do not exhibit a tendency to converge or an appetite for transnational bargaining. Opposition comes from employers and also some trade union quarters.

In the Member States, nurses' wages differ significantly on the basis of several variables. The financial situation of these professionals varies on national lines and with their position, power, gender, and practice setting, to cite some elements. As is evident from the materials presented here, throughout the EU, there is much diversity in nurses' pay determination. There is no general formula which applies to all or even to most of them. However, one thing is certain. Utilization of the various noted allowances and other means to enlarge their stipends represent efforts to make nurses' salaries more competitive. This is important because remuneration methods relate to work performance, quality of care, efficiency, equity, effectiveness, and patient satisfaction. They can guide these elements in a positive or negative direction. Matters concerning salaries have become quite complex. Florence Nightingale made it seem so simple when she wrote: "after ten years good service . . . raise nurses' wages; after a second ten years . . . raise them further" (Nightingale 1954c, p. 10).

As noted, from a comparative perspective, nurses' salaries are low. This contributes to a sense that these professionals are assigned an inferior status and they are undervalued. Moreover, it reinforces the portrayal of nursing as a vocation and not a profession or a career (Lane, Antunes, and Kingma 2009). However, there are some features of the workplace that potentially could compensate for or, at least, temper the impact of these low levels of pay. At the same time, there are others that can only make matters worse. The next chapter will focus on other elements in nurses' working world.

3

The World of Work: Basic Organizational Features

Working Time

Member States feature a galaxy of laws and regulations concerned with the world of work. To a large degree, these have been constructed under the influence of the minimum standards established by the EU. Traditionally, employees have been subjected to mandates governing their working time. In fact, in many Member States, determination of this matter has been a central issue in industrial relations and in nurses' collective action. It is of particular importance in the health sector, given that services must be offered on a continuous basis in many workplaces. In an environment characterized, to a large extent, as noted, by a shortage of staff, particularly nursing personnel, and increased demand, most recently, health-care institutions have been pressured to reduce costs, become more efficient, and raise the quality of care. These and many other issues in the health arena are related to working time and work organization. Thus, time is a key organizational factor from several perspectives. It is a major issue in patient care units because it determines the entire organization of the work day and the manner in which services are delivered. Time management provides a potent mechanism for the regulation of workload and definition of the allocation of tasks, among other things (De Troyer 2001; Mermet and Lehndorff 2001; Pillinger 2000).

Establishing a limit on the number of hours a person works has traditionally been a singular trade union concern that has been acknowledged by the EU since its birth. More specifically, Article 2 of the 1961 European Social Charter made reference to "reasonable daily and weekly working hours," and it also stated that "the working week be progressively reduced to the extent that . . . relevant factors permit." Moreover, in 1975, the EU attempted to regulate working time with a

Recommendation for a forty-hour work week and four weeks of annual paid vacation. In the 1989 Community Charter on the Fundamental Rights of Workers, the issue of working time was recognized as significant to the improvement of living and working conditions. Also, the Charter of Fundamental Rights of the European Union concluded in 2000 made reference to workers' right to a limitation on maximum working hours, daily and weekly rest periods, an annual period of paid leave, and working conditions that respect health, safety, and dignity.

Some of these and other EU initiatives culminated in the Working Time Directive (Council Directive 93/104/EC) adopted in 1993 and its consolidated version of 2003 (Directive 2003/88/EC). This document has been labeled "the single most dramatic factor to impact upon the working environment" (Gunnarsdóttir and Rafferty 2006, p. 168). It was heralded by health-care trade unions throughout the Member States, but not necessarily by other stakeholders. The measure was passed on the basis of Article 118a (now Article 138) of the 1957 Treaty Establishing the European Community. This provision affirmed that Member States should undertake efforts to encourage improvements in the general climate at work and specifically, the health and safety of workers. In addition, it was indicated that these nations should attempt to harmonize conditions in this sector. As an aid in these tasks, bearing in mind, the conditions and technical rules of individual Member States, the Council was to issue directives establishing minimum requirements for implementation.

The aforementioned directive is significant because it provides for a limitation on the maximum number of working hours per week, mandatory rest periods, and paid annual vacations for workers in the EU. In addition, there are provisions related to night work, shift work, and general patterns of work. In spite of the exceptions and derogations found in the document, implementation creates for the first time a common European standard. In an effort to ensure a satisfactory climate at the workplace, the Working Time Directive establishes a basic framework of legal rights for employees. More specifically, it affirms that workers are entitled to a rest period of eleven consecutive hours on a daily basis, a twenty-minute break after having worked for six consecutive hours and on a weekly basis, a minimum uninterrupted rest period of twenty-four hours. In addition, the maximum weekly working time is established at forty-eight hours, including overtime averaged over a reference period of four months or potentially longer.

In an attempt to protect night workers, their working time has a limit of eight hours. Individuals may voluntarily select to exceed this

114

limitation. However, those refusing longer hours may not be penalized by employers. Moreover, these workers are entitled to regular free medical examinations and if health problems are found, they are entitled to take up day work. Added protection for night workers is a mandate that they must not perform work involving heavy physical or mental strain for longer than eight hours. Another important provision relates to paid annual leave of at least four weeks with no opting-out or carrying over of pay in lieu, except on termination of employment.

Of all the provisions, it is the exemption and derogation possibilities that provided a source for intense debate. In addition to a complete derogation from the directive, if workers concerned are allowed equivalent periods of compensatory rest, or if this is not possible, appropriate protection, derogations are permitted. In this context, the document specifically refers to hospitals or like facilities and the activities of doctors-in-training. This reference is of significance for all health-care personnel and especially, the nursing profession. Believing every employee should be able to limit their working time, EFN favors phasing out these derogations that offer flexibility and freedom of contract to both employers and employees. They reach into many facets of working time regulation, such as consent to work beyond the established limit of hours, record keeping, etc. They were adopted, for the most part, to satisfy the wishes of the United Kingdom who has used or, some would say, blatantly abused them (European Trade Union Confederation 2008). This nation, over and above the opposition of the Royal College of Nursing, immediately chose to opt-out of a forty-eight-hour week to work longer hours at least for the time being. In addition to the United Kingdom, Bulgaria, Estonia, Cyprus, and Malta opted-out of the forty-eight-hour work week as a possibility for all its workers. On the other hand, the Czech Republic, France, Germany, Hungary, Luxembourg, the Netherlands, Poland, Slovakia, Slovenia, and Spain chose to extend schedules beyond the forty-eight-hour limit only for those professions that rely on long duty arrangements. For example, in Hungary, in addition to the statutory forty-hour work week, it is possible for health-care workers to opt-out and voluntarily work up to twelve extra hours per week. Thus, adding overtime and voluntary hours, maximum weekly working time can reach sixty hours. In fact, in Latvia, nurses have routinely worked an average of sixty hours per week. In some nations, a special pay rate encourages employees to select this option. Doing so, they earn 50 percent more than the overtime rate. Moreover, these voluntary hours have been considered as an extra service period in calculating retirement pensions (Alford 2003; Neumann 2004).

The Working Time Directive's legal basis was sown by provisions already in place in Germany, the Netherlands, and Belgium. Legal instruments found in Greece, France, Italy, and Portugal lent themselves to the notion of derogations. Basically, a compromise measure, the Working Time Directive applies to all sectors of activity, both public and private. Also, of note is the fact that for their implementation, many of the important provisions in the document require the involvement of trade unions and collective bargaining and/or national legislation. The directive turned out to be one thing in theory and another in practice. Being a complex piece of legislation, due, among other things, to its exemption and derogation possibilities, difficulties in implementation arose, especially in the health sector (Adnett and Hardy 2001; Falkner et al. 2005). The United Kingdom asserted working time was not a health and safety issue, but rather an employment rights matter. Thus, it argued that another legislative process should have been utilized in dealing with the document. It was of the opinion that it should have been adopted by the Council with a unanimous vote, rather than a Qualified Majority Vote. Doing so would have probably guaranteed its defeat. However, such an argument did not stand with the CJEU.

In addition to having consequences for the quality of services, the Working Time Directive impacted all health-care providers in terms of their employment conditions, their professional roles and boundaries, the organization of their work, and the division of labor. In short, it created staffing problems, particularly, for the many units responsible for offering services around the clock and those in small communities. The United Kingdom, Ireland, and the Netherlands were among those nations that negatively evaluated the directive because it nurtured capacity problems for their health-care delivery systems. Implementation of the instrument throughout the Member States evidenced a variety of managerial approaches that had implications for the nature of its application (Mahon and Young 2006). It fostered an acute examination of staffing, infrastructures, skill mix, and the quality and safety of service delivery, in addition to work practices in the various health-care professions, among other critical elements. The task was complex and became even more so because of decisions taken by the CJEU concerning on-call work defined as "work done on an 'as-needed basis,' whereby workers must be available at certain times to be called into work when required by their employer" (Carley 2007,

p. 34). In some countries, such as Germany and Sweden, on-call duty was not considered a part of overall working hours. In others, such as Denmark, this work arrangement was a component of normal working time. In the Simap (Case C-303/98;ECR I-7963) and the Jaeger (Case C-151/02;ECR I-8389) cases, in 2000 and 2003, respectively, the CJEU ruled that on-call duty and stand-by time should be classified as a part of overall working time. Such decisions have garnered support of the EFN. These judgments increase the overall significance of the Working Time Directive for health-care professionals.

Among the Member States for which information is available, there are diverse conceptions of and practices concerning on-call duty. Furthermore, the concept is not defined or not used in Cyprus, Greece, Latvia, Malta, Portugal, Romania, and Spain. Thus, comparison is difficult. However, it is evident that this work arrangement is most prevalent in the health-care sector. In many Member States, such as Austria, the Czech Republic, Estonia, Finland, France, Hungary, Lithuania, Poland, and Slovakia on-call work is viewed as an additional or integral part of working time. In other words, it counts as working time. On the other hand, it is considered a form of employment or employment contract in Belgium, Italy, and the Netherlands (Carley 2007). The aforementioned rulings have not afforded uniform practices. Some Member States, given these judgments, have used them as an excuse to invoke the opt-out possibility. Interpretation of the CJEU's decisions raised considerable difficulties. The European Commission attempted to revise the Working Time Directive, but to no avail. Consensus was not realized. In June 2008, the Council achieved an accord related to on-call duty. It was agreed that inactive on-call time has to be viewed as working time, unless stipulated differently by national law or collective agreements. However, in the conciliation process, the EP and the Council failed to reach a compromise. It is generally agreed that problems have resulted from the failure to achieve consensus and from the fact that the CJEU's interpretation of working time differs from that held by many of the supporters of the original directive (Peeters, McKee, and Merkur 2010).

Implementation of the new regulations had multiple implications for management of nurses' working time. In the first place, the forty-eight-hour limit posed a problem in that many nurses worked regular long hours through overtime. In addition, the duration of shifts became of concern because many members of the nursing staff preferred longer and, therefore, fewer shifts. The requirement of an eleven-hour minimum daily rest presented an obstacle, due to variations in shifts. For example, if a nurse worked a late shift followed by an early one, this requirement posed a problem. In addition, the new restrictions on working hours potentially threatened a considerable increase in personnel costs for any given health-care facility.

Implementation of the directive triggered new working methods and work flexibility became the motto of the times. Managers resorted more and more to working time flexibility, meaning utilization of those arrangements that permit a closer match between labor input and production needs (Evans, Lippoldt, and Marianna 2001).This approach paved the way for marked growth in variable hours, part-time, temporary, and short-term work arrangements, along with job sharing and annualization of working time, to cite some schemes. Many of these initiatives, being based on new management techniques and the concept of the flexible form, had their origin in the private sector and then were applied more widely (Arrowsmith and Mosse 2000; Commission of the European Communities 2000; Pillinger 2000).

The nursing role underwent a reevaluation that not only responded to the requisites of the directive, but to economic pressures as well. More efficient use of nursing personnel received attention. There were changes in the provision of care. Staff reductions, cross-training of personnel to carry out additional responsibilities, changes in the mix of nursing staff, and a redistribution of patients across nursing units were some of the innovations realized in various institutions. Moreover, new patterns of patient care and managerial and patient care staff responsibilities emerged. In certain situations, when it contributed to the quality of care, nurses experienced an expansion of practice. Many tasks formerly performed by higher paid physicians were reallocated to nurses, representing a cost savings. Other new developments in nursing roles included an expansion in nurses' prescribing privileges and the use of nurse-led night teams and nurse practitioners. New responsibilities assumed by nurses involved more clinical leadership, the performance of minor surgical procedures, the ordering of tests, and admitting and discharging patients, among other duties. Changed organizational practices included supervised multispecialty handover in the evenings, bleep filtering, and switching nonurgent work to other parts of the day from nights, to cite a few.

A major innovation developed by the National Health Service in the United Kingdom was the Hospital at Night model which redesigned the workforce, service, and productivity. To meet the requirements of the Working Time Directive and the immediate needs of patients, this model offers a multiprofessional team with a full range of skills and competences. The team possesses the necessary requisites to cope with a wide variety of needs and has the capacity to obtain specialist expertise when required. This model for delivering care at night and out of hours has created a more nurse-led and multidisciplinary work pattern. It has proven most successful and has received approval from the Department of Health, the British Medical Association, and the royal professional colleges. With schemes, such as this one, as well as others, nurses have been assigned more responsibility and clinical decision-making. The Working Time Directive presented a galaxy of new possibilities for them. To enable the demand and supply of services to be matched according to its restrictions, many changes resulted in nurses' working methods, their scope of practice, their work organization, and the barriers between professional roles.

Even though many nurse leaders and other health-care professionals welcomed opportunities afforded the profession as a result of the directive, nurses' unions were only cautiously positive and, according to surveys, nurses themselves remained divided. Typical are surveys of these professionals in the United Kingdom carried out by the British publication, *Nursing Times*, which revealed that approximately two-thirds of the respondents were of the opinion that they were not ready for the challenges presented by the Working Time Directive. A significant share was not comfortable with the additional level of responsibility assumed which led, they claimed, to increased pressure on nurses and expectations for them to make clinical decisions. Only 24 percent evaluated this situation in a positive manner. One-third felt their training was lacking. For the most part, nurses viewed use of the extended role as an opportunity for junior medical staff "to dump" much of their routine work on them. On the positive side, 56 percent of those surveyed indicated they were more inclined since the issuance of the Working Time Directive to challenge medical staff (Ford 2009; Santry 2010). Evidently, the instrument provided assertiveness training. Consistency in responses seems to be lacking.

In addition to participating in these and other formal surveys undertaken in the United Kingdom, many nurses offered comments concerning the new arrangements on various nursing websites and in other publications. From these remarks, it is evident that a multitude failed to grasp the many opportunities and benefits afforded to nursing development. It only saw more work, not a realization of responsibilities

119

along with other changes. In short, it failed to think "outside the box." Moreover, the tone of many comments was biting, intense, inflexible, and often colored with anger. This was particularly true in opinions related to physicians that most definitely reflected the traditional friction between these professionals and nurses.

Throughout the Member States, working time is governed by national legislation, collective bargaining, or a combination of the two. In some countries, such as France, Portugal, Spain, and Sweden, the influence of legislation has been dominant, whereas in others, for example, Denmark, Germany, and Italy, collective bargaining has been of great significance. Belgium, Greece, Ireland, and the Netherlands exemplify mixed systems. In terms of comparing actual working time throughout the various Member States several problems arise. In the first place, various definitions are assigned to the term. Also, there are diverse legal, political, and collective bargaining procedures related to its determination. Data collection varies in such a way that comparison encounters major obstacles. In that universal guidelines are not used, comparable data are not collected (Carley 2007; Pillinger 2000).

Restrictions on working hours are important to all health-care providers, especially given the impact of working time on the quality of services, which, in turn, influences the safety, well-being, and health of the population. Innumerable studies have demonstrated the negative interplay between extremely long working hours, the health of nurses, increased risk from occupational hazards, and risks to patient safety. In addition, it has been concluded that when these professionals work more than forty hours per week, or overtime, or in shifts greater than twelve hours, the risks of making errors multiply (Geiger-Brown and Trinkoff 2010; Keller 2009; Rogers et al. 2004). However, a recent report ("What are 12-Hour Shifts Good for?" 2013) affirms that there is insufficient evidence to determine the impact of shift length on practitioners and the quality of care rendered to patients.

A document issued by the European Commission (Commission of the European Communities 2000) noted that after salaries, the next most important subject for any collective bargaining endeavor is that of establishing work time. This is of utmost significance, given its enunciated influence on various facets of health and job satisfaction. Certain elements of work time have been assigned particular importance. They are: the number of hours worked in a given week, the organization of these hours, the predictability of and amount of flexibility related to them, and the employee's control over this work time (Hasselhorn,

Müller, and Tackenberg 2005). Given the aforementioned difficulties related to data, plus the fact that the work time behavior of nurses differs not only from one Member State to the other, but also between health-care institutions, working hours will be presented in a general framework.

Establishment of the length of working time must be done within the parameters of rules concerning maximum working hours. Needless to say, these should meet the requisites of the Working Time Directive. In terms of the maximum number of working hours per week, Member States fall into three categories. Sixteen (Cyprus, Czech Republic, Denmark, France, Germany, Greece, Hungary, Ireland, Italy, Lithuania, Luxembourg, Malta, the Netherlands, Romania, Slovenia, and the United Kingdom) have set their limit at forty-eight hours as specified in the Working Time Directive, eleven (Austria, Bulgaria, Croatia, Estonia, Finland, Latvia, Portugal, Poland, Slovakia, Spain, and Sweden) opted for forty hours and one (Belgium) for thirty-eight hours. In addition, each country also has rules concerning the maximum number of hours in a work day. In this case, the classification is not as homogeneous. Member States divide into six different categories of daily maximum hours as follows: thirteen (Cyprus, Denmark, Ireland, Italy and the United Kingdom), 12.5 (Malta), twelve (Greece, Hungary), ten (Austria, France, Luxembourg, Slovenia), nine (Czech Republic, the Netherlands, Slovakia, Spain), and eight (Belgium, 'Bulgaria, Croatia, Estonia, Finland, Germany, Latvia, Lithuania, Poland, Portugal, Romania, Sweden). It must be remembered these limits may be exceeded as permitted by the Working Time Directive. Unfortunately, these figures cannot be compared due to the complex nature of the regulations that apply to overtime and variable working hours. The application of these rules might mean that the actual differences between the categories, for example, between those Member States with a forty-eight-hour week maximum and those with a forty-hour week, in actuality, might not be that great (Carley 2007). Still, these figures are of use in terms of affording the reader a general overview of the working time situation in the Member States.

In 2006, for the first time, the European Industrial Relations Observatory reported on agreed upon nurses' working time in public sector hospitals in twenty-one Member States. Data were not available for the entire community. The average weekly working time for these professionals was 38.1 hours, 0.6 hours less than the Member States' overall average for the whole economy. In the EU15, the number of Member

States in the organization prior to the accession of ten candidate nations in 2004, Greek nurses, agreeing to forty hours, had the longest work week, whereas the French and Portuguese at thirty-five hours claimed the shortest. The thirty-five hour work week in France was optional, but adherence was quick to be secured. Hospitals enforcing this standard were allowed a 10 percent reduction in their obligatory social security contributions for employees. In addition, according to the 6 percent rule, with the scope of increased productivity, they could employ an additional 6 percent of staff. In Italy, Luxembourg, the Netherlands, and Portugal, nurses' normal working hours are significantly less than the national average for the whole economy. As for the other Member States, working hours for these professionals are not often much higher than this average. The average agreed upon work week for hospital nurses in the EU15 stands at 37.4 hours which is below the average for the whole economy by 0.5 hours. In fact, among the various occupational sectors, the lowest amount of normal working hours has been found among public hospital nurses (Carley 2007; Wait 2006).

In the newly acceded Member States for which information is available, the average consented to weekly working hours for hospital nurses, registering at 39.2 hours, is 0.4 hours below the average for the whole economy and 1.8 hours above the EU15 average. In Cyprus and the Czech Republic, hospital nurses' average weekly working time has almost reached the EU15 average. In Slovakia, these hours total 38.6 and the other Member States in this category have a forty-hour work week. The latter's weekly hours for nurses are the same as the average for the whole economy, whereas in Cyprus, the Czech Republic, and Slovakia, they are below this average. For the most part, throughout the EU, basic weekly working hours for full-time nursing staff are set at between thirty-five and forty hours per week, but this does not mean they do not work more. In the EU15, normal agreed upon weekly hours have, for the most part, tended to decrease in recent times, leaving a gap of approximately 1.7 hours or 4.5 percent between these nations and the newly acceded Member States (Carley 2007). In the latter, with the exception of Cyprus, the Czech Republic, and Slovakia, hours have been stationary at forty for an extended period of time. In addition, collective agreements in these countries do not tend to deviate from the statutory norm of forty hours.

The existence of different ways of calculating work time with annual, rather than weekly measures, has become increasingly common. One flexible work practice that has been introduced in some Member States' health-care arena is that of annualized working hours. They have been incorporated into public service agreements or legislation in several European nations, excluding principally the newly acceded countries. Basically, this practice, as exemplified by Finland, allows for a one-year leveling period in establishing work hours, subject to the regulation of the duration of the work day and week. Thus, it is possible to divide working hours in different ways over the period of a year. In fact, given the provision of the Finnish Working Hours Act and the nature of collective bargaining agreements, it has been possible to invoke annualized working hours at the local level with specificity, meaning by health-care facility. This option, of common usage, has been in effect for some time (Finland: Ministry of Labour 2003). The purpose of this practice is to enhance the congruence of demand and supply of services. Cost is also of importance. As one can imagine, the institutional objective is to reduce expenditures. There are advantages for the health-care professional as well. Utilization of a longer leveling period, rather than shorter ones, allows for greater recognition of employees' desires and needs, as far as working methods are concerned.

From the employees' perspective, this method of planning work time has proven popular in that they have been able to enjoy longer periods of uninterrupted free time. The United Kingdom has also adopted this practice of annualized working hours, at first, on an experimental basis, and then, as a permanent policy. Nurses and trade unions fully supported the project. Annualized hours have been introduced in French hospitals as well. They have become a feature of several health-care delivery systems across the EU. A variation of the same principle has been applied to lifetime working hours. Sweden, Denmark, and Finland have adopted this model which provides for individually negotiated flexibility over the life cycle, including part-time arrangements, education/training leave, and partial early retirement, among other matters.

Overtime

At one time, overtime was not a prominent feature of nursing in many of the Member States. In fact, in some, it was exceptional. However, it has become commonplace in both the public and private sectors. Primarily, it has been used to confront the downsizing of nursing departments, the general shortage of nurses, and problems related to cost control. Throughout the EU, not only are there different regulations defining the maximum hours one may work, but overtime differs in its nature as well. In some cases, it is mandatory. The employee has no choice whatsoever, but to accept the obligation. On the other hand, overtime may be voluntary, meaning that the employee may decide whether or not to engage in the extra work. Nurses in the Member States that have implemented the Working Time Directive are protected by law from obligatory overtime. More specifically, in Finland, the consent of an employee is required each time one is expected to work overtime. Within the EU, overtime and extended unpaid hours are important facets of health-care staffing, in general, and, particularly, nurse staffing. They contribute heavily to the nature of services delivered. Being regulated by rules, legislation, and/or collective bargaining frequently related, in turn, to other instruments concerned with working time, regulation is quite complicated.

As in other instances, data problems present difficulties in terms of cross-national comparisons. In the first place, in some cases, national statistics on overtime are not available. Second, when data have been elaborated, definitions, measures, and populations covered, among other variables, vary greatly. Most recently, the Royal College of Nursing Wales, in exasperation, underscored the need for an effective way to measure the hours, and especially, the excess hours, that nursing staff work. Detailed analysis of overtime is impossible. However, some generalizations may be made.

As opposed to the situation in the United States, where overtime for a nurse is not federally regulated, in the EU, every Member State permits certain levels of overtime to be worked in addition to normal or regular contracted hours. For example, Croatian law (Croatia: Ministry of Economy, Labour and Entrepreneurship 2011, Article 48) permits overtime work, but daily work with a collective agreement is limited to twelve hours. In this context, it must be reiterated that not all EU countries recognize the limits established by the Working Time Directive. For health-care workers, in general, and nurses, in particular, often these ceilings, set by law or collective bargaining, are considerably higher than those in other lines of work. Illustrative of the situation are annual limits of 120, 150, 200, 220, 250 and 300 or 400 hours per year in Lithuania, Poland, Spain, Sweden, France, Finland, and Hungary, respectively (Federation of European Employers 2004, 2011; Kowalska 2007; Lovén 2009; Neumann 2004; Spain 2003). In addition to annual restrictions, sometimes these overtime hours are regulated on a daily, weekly, or monthly basis, as in Poland, the Czech Republic, and Sweden. Moreover, often conditions related to overtime can be compromised via collective bargaining. It is noteworthy that in some nations, in situations where more work time is necessary, these hours may be extended, if individual employees voluntarily consent in writing. Also, usually provisions exist for emergency work. Obviously, in emergencies overtime is not limited.

Many health-care providers undertake excess work hours. Studies have revealed that in Europe, approximately one-third of nurses interviewed asserted they had to work overtime. More specifically, in Germany and Italy, a majority responded likewise (Hasselhorn et al. 2005). The same holds true in the United Kingdom (Ball and Pike 2007). Overtime is also extensive in the newly acceded Member States, particularly Bulgaria and Latvia. Also, in the confines of the EU, there are not great differences between the public and private sectors in terms of the percentage of nurses that undertake excess hours. Their numbers demonstrate that nursing professionals are being overstretched. In addition, they indicate that health-care institutions are not adequately staffed and that many service providers need to generate extra income to offset poor wages. In several of the newly acceded Member States, as exemplified by Bulgaria, they reveal "formation of a pattern of health worker exploitation and self-exploitation" (Daskalova et al. 2005, p. 44). For the most part, staff nurses, and not those in leadership roles, assume overtime responsibilities. As in the case of the extent of general overtime working, for nurses' excess hours there is not a clear division between the newly acceded Member States and the older ones.

Part-time

As noted, in the health-care sector, in recent times, much use has been made of nonstandard forms of employment. In the case of nursing, use of part-time work has come into vogue and grown more rapidly than full-time. Research has concluded that the market environment determines how much a nurse works, meaning full-time or part-time, rather than whether she works (Brewer et al. 2006). Not only do definitions of part-time employment vary from country to country across the EU, but its prevalence does as well. Just before the turn of the century, part-time arrangements for nurses were not a common feature of European health-care systems. They were widespread in Belgium, the Netherlands, and the United Kingdom. In the Netherlands, they were extremely popular, being selected by 74.3 percent of the professional nursing staff. In fact, in this country, the share of nursing part-timers in hospitals was higher than the percentage of part-time employment in the total workforce. On the other hand, in Sweden, it was lower than average in the health-care sector. In Italy, Spain, Portugal, and Ireland, the level of part-time work was negligible. In many Member States, it occurred only in certain sectors. For example, in Greece, it was only witnessed in private health-care facilities. Very often, there was no real choice between full-time and part-time work. The former was imposed by rigid work contracts (Bouten and Versieck 1995; Mermet and Lehndorff 2001; Versieck, Bouten, and Pacolet 1995).

The prevalence of part-time work is related to the employment rate of a nation. With the notable exceptions of Cyprus, Portugal, and Finland, it tends to be more prevalent in those countries with an employment rate exceeding 67 percent. In nations with lower employment rates, such as Greece, Hungary, and Slovakia, utilization of part-timers is much less frequent (Vandenbrande et al. 2007). These generalizations are, for the most part, applicable to nursing staff. However, it is of note that there has been limited availability of part-time work for nurses in Austria. Given economic conditions, part-time employment is not used as much in the newly acceded Member States, although it is on the increase (European Foundation for the Improvement of Living and Working Conditions 2007a; Lethbridge 2004; Marion 2007). Health-care staff in these countries, for the most part, do not engage in part-time arrangements. In that the nursing profession consists of an overwhelming percentage of females and given the general relationship between part-time arrangements and women's employment in many West European health-care delivery systems, this phenomenon is striking.

Complete and comparable data are not available for the extent of part-time work in the nursing profession in the EU Member States. Suffice it to say, it is more developed in Western Europe. In Denmark, 54 percent of nurses work part-time. These professionals are joined by 40 percent of their colleagues in Germany and 37 percent of those in the United Kingdom. The rates for Ireland and Sweden are 26.3 percent and 20 percent, respectively. Also, it has been reported that 45 percent of Belgian hospital nurses are part-timers. Across the Member States, the proportion of employees working part-time registers at 38 percent for females and 12 percent for males (European Foundation for the Improvement of Living and Working Conditions 2009c; European Working Conditions Observatory 2014; International Council of Nurses Workforce Forum 2013).

Issuance of the Working Time Directive planted the seeds for a variety of diverse work patterns among which part-time employment occupied a prominent place. In many Member States, it was perceived as a solution to human resource problems. In addition to workplace requirements, employees' changing lifestyles and expectations, among other elements, enhanced its growth. In the health sector, it went hand in hand with increased flexibility. Human resource managers, in an effort to alleviate their burden, very often, encouraged part-time employment of which there are many varieties, ranging from working four-fifths of full-time hours in France to the provisions of the Abvakabo Agreement in the Netherlands that allows female employees working on a part-time basis to develop their own schedules to cover needed services.

From the managers' perspective, part-time arrangements lower payroll requirements. To a large extent, such employees have a lower salary rate than those working in a full-time capacity. For example, in Austria, part-timers earn 24.2 percent less than full-timers. This difference is less pronounced for health-care providers, but it exists. Generally the practice is "the fewer hours worked, the lower the rate of pay." This situation is not limited to a particular country (Allinger 2014).

In the health-care sector, Italian collective agreements have restricted part-time contracts by not allowing them to exceed 25 percent of the total number. It has been demanded that use of such arrangements be strictly related to need and that periodic evaluations be undertaken. Furthermore, such contracts have been limited to employees without managerial duties. This is a practice found in other Member States, for example, the United Kingdom and Sweden. Such a practice only reinforces the glass ceiling for many in a predominantly female profession. These part-time agreements in Italy are of two types: horizontal part-time contracts and vertical part-time contracts. The first category consists of agreements featuring fixed work days and hours. The second includes a variety of accords. There are fixed ones providing for work in three eight-hour days per week. Variable ones, as implied by the name, rely on eight-hour days distributed in a variable way and the modular model refers to total hours calculated for the month and distributed in a variable manner (B 2007; Bach n.d.-a, n.d.-b; Mermet and Lehndorff 2001). There are many options.

Diverse mechanisms aided the attractiveness of part-time hours. For example, in France, salary increases along with improved promotion and career development opportunities for part-timers led nurses to select this option (Arrowsmith and Mosse 2000). On the other hand, in Belgium, it was the nurses who fought fiercely for recognition of part-time work arrangements. Even though they were rapidly increasing, the labor movement for many years refused to confront the issue. It was unwilling to discuss part-time workers' terms and conditions of employment. The increase in part-timers was so great, it was feared that labor costs would rise as well. To abate this alarm, bonuses in the form of time off or extra pay were offered to nurses selecting full-time. Such a measure only infuriated these professionals beyond question. They threatened resignation, if denied part-time work opportunities which were so widespread that trade unions could no longer fail to become involved with standards concerning their status (ILO Sectoral Activities Program n.d.; Mermet and Lehndorff 2001).

In many Member States, it is difficult to secure a transition from part-time to full-time employment. Such a happening has been comparatively rare. However, in Sweden, where the Swedish Health Care Union (SHSTE) made this a priority issue, it has been commonplace. Moreover, it is considered a right to make a temporary transition in the other direction, that is, from full to part-time arrangements, as well. Rights of this kind are also found in the Netherlands. In Belgium, in the Flemish not-for-profit health-care sector, a similar transition that enables staff to gradually shift into retirement has been available. Known as the "landing strip," it allows employees over fifty years of age with at least twenty years of service in the sector to change their status to part-time with reasonable income (*Flexible Career Options* 2000). Also, in Belgium, there have been other schemes to progressively reduce working hours before retirement that practically amount to transitioning to part-time. From age forty-five, nurses have been allowed to take off one day per month, those over age fifty, two days and after age fifty-five, three days. Many Belgian collective agreements affecting these practitioners have reduced working hours based on age. For example, in 2000, the work week for nurses over age fifty-five was reduced by six hours and by two hours for those over forty-five. Working hours for these professionals have been decreased by up to 15 percent (Safuta and Baeten 2011).

There is a dearth of studies concerned with part-time employment in the nursing profession in the Member States. In that the profession is overwhelmingly feminine, there are few nuances in terms of part-time arrangements and gender. However, it can be noted that, in the United Kingdom, more male nurses have opted for part-time work than in the past. In general, the share of this type of employment for nurses is related to the practice site and the specialization involved, if any. For example, in France, it was found that nurse specialists work part-time less frequently than their staff colleagues. Those professionals hired on the basis of the aforementioned 6 percent rule in France tended to be awarded part-time contracts. Fewer nurses working in a hospital setting tend to select part-time. On the other hand, their counterparts employed in the social sector manifest the opposite tendency. Part-time has been known to be more prevalent in sectors that nurses experience late in their work life, such as physicians' offices, the community, or agency/bank nursing. For the self-employed nurse, part-time has been minimal (Audric et al. 2001; Segrestin and Tonneau 2002).

Responsibilities for dependents and/or children, as well as other factors, have also been known to influence selection of part-time employment. In terms of age, diverse tendencies are evident. In France, it has been reported that part-time work was becoming more popular with older nurses than younger ones, whereas the exact opposite has been noted in the United Kingdom. Working hours have also been related to ethnicity and nationality. For example, in the United Kingdom, black minority ethnic nurses and those recruited from abroad are less likely to work part-time than their white colleagues. This fact has served to raise the subject of discrimination in connection with access to part-time arrangements. Also, the situation has been attributed to age. In the United Kingdom, these nurses have been among the younger in the profession (Ball and Pike 2006a; Pike and Ball 2007; Royal College of Nursing 2007; Segrestin and Tonneau 2002; Vilain and Niel 1999). The matter of part-time employment in nursing is a subject that merits investigation and on a comparative basis.

Part-time employment results from a variety of situations, such as a weak labor market or unfavorable labor conditions. It carries advantages for both employer and employee and, at the same time, perils for both groups. Given that the nursing profession is exceedingly feminine in nature, very often, gender relates to the selection of part-time employment. It is the traditional European gender division of care and domestic responsibilities at home that often generate such a choice. Gender inequality definitely characterizes the distribution of tasks affiliated with the home. For the professional nurse part-time work stands to enrich work–family compatibility. It affords flexibility in terms of fulfilling daily responsibilities. However, this comes at a price: the price of underemployment, reduced opportunities for career advancement, and unpaid domestic workloads accounting for a part of the large mass of gender inequality (European Foundation for the Improvement of Living and Working Conditions 2007b).

Research has demonstrated that part-time nurses have tended to be more flexible and more reliable in terms of showing up for work than their full-time counterparts (Edwards and Robinson 2004). Thus, they have often been used more frequently than full-timers for inconvenient shift work, such as nights and weekends. Furthermore, they are expected to be more mobile and, therefore, they have exhibited a tendency to frequently change work sites as opportunities for task flexibility are exploited (Bach n.d.-a, n.d.-b). Frequently, these practices signify that nurses, working and covering such important in-service demands, could be exposed to greater social risks than full-timers. In several respects, part-timers operate at a disadvantage in the professional hierarchy. This is reflected in the fact that very often they are not given performance evaluations on a regular basis and career-oriented training opportunities available to their counterparts are denied to them. This training is delivered in the form of formal courses, private lessons, workshops, long-distance learning opportunities, and other forms of structured learning. Obtaining further qualifications through these instruments and lateral job moves are requisites of career advancement.

A study (Edwards and Robinson 2004) evaluating part-time employment of nurses in the United Kingdom from the line managerial perspective indicated advantages. Many of these related to retention and the quality of the professional. Retention was perceived as the most important benefit. This is understandable, given the extreme shortage of nursing personnel. Moreover, the staff that was retained was labeled in rank order as mature, with family experience, more experienced and more flexible, more enthusiastic and more hard-working, better qualified, producing better quality of work, and more creative. Another significant advantage for this group was recruitment, but other evidence has indicated the part-time role in facilitating recruitment is limited. In Italy, research has concluded that the efficacy of part-time arrangements as a means of recruitment is negligible. They did not attract more nursing students, nor did they entice nurses to return to work (Mermet and Lehndorff 2001).

Communication and information flow were deemed problems by these line managers as far as part-time nurses were concerned. Problems related to the giving and receiving of information were identified along with those concerning communication with a team and other staff, patients, their families, supervisors, and subordinates. Basically, there were difficulties in interacting with various actors in a health-care delivery system (Edwards and Robinson 2004). Such could result from the part-timers' role in the professional hierarchy and also, from a lack of continuity in service and limited presence.

Line managers also identified managerial and supervisory disadvantages related to the part-time employment of nurses. From this perspective, these nurses, it was claimed, being more difficult to supervise, required more managerial time. Obviously, this means an increase in costs. Problems with assuming and/or completing tasks were identified along with work scheduling difficulties and those related to developing the team chemistry, impediments encountered with full-timers and part-timers. Furthermore, it was indicated that part-time nurses demonstrated less institutional and professional commitment as manifested sometimes in a lack of desire to achieve promotion and to assume new tasks and roles. Significant differences between nurses undertaking part-time work and those involved with full-time arrangements concerned their engagement related to the nursing activities they carry out, the nature of these activities, their interests, the extent of their assumption of responsibilities, and the scope of their practice experience.

Even though these line managers identified beneficial attributes with part-time nurses, it is clear they also had significant reservations. The same holds true for the nurses surveyed. Approximately one-third indicated they were unhappy with their part-time employment. In that part-timers' engagement is related to the activities they carry out, it is evident that modification of work patterns are necessary, so as to reap full advantage from the skills of an important part of the nursing population—the part-timer. At the same time, the chemistry of the entire nursing team must be developed. To date, part-timers, in general, have felt isolated and thus, not able to fully exercise their power. Moreover, they have been of little interest to trade unions, as noted previously, was the case in Belgium. Passive acceptance of the nonstandard labor market for nurses will not lead to a change in work patterns and an enhancement of nursing resources.

It is quite evident that there are advantages to part-time employment. At the same time, it is quite clear that problems are perceived from both the employers' and employees' perspective. These have been recognized by the EU. The Council concluded a multi-organizational framework agreement related to part-time arrangements that was presented in Council Directive 97/81/EC of 15 December 1997. This instrument, to a large degree, focuses on discrimination against part-timers. It establishes general principles and minimum requirements concerning this type of employment. It underscores the need to facilitate access to part-time work via measures allowing for preparation for retirement and the reconciliation of professional and family life. In addition, it stresses the importance of part-timers' participation in training and educational opportunities for the benefit of employers, themselves, and the place of work. Such participation is to enhance career opportunities and professional mobility. It also benefits the profession and the consumer population. In that part-time hours are not usually available to senior-grade workers, it assigns employers responsibility for ensuring access to them as far as possible. Moreover, these workers are to receive the same protection as their counterparts. Meeting the requisites of this directive would mean, in this case, that across the Member States, nurses in part-time employment would no longer be on the periphery of the nursing staff, but would be included in the mainstream of the nursing labor market. It is obvious that the quality of part-time arrangements requires finetuning and, at the same time, expansion to include nurses in senior grades and management.

Work Patterns

The scheduling process reflects the health-care setting, the adopted care delivery model, the field of practice and type of care being provided, patient complexity or acuity, the time of day/night, the physical layout of the unit, the skill level and the mix of the available nursing staff, as well as professional nursing standards, to cite a few important variables. Not only do work hours frequently vary from one nation to another, but the same variation applies to the manner in which they are distributed. This diversity is evident as it relates to the nursing profession across the EU Member States. In some instances, the work day is uniform for all personnel without exception. In others, it is identical for all health-care professionals, but diverse for the remainder of public and private health-care employees. In still others, work time depends on the specific health-care profession. Sometimes, work arrangements can be structured to suit the institution involved. For example, in Lithuania, such is the case. Heads of individual health-care facilities decide working hours of all personnel. And, in Sweden, collective agreements can tailor work schedules to specific work places in the same fashion (Jones 2007; Mermet and Lehndorff 2001; Padaiga et al. 2006). One thing, however, is clear. Health-care providers work more atypical hours than those employed in other sectors.

Although scheduling is only a single phase of the staffing function, it is pivotal for unit productivity and employee morale. In essence, nurses' schedules, reflecting the nature of the employer institution, depend on the site of employment. Moreover, work requirements often differ from one service to another. In spite of these diversities, as noted, a recent trend related to work organization in many Member States has been the use of atypical arrangements. This tendency pervades the health-care sector, including nursing. New employment models based on flexible contracts and the transfer of personnel to alternate employers can destabilize job security. Often, a series of nonstandard working methods, including part-time, short-term contracts, multiple employment, and independent contracting, constitute part of the new age. Capacity-oriented variable working hours, work-on-call, and, especially, flexi-time schemes have come into fashion (Dubois, McKee, and Nolte 2006; Mermet and Lehndorff 2001; Padaiga et al. 2006). Times have changed. Flexibility lies at the base of nurses' work methods. This flexibility results, in part, from a strategy aimed at enhancing retention and enriching the work–life equilibrium of employees. It also includes self-scheduling which promises increased autonomy and job satisfaction.

These new schemes were viewed as instruments that would improve the overall quality of life for employees and would redistribute work to allow them to move at will in and between part-time and full-time arrangements. Moreover, recognizing the importance of having desirable work schedules, such schemes were to enhance individual choices concerning when and where people work. In addition to affording equal opportunities and serving as an aid in the reconciliation of family and work and the development of family-friendly policies, the new flexibility was to improve work conditions and reduce stress and ill health at the workplace. However, it is to be noted that flexible working provisions have given rise to particular drawbacks. For example, for many older nurses, free of active caring obligations, they have presented problems in that these practitioners are forced to accommodate the flexible working requirements of their colleagues with caring responsibilities. Such a situation can lead to an inflexible workforce (Bennett, Davey, and Harris 2007; Pillinger 2000).

Given that in many facilities health care has to be provided around the clock, the most common and traditional work mode for nurses has been the shift arrangement, an important part of the profession's life. It has gone hand-in-hand with shift work. Over time, this has meant

133

dividing the day into a number of work periods, usually equal in terms of number of hours. Traditionally, in most countries, as in the United States, there were three shifts per day, each consisting of eight hours, and in the United Kingdom, they were referred to as "earlies," "lates," and "nights." Published in 1995, a quality study (Bouten and Versieck 1995) of extensive scope on the nursing profession in the European Community revealed that the most prevalent shifts consisted of eight hours each as in Italy, Portugal, Luxembourg, and Ireland. Moreover, shift work often took place on a rotating basis, as in Ireland. However, rotation was not standard in all cases. Some countries followed the example of the United Kingdom where arrangements were not centrally decided. Individual employing authorities could determine what system was best in terms of meeting local needs. Moreover, in a few instances, as exemplified by Portugal, rotation not only varied from hospital to hospital, but service to service. Then, another option was the practice of permanent night shifts, as in the United Kingdom and France. In most hospitals over a certain size at that time there were flexible day shifts and a permanent night shift. Forty-six percent of the nurses worked only days, 26 percent only nights, and the remaining 28 percent a combination of shifts.

Many Member States, such as Finland, Germany, Slovakia, Belgium, Italy, and Spain, still cling to the classical shift system, even though the ending and beginning clock times might be diverse ("Editorial" 2008; Flinkman et al. 2008; Hasselhorn, Müller, and Tackenberg 2005; Mermet and Lehndorff 2001). Not only is the practice of shift rotation prevalent in several Member States, but it is often accompanied by internal mobility between different services. Exceptions are provided by those countries where rotation is not universal. For example, frequently in France, as noted, and in Denmark and Germany, there are permanent night shifts. Many nurses accept these voluntarily for reasons related to family and/or social responsibilities. In France, these night duty nurses have had reduced hours, working only thirty-two and not thirty-five hours per week. In addition, they have only worked three nights weekly which is definitely an important factor in their work–life balance. On the other hand, some facilities in the United Kingdom have eliminated this practice. Claiming that nurses would be exposed to a broader variety of responsibilities, elimination of permanent night shifts was justified on grounds of professional development. Diverse duty periods relate to different work demands, disparate experiences, and collaboration with other sets of coworkers. For example, some types of nurses, as well as other categories of health-care employees, are not included in certain shifts. Moreover, the needs of patients and the nature of the work required differ from one part of the work day to the other (Arrowsmith and Mosse 2000; Hasselhorn, Müller, and Tackenberg 2005). Internal mobility between different services is justified in the same fashion. Nurses garner diverse experiences and also, this practice aids in solidifying institutional identity on the part of staff members. It is noteworthy that the Croatian Labour Act mandates shift rotation and affirms that night shifts may be undertaken at most for one week (Croatia: Ministry of Economy, Labour and Entrepreneurship 2009, Article 50).

Even though a study of the nursing profession in several Member States revealed that a majority of nurses worked a full rotation of shifts, it should be noted that in many places, it is possible to undertake only day shifts. However, alternating shifts have a role in Austria, the United Kingdom, Belgium, and the Netherlands to mention a few nations. Even though nurses in several Member States consider shift work with night duty to be the least attractive work mode, often it happens to be the prevalent practice. For example, in Belgium, 83 percent of nurses are involved in this type of work. When it was introduced, especially in Germany and the United Kingdom, it did not receive a warm reception, principally because it was known to be linked with domestic and health problems. Studies have confirmed that nurses who work rotating shifts experience the most job-related stress. They are followed, in turn, by colleagues working afternoon, day, and night shifts (Chan and Lai 2010; Dubois, McKee, and Nolte 2006; Hasselhorn, Müller, and Tackenberg 2005).

Within Member States, sometimes, there is a difference in practice between the public and private sectors. In this respect, in the United Kingdom, in the private or independent sector, fewer nurses are involved in internal rotation shift patterns. Moreover, in this arena, more nurses work permanent night shifts. And, even though difficulty has been encountered in Spain, in attempting to change the classical three shift system, more flexibility is evident in the private sector. This difficulty can be attributed to the fact that in Spain, employment regulations are quite rigid and inflexible. Ignoring regional differences, they afford sparse autonomy to human resource managers and they create obstacles to the implementation of modern personnel policies. Moreover, as noted, it is difficult to coordinate the centralized regulation of resources with the decentralized delivery of health-care services (Ball and Pike 2007; "Editorial" 2008; López-Valcárcel, Quintana, and Socorro 2006).

In many Member States, in the 1990s, health-care reforms enhanced the authority of local management. With the locus of decision-making at this level a change in shift patterns was realized. In many places, the traditional shift system underwent a transformation related to the number of working hours in each duty period. Diverse and individual-ized programs replaced the traditional ones or were incorporated into them. In several cases, the twelve-hour shift allowing for two per day, if adopted exclusively, was utilized. This duty period is used in Hungary, Belgium, Austria, and the United Kingdom, among other Member States. Longer shifts were welcomed by many a nurse. In fact, in the United Kingdom, they were enforced immediately in disparate services in over two-thirds of the health-care facilities. This arrangement was viewed as a method to enhance the working life of staff as well as the quality of time away from work. Studies have demonstrated a positive effect on the planning and prioritizing of nursing care, shift hand over sessions, and patient–family relationships. Not all evaluations have been completely positive. However, the same issues have been identi-fied in diverse services. Many of these relate to motivation of staff and fatigue (Richardson et al. 2005).

Given the impact of flexibility on work patterns, plus the fact that often they can be negotiated within a team and/or with a manager, it is not surprising that there are a variety of shift lengths. For example, in the United Kingdom, approximately 46 percent of all nurses have worked shifts of eight hours or less. Nineteen percent have had nine- to ten-hour duty periods. Eleven- or twelve-hour shifts have been worked by 19 percent of the nurses and 15 percent have worked those of more than twelve hours. In Northern Ireland, more nurses have had nine- to ten- and eleven- to twelve-hour periods than occurs elsewhere (Ball and Pike 2005). Variety is definitely the name of the game.

The relationship between the various shifts is also of interest. Some Member States, such as Belgium and France, feature overlapping shift systems. For example, Belgium has used the practice of having nurses work eight-hour shifts with a two-hour overlap between shifts. Work intensification led to an increase in part-time employment which modified this arrangement. The overlap between shifts was reduced with detrimental effects, especially on the decline of sociability and personal relationships, given an increase in stress (De Troyer 2000). The lack of standardization in nursing shift patterns and rotation must be underscored. Given the aforementioned decentralization, among other factors, diverse modes have developed in France in such a manner that this is the case. In the Danish health-care sector, working time is mostly nonstandard. The largest part of shift workers has irregular duty periods (Ballebye and Nielsen 2009). These cases are typical.

The type of contract and the working time system have consequences for an individual's well-being and health. Although the shift system is fundamental to nursing, it does create adversities for members of the profession. The effects of long shifts and, especially, the resulting physical and mental fatigue, have been well-documented. Prolonged periods of wakefulness and intense work can produce serious performance decrements. There is a significantly increased risk of making procedural and medication errors. Decreased vigilance at work, performance lapses, and occupational injuries, such as needle sticks, are more likely to occur. The risk for making an error almost doubles when a nurse works 12.5 or more consecutive hours. Moreover, working more than forty hours per week augments errors as well as near-errors. Safety and performance levels definitely suffer. In addition, outside of the workplace, the professional is more apt to experience a mishap, especially on the commute home. According to some researchers, there was a lack of clarity as to whether long shifts impacted negatively on health alone or in combination with other factors. Thus, a recent study explored how these work characteristics related to nurses' work-related injuries and illness over and above long work schedules. It was concluded that nonday shifts and mandatory overtime may have a negative impact on nurses' health independent of working long hours. These work characteristics do affect health, nurse-to-patient ratios, as well as work–family balance (de Castro et al. 2010; Institute of Medicine of the National Academies 2004; Lockley et al. 2007; Scott et al. 2006).

Rotating shifts have garnered their share of research efforts. Changes in sleep patterns, sleep deprivation, cardiovascular and gastrointestinal disorders, mood fatigue, irritability, and disruptions in social and family life, as well as increased alcohol intake, have been associated with this work pattern. Other difficulties include reduced alertness and performance, less satisfactory psychological health, and an increased incidence of cancer, especially breast and colorectal cancer in women. Over time, there has been a significant increase of the latter in this population. Moreover, changes in nurses' secretion of hormones have been attributed to this work pattern. Thus, it has been concluded that ergonomic shift schedules congruent with the body clock and nurses' preferences should be preferred in order to temper the adverse impact on health. In terms of the best benefits for health and productivity, permanent evening or night shifts, according to some people, seem to offer the most (Hegedus 2002; Korompeli et al. 2009).

The important impact of work patterns and especially, shift work on the individual nurse, the immediate professional health-care delivery team, and the services delivered, has been recognized by the ICN. This organization issued a call for an information campaign on all types of rota and best-practice management. The objective was to educate practitioners on the various facets of the themes, so they could cope with the consequences and undertake meaningful participation in multifaceted policy making on the matter. An active role was envisioned for national nurses associations as well (ICN 2007a).

As in other professions, nurses have reacted differently to their schedules. Some are very concerned about them, whereas others are not. Very often, the reaction to them relates to age, as in Belgium, Germany, Finland, France, and Italy. In these nations, the youngest and oldest professionals have been less worried about getting an unsatisfactory schedule than their colleagues in other age groups. On the other hand, in Great Britain, concern has increased with age. And, in the Netherlands, nurses under thirty have tended to pay less attention to this matter. In general, it may be stated that as a rule, among European nursing staff, work schedules have been of more concern to those professionals between the ages of twenty-five and fifty than to older or younger ones. Such a trend is understandable for the simple reason that people in that age bracket have more family obligations. The type of employment contract has also related to this subject. For example, in Belgium and France, nurses working on a permanent basis, as opposed to those employed on temporary arrangements, have been more preoccupied about getting a less than desirable schedule (Laine and the NEXT Study Group 2003).

Job satisfaction is closely related to the degree of influence an individual nurse has on the planning of work schedules. This has been found to vary greatly between Member States. Research has revealed that nurses in the Netherlands and Great Britain have exerted greater influence on the matching of their work schedules with their individual desires and preferences, than their French and Slovakian colleagues. More specifically, studies of the nursing profession in Europe (Hasselhorn, Müller, and Tackenberg 2005; Ogińska et al. 2003) have noted that in Poland and Belgium, one of two nurses reported having little or no influence on this matter and in Italy, France, and Slovakia, two of three nurses reported the same.

The unpredictability of work schedules is one factor that causes nurses to consider leaving the profession. The predictability of these schedules and opportunities to change them assume a special importance. In England, information concerning the rota has become available only one month in advance. At the other extreme, in Spain, it has been posted a year in advance. Obviously, it is easier for nurses to organize their lives in the latter circumstances. Moreover, in Spain, if nurses have inconvenient working times, they may change them among themselves or request a certain day off. On the other hand, in the United Kingdom, one study reported that over 50 percent of nurses working shifts claimed they could not change their schedule, if they so desired, but colleagues doing agency or bank work probably could (Ball and Pike 2006a, 2006b). Such practices engender friction and animosity. In fact, part-timers have been more satisfied than full-timers with their control over and choice of hours. Practices concerning these matters are significant, especially in this age marred by a severe nurse shortage. The degree of influence an individual nurse holds in the planning of schedules and possibilities to change them impinge heavily on evaluation of working hours which, in turn, is related to one's commitment to an institution and to the profession (Ball and Pike 2006a, 2006b; Hasselhorn, Müller, and Tackenberg 2005; Martinez and Martinez 2002).

Shift patterns differ as to their mode of operation, but certainly not in terms of significance. They establish the staffing level to meet patient need in a given service at a given time. Due to the value of this function, the ICN underscores the importance of rostering, especially its role in determining the level and skill mix of the nursing team and thus, the quality of service provided, as well as nurses' well-being and health (ICN 2007a). Effective use of personnel is central to the achievement of a health-care delivery system's objectives.

Annual Paid and Additional Leaves

Employees' annual amount of working time is heavily affected by the length of the paid annual leave to which they are entitled. In its social agenda, the EU has included provisions that create a minimum safety net of protection for workers. In addition to the limitations on working time discussed above, this agenda also establishes a right to paid annual leave. More specifically, the aforementioned Working Time Directive establishes a vacation floor by specifying that workers are entitled to a paid minimum annual leave of at least four weeks or twenty days.

The latter figure is harmonized on the basis of a five-day work week. Such a proclamation certainly contrasts with the American scene. The United States is the only nation with an advanced economy that fails to mandate paid annual vacations for its workers. It is definitely atypical. In contrast, all EU Member States feature a statutory minimum period of paid annual leave. In some, the entitlement increases with length of service.

In a majority of these countries (Belgium, Bulgaria, Croatia, Cyprus, the Czech Republic, Estonia, Finland, Germany, Greece, Hungary, Ireland, Italy, Latvia, Lithuania, Netherlands, Poland, Romania, Slovakia, and Slovenia) the floor established by the EU statute is utilized as the national minimum. This category includes all the newly acceded Member States, except Malta. Another set of nations has adopted a higher legal requirement as to minimum paid leave measured in days. Both Portugal and Spain have adopted twenty-two days as their statutory minimum. Malta and the United Kingdom have set their mark at twenty-four days and Austria, Denmark, France, Luxembourg, and Sweden established theirs at twenty-five. It is to be noted that these figures can be and often are augmented through collective agreements. Thus, in some Member States, such as France, the requirements are actually greater than the established minimum (Cabrita and Galli da Bino 2013; Carley 2007, 2009).

In the Czech Republic, Denmark, Finland, Germany, Ireland, Italy, the Netherlands, and Sweden, the average collectively agreed upon annual leave passes the statutory minimum by at least four days. Such situations indicate that the law serves basically as a safety net. On the other hand, circumstances are diverse in Austria, Cyprus, Estonia, Romania, Slovakia, the United Kingdom, and most of the other newly acceded Member States where average collectively agreed upon annual leaves and statutory minima are similar or identical. Such a phenomenon portrays a more incisive role for the law. In general, workers in the EU are entitled on average to 25.3 days of annual paid leave (Carley 2009; "Increase in Statutory Holiday Entitlement" 2007). The entitlement varies significantly from nation to nation and reaches thirty or more days in some cases.

It is also noteworthy that in some nations certain groups of workers receive additional time off. Such frequently occurs when they reach a certain age. Recently, Danes extended the rights of senior workers by introducing special "senior days" into the world of work. Employees at age sixty now receive two extra days off per year at full pay. Those aged sixty-one get three and those that are sixty-two have four. Similar practices take place in Hungary and Slovenia. In the former, ten days are added to the statutory minimum paid leave after age forty-four and in the latter, three extra days are due older employees (Carley 2009; European Foundation for the Improvement of Living and Working Conditions 2009b; Federation of European Employers 2004, 2011).

Seniority also serves as a basis for extending paid annual leave in some Member States. Finland, Austria, Greece, and Poland serve as examples of this practice. In Finland, after completing a year of work, employees are given an extra week of leave. In Austria, six additional days off are awarded to workers with more than twenty-five years of service. After three years with an institution, Greek workers are granted two extra days of annual leave. Then, time off is increased by one work day for each year of employment after that. Polish counterparts in a similar vein receive extra days of leave time after ten years of service. Leave entitlement is increased for workers with longer service in several other nations as well. Difficult work schedules, depending on how often they are undertaken, are also rewarded with extra days of leave in some countries. Such occurs in Austria, where two to three extra days of leave time are granted for shift work (Carley 2009; European Foundation for the Improvement of Living and Working Conditions 2009a; Ray and Schmitt 2008).

There are differences among the Member States in terms of the timing of one's leave. In Sweden, Hungary, and the Czech Republic, there is a requirement that the matter be a subject for consultation or bargaining with employees or their representatives. Other nations guarantee workers the opportunity to use at least some of their time off during the summer months. The Netherlands is the most specific in its mandate that workers be granted leave in a single block between April 30th and October 1st. Other nations, such as Finland, Denmark, France, Portugal, and Austria, utilize a summer block system as well for scheduling leaves, but each block includes only a portion of the total vacation time (Ray and Schmitt 2007, 2008). Even though it is mandated in Austria, Sweden, Germany, and the Netherlands, entitlement to vacation pay higher than the worker's normal remuneration is not a prevalent practice throughout the Member States.

Many nations feature regulations that ensure annual paid leave is used in the year in which it is awarded. Such is the case in Denmark, Ireland, Portugal, and Spain. To guarantee that a leave is taken in appropriate fashion, according to Article 7 of the Working Time Directive, it is illegal for employers to offer extra remuneration in lieu. An exception prevails in the case of termination of employment. In addition, in some instances, it is not possible to carry over leave time from one year to the next. Only in some situations may part of a leave be carried over and often, as in Croatia, it must be used by a specific date in the following year. The CJEU in *Federatie Nederlandse Vakbeweging v. Staat der Nederlanden* (Case C-124/05) recognized that paid annual leave, a prime component of EU social law, cannot be replaced by financial measures and that other types of provisions should not discourage or prevent individuals from taking it.

In some Member States, there are occasions for time off in addition to paid annual leave. Workers qualify for this when carrying out trade union responsibilities or civic duties, such as jury duty in Sweden and to change residence in Spain. The French allow unpaid leave for community service, in addition to a specified number of days for representing an organization and a block of months for tasks related to international solidarity. If travel is involved, in Greece, workers have been granted three days off for electoral purposes. It is to be noted that practices for absentee voting in the confines of the EU are often diverse from those in the United States or nonexistent.

Public Holidays

Public holidays, national and local, are another benefit enjoyed by many European workers. This time off is offered in addition to paid annual leave. Statutes in Austria, Portugal, and Italy mandate that employees be awarded thirteen paid holidays. Those in Spain require twelve, while those in Belgium authorize ten. The numbers are nine, six, and one for Denmark and Ireland, Greece, and France, respectively (Ray and Schmitt 2008). Typical of these holidays, some of which are not celebrated in the United States, are New Year's Day, Good Friday, Easter Monday, Labor Day, Assumption Day, All Saints' Day, and Christmas. Member States then add their own variety to this list to create a national flavor. For example, the Italians add Epiphany, the Anniversary of the Liberation from Fascism, the Anniversary of the Birth of the Republic, Immaculate Conception Day, Saint Stephen's Day, and the festival of the specific local patron saint which, obviously, differs from locality to locality. Each Member State establishes its own dates for public holidays. However, in Germany, the decision is made at a subnational level, that of the Land. In some nations, employers have the option to schedule workers with the stipulation they pay a wage premium or offer time off at a later date, as in Greece. Moreover, in some places, for example, the United Kingdom, full-time workers have not enjoyed the legal right to avoid working on a public holiday, if so requested ("UK Workers Get Least Paid Leave" 2007).

The total of annual leave days plus public holidays varies significantly throughout the Member States. The top rung of the EU's entitlement table is reserved for Sweden with its offer of forty-three days off. The bottom step belongs to Estonia and its award of twenty-six days. The difference is approximately 65 percent or almost 3.5 work weeks. In addition to Sweden, other nations that feature higher rates include Germany (forty days), Italy (thirty-nine days), Luxembourg (thirty-eight days), Denmark (thirty-eight days) and Austria (thirty-seven days). If one adds Malta, Portugal, France, and Finland to this list, it could be asserted that these nations all have guaranteed workers a minimum of thirty-five days leave per year. On the other hand, especially low leave rewards are affiliated with Ireland (twenty-nine days), Hungary (twenty-eight days), Latvia (twenty-seven days) and Estonia (twenty-six days). The average for the Member States has been calculated as 33.7 days per year (Carley 2007). This figure certainly underscores the American record in this area.

Maternity and Parental Leaves

To have an adequate notion of leave policies in Member States, mention must be made of the protection of pregnant employees and the practice of maternity and parental leaves along with childhood provisions as part of the social arrangements. These leaves represent opportunities that allow parents to be absent from employment obligations for reasons related to childbirth, while retaining job security and a minimization of the risks of losing one's work. Legal rights in these areas have impinged, and often in negative fashion, on European nurses' intent to leave the profession (Stordeur et al. 2003a).

An important initiative at the European level, is Council Directive 92/85/EEC of October 1992 on the introduction of measures to encourage improvements in the safety and health at work of pregnant workers and those who have recently given birth or are breastfeeding. Being concerned with the safety and health of workers, the document's legal basis lies in Article 118A of the Treaty Establishing the European Community. Minimum protection standards for pregnant women are established and employers are obliged to assess risks in the workplace that might be harmful to this population and those who have recently given birth. These workers are afforded protection from exposure to dangerous agents, hazardous procedures, and night work. Moreover, there are provisions for a maternity leave of at least fourteen weeks with an adequate allowance and a prohibition of dismissal for reasons affiliated with the pregnancy. In addition, most recently, agreement has accorded self-employed female workers the same access to maternity leave as salaried workers (Carley et al. 2010). The aforementioned directive also stipulated that Member States should implement these minimum provisions or more favorable ones within two years, either with national laws, regulations and administrative provisions, or collective agreements.

Currently, maternity leave available to nurses practicing in Member States varies considerably, according to an ILO report ("Maternity Leaves" 2012). It ranges from the established minimum of fourteen weeks to a maximum of sixty weeks. Sweden wins the prize for the longest maternity absence in the EU, the maximum. It is followed by Denmark and the United Kingdom who offer fifty-two weeks. In terms of length of leave, an overwhelming majority of the Member States (20) fall within the range of fourteen to twenty weeks. Of these, most offer absences of sixteen weeks. Much longer leaves are accorded in Hungary and Croatia (twenty-four weeks), Ireland (twenty-six weeks), and Slovakia and the Czech Republic (twenty-eight weeks). It is noteworthy that, in some Member States, there is a difference between the public and private sectors regarding the number of weeks allotted and some nations make a distinction between leaves related to the first birth and those following. They are usually longer in the latter case. Most recently, in action related to the Commission's proposal to review the directive noted above, the European Parliament (EP) exceeded the Commission's suggestion and approved an extension of the minimum maternity leave from fourteen to twenty weeks with full pay. In addition, it sanctioned the introduction of two weeks of paternity leave for fathers. These amendments were not welcomed by most Member States due to the costs involved (Associated Press 2010; "Bulgaria" 2008; European Parliament: Press Service 2010; Plantenga et al. 2008).

Not only do lengths of maternity leave differ among the Member States, but payment arrangements do as well. These are established either by law, or collective agreements, or both. In fifteen nations, women on leave receive 100 percent of their salary for the entire period. In eleven, the payments range between 50 percent and 90 percent. Two Member States use split sums, meaning part of the period is covered with a payment that at a certain point is reduced. These nations have adopted a sliding scale. Also, often a maximum daily rate has been established. In terms of nurses in the Central and East European Member States, it must be remembered that they experienced a severe decline in the worth of their benefits, caused by the falling value of health-care stipends that automatically decreased the worth of paid leave. Then, it is also noteworthy that these nurses absent from work for maternity or any reasons are isolated from the aforementioned gratitude or informal payments. Their loss during such leave, compared to that of any colleagues from other nations, has been greater. In its approval of an extension of the minimum maternity leave, the EP also resolved that leave payments to individual workers must be equal to 100 percent of their monthly salary or their average monthly salary (Alford 2003; European Parliament: Press Service 2010; Plantenga et al. 2008; "Social Security" 2010).

Over and above maternity leave, other leave arrangements, principally parental leave, are available to parents in EU Member States. This type of absence from work represents an effort to transform the division of labor in the home by affording time off to the father of the child. It is a unique practice in that it attempts to change the behavior of males, not females, and it acknowledges that women are not able to participate in the labor market on equal terms unless men share caring for children (European Parliament-Directorate General for Internal Policies 2010; Weiler 2005). The male role in parenting was recognized for the first time with the issuance of Council Directive 96/34/EC which was substituted with Council Directive 2010/18/EU. The more recent document, as the previous one, recognizes that males have an important role in parenting and that the law should reinforce this position. Traditionally, the law concerned with parenthood has frequently given rights and opportunities to females, but not to males (Shaw, Hunt, and Wallace 2007).

The new directive, based on a Framework Agreement between the three European general cross-industry social partner organizations (the European Trade Union Conference, the European Centre of Enterprises with Public Participation, and BUSINESSEUROPE, an organization of forty central industrial and employers' federations), provided that male and female employees, regardless of the type of their employment contract, are entitled to an individual right to parental leave of at least four months which can be taken at any time until the child turns eight. In an effort to encourage fathers to participate in this program, it is stipulated

145

that at least one of the four months is to be labeled "nontransferable." Thus, it cannot be transferred to the other parent. In other words, it is lost, if not taken. In addition, provisions that guarantee employment rights and nondiscrimination are included in the document. Of significance is that all matters related to income during the leave period are left for the agendas of the individual Member States. Giving a right to a leave, but not to one with pay, fails to confront factors impinging on use of the practice. Member States were given two years to implement the directive as issued or with more favorable conditions.

Given the date of the latest directive on the subject of parental leave, existing arrangements are still and for a while will be based on the previous legal basis. In nine of the Member States, parental leave is considered an individual as opposed to a family right. Its duration varies throughout the region. It ranges from a minimum of twelve weeks to a maximum of one hundred fifty-six weeks with nine countries offering a leave of one hundred forty-four weeks or thirty-six months valid to the child's age of three. An almost equal number falls between leaves of twelve and twenty-six weeks. The remaining Member States lie between these two groups. In terms of total parental leave, sometimes, the duration is lengthened, if both parents participate. Often, as in Slovakia, time limits are placed on this type of leave. In the noted nation, it must be used within a five-year period. In a majority of the Member States, those taking advantage of parental leave are reimbursed in some manner for their loss of income. Like other facets of the program, payments differ. They represent a flat rate, a percentage of salary, and a means test. Also, sometimes, remuneration is received only for part of the leave or it changes, being linked to the specific period of a leave. Furthermore, distinctions have been made according to the number of children in the family. In nine Member States parental leave is unpaid. Other particulars in national agreements, such as those related to entitlement and flexibility, differ as well (Cziria 2012; Kovács 2009; Plantenga et al. 2008; "Social Security" 2010). News broadcasts have made known that, to a large extent, males have not taken advantage of this leave opportunity.

Childcare

Closely related to maternity and parental leaves and working time, are the personal services which are of significance to employees responsible for raising children. It is generally acknowledged that such responsibilities affect the work and turnover habits of nurses. Of these personal services, childcare is of prime importance. It is especially of interest to the nursing profession, given the number of women included in its ranks and the magnitude of the current nursing shortage. As opposed to the American scene, childcare outside of the home is a recent ingredient in European public policies. The women's liberation movement served as an impetus to the placement of this issue, in general, and specifically, that of the provision of appropriate daycare facilities, on the public agenda (Radulova 2009).

The literature has revealed nurses' difficulties with childcare. Facilities have been described as "patchy and insufficient," creating a problem of availability. In many instances, accessibility is labeled difficult as well, given the cost. Focus groups have noted the lack of affordable childcare for nurses' children. Quality has also been underscored as an important factor that sometimes leaves to be desired. In addition, opening and closing times have posed a problem. The lack of fixed regular work schedules experienced by nurses is not always conducive to appropriate childcare arrangements. Also, it has been demonstrated that the higher incidence of single parent families among established minority ethnic nurses means these professionals bear a greater burden than many of their colleagues. Moreover, the internal rotation shift system is particularly difficult for professionals in terms of arranging childcare. The fixed system is easier as far as organizing one's domestic life is concerned. In spite of these common troublesome areas related to availability, cost, and quality, it is to be noted that the provision of childcare is diverse from one Member State to another. Such differences include the nature of the structures, the national approach adopted, and the priority assigned to the matter, among others (Commission of the European Communities 2008; Dhaliwal and McKay 2008; Estryn-Behar et al. 2002; Versieck, Bouten, and Pacolet 1995).

EU actors have been sensitive to this issue. In 1992, the Council issued a Recommendation on childcare (92/241/EEC) that stressed "the sharing of occupational, family and upbringing responsibilities arising from the care of children between women and men" (Article 2(4)). A goal was to "achieve a more equal sharing of parental responsibilities between men and women and to enable women to have a more effective role in the labour market" (Article 6). In addition, it was recommended that services be offered at affordable prices, that they be distributed in appropriate fashion to meet the needs of the population, and that financial support from the public, private, and third sectors be explored.

At this time, in the eyes of the decision-makers, childcare was primarily linked to the problem of gender inequality. However, with the 1997 launching of the European Employment Strategy, aimed at coordinating national employment policies via the Open Method of Coordination, the orientation was readjusted. Gender equality concerns were no longer dominant. Economics and an increase in the female employment rate received prime attention. The European Employment Strategy guidelines viewed the sharing of family responsibilities and the provision of childcare to be crucial to entry into and continued participation in the workforce. They were linked to low female labor participation which was and is still useful to the nurse shortage. Childcare became an instrument to stimulate the female labor market, an important component of the EU's reconciliation policy mix (Radulova 2009). In 2002, at the Barcelona Summit, the Council polished the objectives of the European Employment Strategy and established targets for the provision of childcare. It was agreed that by 2010, childcare would be provided throughout the Member States to at least 90 percent of the children between the age of three and the mandatory school age and to 33 percent of those under three years of age.

Action has been undertaken in the various Member States in this regard. Recognizing that often the costs of childcare are prohibitive, several initiatives are noteworthy. In the Netherlands, employers are now obliged to contribute to their employees' childcare costs. In Estonia, also, financial benefits are available for these purposes and payments by Maltese employers for childcare services are no longer considered taxable fringe benefits. Furthermore, the Austrian government has introduced a so-called household service check, the name of which makes the item self-explanatory. In the National Health Service of the United Kingdom, all component organizations are required to take part in Improving Working Lives, an accreditation process which contains benchmarks to assess the extent to which stellar human resources practices are being followed. Childcare provision is an important spoke of the program (Buchan and Maynard 2006; Malhotra 2006). A more recent effort by the National Health Service Staff Council deals with multiple facets of childcare. It refers to availability, extended and unsocial hours, culturally competent providers, accommodation of the needs of black minority and ethnic families, children with special needs, before and after school clubs, and holiday and play schemes (NHS Staff Council 2009). The perspective is a serious one and quite broad in scope.

These activities are representative of the many that have been undertaken. In addition, the European social partners have been active in efforts related to cost and the availability of facilities. Moreover, monetary assistance from Structural Funds, financial instruments that allow the EU to aid in the resolution of structural economic and social problems, and the European Agricultural Fund for Rural Development have been committed to multifaceted childcare endeavors (Commission of the European Communities 2008; Vandenbrande et al. 2007; Weiler, Newell, and Carley 2007). In spite of these efforts and others, Member States are far away from reaching the so-called Barcelona targets. As far as the younger age group is concerned (zero to three years old), only five Member States (Belgium, Denmark, the Netherlands, Sweden, and Spain) have achieved the 33 percent coverage rate. In terms of children between the age of three and the mandatory school age, the performance record is somewhat better in that eight Member States (Belgium, Denmark, France, Germany, Ireland, Sweden, Spain, and Italy) have surpassed the 90 percent coverage rate (Commission of the European Communities 2008; European Commission 2008). It is noteworthy that none of the newly acceded Member States are included in either group. It is obvious that there is a need for concerted efforts on the part of many parties. Although the Commission has no formal powers in the field of childcare, it is committed to encouraging achievement of the Barcelona targets via support and monitoring activities.

It must be remembered that very often childcare facilities throughout the EU operate on a part-time basis only. This issue is significant in the Member States featuring diverse working time patterns (Plantenga et al. 2008). Moreover, as noted, often services are not always affordable and their hours are not congruent with work schedules involving atypical hours. Given this situation, one can appreciate the difficulties experienced by many nurses in constructing appropriate childcare arrangements. Years ago, Versieck, Bouten, and Pacolet (1995), convinced that much remained to be done as far as childcare for nurses' children was concerned, issued a call for childcare facilities available to nurses to be open around the clock at reduced prices. It is quite evident that their words have not been heeded. Rather, in the interests of costsavings and efficiency, very often, many childcare services have been reduced or canceled. However, it is instructive that one small hospital in Malta has been staffed entirely by nurses, enticed, in part, by the existence of a childcare center, to rejoin the working world (Muscat and Grech 2006). Such an incentive helps to garner and retain labor market participation of female nurses with offspring. This is especially cogent in this day and age, given the shortage of these qualified professionals in many Member States.

Childcare policies and leave opportunities, such as maternity and parental leaves, facilitate the reconciliation of work and family life. They support parents in their efforts to combine work obligations and ambitions with family responsibilities. This, as noted, is of particular importance to nurses, given the nature of some of their work conditions. Via these measures, families have the possibility of offering offspring a propitious start in life. Moreover, they facilitate the work–family equilibrium and protection of the health and well-being of parent and child. However, benefits accrued from these instruments go beyond the realms of family and specific work environments. They contribute to the resolution of demographic and economic problems, among others. These policies incorporate a strategy to enhance female labor market participation as well as promotion of employment opportunities. With an eye to the future, they encourage people to have children and thus, counter current low birth rates that endanger economic productivity (European Parliament-Directorate General for Internal Policies 2010). Their benefits are multifaceted. This discussion has underscored national variations in the implementation of these policies whose importance to nurses is monumental. Such variety has resulted from the diversity of social, economic, and political instruments found in the Member States and the different cultural interpretations and understandings of the family, its structure, and its various components. Of all these policies, as far as nurses are concerned, it would seem that childcare is the area for greatest concern.

Absenteeism

Since the end of World War II there has been an increase in nurses' absences from work. There are several explanations for this phenomenon. From an economic perspective, it can be explained on the basis of more than ample income and generous fringe benefits. In addition, absenteeism has been presented from a psychological viewpoint. Experiencing job dissatisfaction or need deficiency, the employee fails to meet work obligations. It is also known that, according to jurisprudential theory, workers' job attendance is heavily influenced by organizational personnel policies. Sociological explanations refer to the galaxy of societal, organizational, and work group factors that impact on employees' capacity and will to engage in work. In terms of disability theory, absenteeism is caused, for the most part, by illness or injury that physically prevents people from working. Also, a decline in the work ethic has been cited as a major contributor (Gillies 1994). Absenteeism rates vary throughout the confines of the EU. One end of the continuum is occupied by the Scandinavian countries which claim the highest rate and the other end is inhabited by the newly acceded Member States with the lowest measure. More specifically, Swedish nurses, in comparison to their colleagues elsewhere, are more prone to absenteeism. This has been attributed to the large number of these professionals over fifty years of age and to the elevated frequency of gainful employment among women (European Foundation for the Improvement of Living and Working Conditions 2009a; Josephson et al. 2003; Peña-Casas and Pochet 2009).

Absentee figures for the newly acceded Member States have generally tended to decrease over time. In part, the situation reflects a decline in absences due to injury or disease and a reduction in annual and other types of leave. Scholars, however, have claimed that official statistics fail to completely portray reality. Custom and practice have been modified as these nations joined the democratic community. Prior to transition, personnel took full advantage of any and all types of leave or absences. However, circumstances have changed as job security has declined, a result of attempting to harmonize practices with those of the EU. It is noteworthy that transition and health system reform have meant that in Bulgaria, the positions available for nurses were reduced 1.9 times (Tomev, Daskalova, and Mihailova 2005) and the unemployment rate in Poland settled at 20 percent (Krajewski-Siuda and Romaniuk 2006). Similar situations, in other nations in this group, have illustrated that work security is tenuous at best. Consequently, staff show up for work under any or most circumstances, a phenomenon labeled "presenteeism." Although there is far less nonproductive time in these countries, these additional factors have caused working time to be sustained at high levels and have accounted for the birth of "presenteeism." With the exception of the Czech Republic, workers have exhibited a reticence to be absent from their site of employment, primarily for fear of dismissal and loss of income. This fear is significant. For example, among health-care workers in Lithuania, it has registered as high as 60 percent (Alford 2003; Gunnardóttir and Rafferty 2006; Rosskam and Leather 2006).

Who is absent from work? Absentee rates for nurses vary from one field of employment to another. It has been established that the extent of absenteeism for those working in cardiology, psychiatry, and retirement homes has been significantly higher than that for those affiliated with obstetrics-gynecology, rehabilitation, surgery, and psychosomatic clinics. Moreover, working conditions that create extreme stress seem to account for higher values of absenteeism. A recent study concluded that being the most stressed of all staff, nurses are almost four times as likely to be absent from work as people with other occupations. In addition, in France, it has been found that absenteeism is greater for nurses working the night shift (Bonitz 2000; Clews 2009; ILO Sectoral Activities Program n.d.).

Absenteeism is costly. It impinges on expenditures, employee morale, the nurse shortage, productivity, and the quality of care, to cite a few elements. It is generally believed that organizational factors, as opposed to employee characteristics, account for most absences. Thus, structural and other organizational changes can temper and they have tempered the extent of the phenomenon. Efforts that have been successful in decreasing absenteeism among nurses have been those that enhance allegiance to the basic work group, increase job satisfaction, and demonstrate appreciation for their efforts and contribution to an institution's mission (Gillies 1994; Josefsson et al. 2007).

Conclusion

The organizational features of the workplace are an important component of job quality. The type of employment contract, the number of hours worked, the nature of the individual work schedule, the degree of choice an employee has in the determination of working time, its pace and intensity, the nature of leave policies, and the availability of personal services, among other factors, are all pertinent to nurses' perceptions of job quality and their attitudes toward their work situation and their profession. These elements also are important to an explanation of female employment. A study (Kangas and Rostgaard 2007) involving EU affiliates found that attitudinal factors, such as work–lifestyle preferences, are relevant to employment decisions, but contextual variables and institutional factors, such as the availability of day care and leave policies, garner more importance. Moreover, various elements of working time, such as duration and arrangement of working hours, have economic and social ramifications as well. Not only do they have implications for the operation of a health-care facility and its productivity, but also for the employees' work-related health outcomes, both physical and emotional (European Foundation for the Improvement of Living and Working Conditions 2007a; Evans, Lippoldt, and Marianna 2001; Hämäläinen and Lindström 2006). These will be set forth in the following chapter in relation to other elements in the work environment and EU social policy in general.

4

The World of Work:
Its Environment

Introduction

Organizational climate is a significant determinant of individual and group behavior within an institution. An extensive literature focuses on the environment in which health professionals work and its impact on them, both personally and professionally. In the health-care sector, work organization and work content have changed drastically and continue to do so on a regular basis. Work structures, procedures, and tasks are transformed or vanish as new technologies develop along with modifications in their context. As a result, the spectrum of work-related morbidity has been modified extensively as well. General morbidity, such as allergies, musculoskeletal disorders, and mental ill health, can be work-related. These ailments have replaced clinical occupational diseases as the prime problem in occupational health ("Working" 2001). Given the nature of their practice, nurses have extensive exposure to biological, ergonomic, chemical, psychological, and physical hazards. The health-care sector is particularly dangerous for workers in terms of the risk of injury. In fact, work-related injuries in health care have been declared 34 percent higher than the EU average and musculoskeletal disorders, the highest of any sector (Dubois, McKee, and Nolte 2006).

Factors that influence the well-being of a health-care staff in the workplace and their perceptions of job quality include the physical conditions in which they work, their exposure to risks and violence, and the psychosocial atmosphere. There are two types of work hazards that impinge on health: physical and psychosocial. The former adopt a direct physical pathway and the latter travel through a psychosocial stress-mediated pathway. These hazards involving occupational injury and work-related illnesses relate to the nature of working conditions. They also influence practitioners' attitudes toward a place of employment and a profession. In the health-care sector, there is a multitude of such hazards. Risks are many in number. Moreover, multivariate analyses demonstrate a clustering of risks. For example, exposure to environmental risk factors aids in an explanation of the likelihood of exposure to diverse ergonomic risks (European Foundation for the Improvement of Living and Working Conditions 2007b).

Physical Conditions

The health-care work environment is especially fast-paced and is becoming even more so. Workloads for nursing personnel have multiplied. Over 80 percent of German, Belgian, Polish, Slovak, and Dutch nurses have reported that their work has become increasingly physically demanding. The percentage for Finnish nurses registers at 61. In the European context, physical workload has been a concern of more than 60 percent of the nursing staff (Estryn-Behar, Le Nézet, and Jasseron 2005; Estryn-Behar et al. 2003b). Quantitative and emotional high work requirements result, in part, from the augmented demands of work organization and enlarged patient expectations. As in the United States, there is no doubt that workloads and work intensity have increased for nurses throughout the EU. Factors affecting these phenomena include shorter hospital stays, increased patient acuity and turnover, the excessive volume of care, reductions in staff, nurse expertise, unit physical layout, the nature of teamwork, changes resulting from new roles, new services, new drugs, and new technology; plus pressure to achieve economic targets, such as those emerging from the recent economic crisis, and additional ancillary duties. These elements have modified and intensified the nursing workload. Its content has drastically changed in terms of its clinical and administrative aspects. How nurses confront their workload is partially determined by the degree to which they are aided by other caring and support personnel and by the availability of supportive facilities (Dawoud and Maban 2008). Physical workload and its health consequences vary from nation to nation.

In the nursing communities of the Member States, the highest mean scores for quantitative demands, that is, the intensity of work, as indicated by a major study of European nurses (Hasselhorn et al. 2005) have been found in Poland, Germany, Slovakia, and Finland. There is a general tendency for quantitative demands to decrease with age in most nations, but such does not hold for Finland and Germany. In the former, the nursing community features a high proportion of older providers and thus, these folks cannot redistribute responsibilities to younger colleagues. In the latter, the situation has been attributed to the long work week of nurses over fifty years of age. Quantitative demands augment with increasing weekly working hours. Their affiliation with burnout and job satisfaction is extensive and less so with general health and intent to desert the nursing profession.

Important features of the work environment are its physical aspects, facilities and equipment, job characteristics, and, as noted, the organization of working time. Having an influence on the well-being and output of staff, the design of health-care facilities is important. Many traditionally designed structures impinge on the performance and well-being of personnel in negative fashion. Inadequate architecture has been cited by 50 percent of French nurses as an obstacle to their job performance. They consider their work space ill-suited to their responsibilities. Dissatisfaction with physical working conditions is greatest in Poland, Croatia, Slovakia, Italy, France, and Germany. Lesser dissatisfaction is displayed in Finland, Great Britain, Belgium, and the Netherlands. Insufficient physical structures have been found to hinder recruitment and retention efforts. Many facilities are not congruent with the health-care delivery system and the role of its providers. It is the nurses' perceptions of the structural characteristics that make a difference in the evaluation of a health-care facility. These perceptions account for the attractiveness of an institution and thus, they affect organizational commitment and job satisfaction (Estryn-Behar, Le Nézet, and Jasseron 2005; Rechel, Buchan, and McKee 2009; Stordeur, D'Hoore, and the NEXT Study Group 2007; Vŏncina et al. 2006).

A major determinant of work insecurity, especially in the Central and Eastern European Member States, is the deteriorating physical environment in which many nurses work caused primarily by a lack of investment in infrastructures. Maintenance and renovation of health-care facilities and equipment are often not given sufficient attention. The necessary funds are not forthcoming. Capital investment has not been a priority and many health-care institutions are products of under-investment or even complete neglect. In addition, medicines, supplies, and materials are not adequate. New technology has been restricted to urban facilities and access to training and utilization of it limited to a select group of providers. These conditions are a significant factor in the determination of how health-care personnel experience work. Moreover, from the viewpoint of job quality, along with the notion of work intensification, they are an important aspect of health and safety

157

outcomes. There is a strong relationship between excessively intense work patterns and poor working conditions, as just described.

As in the United States, a general problem, resulting from increased workloads and work intensification, relates to time constraints which have consequences for patients. For every additional patient added to a nurse's workload, the risk of the patient dying increases by 7 percent. The more patients a nurse is responsible for on average, the higher the mortality risk for each one across the entire range of staffing levels in hospitals. Moreover, increased workloads mean the provision of less nursing time to patients which is affiliated with higher rates of infection, gastrointestinal bleeding, pneumonia, cardiac arrest, and even death from these and other causes, all things to be avoided (Gordon 2005; Page 2004). From Belgium to the United Kingdom, Estonia, France, Sweden, Italy, and Finland to a host of other Member States, complaints of time pressures that place staff under strain are heard.

Time needed to complete normal tasks subtracts from that allotted to patients. For example, documentation is of prime importance in this day and age. It has been estimated that this process consumes between 13 percent and 28 percent of hospital nurses' time. More specifically, in Germany, it has been reported that hospital administrative tasks can account for up to two-thirds of a nurse's working time (Kirpal 2003; Page 2004). A Belgian project has attempted to temper the burden of these responsibilities by providing nurses with portable pocket personal computers so patient data can be recorded at the bedside. Practitioners agreeing to participate in the project were offered a single monetary award by the Belgian National Institute for Health and Invalidity Insurance.

Time constraints limit exchanges among colleagues. As noted, of particular importance is the concern of many nurses that there is no time to discuss patients' problems with colleagues or to reflect on their practice. Work intensity and resulting pressures do not allow for this. This is a preoccupation, not to be overlooked. Such reflection and time for discussions are of utmost importance. More than 12 percent of Polish, French, and Italian nurses have indicated that, frequently or very frequently, they experience uncertainties about the operation and functioning of specialized equipment. In France, 93 percent of nurses and in Europe, 68.7 percent of these professionals have reported major concern about committing errors in the provision of care (Estryn-Behar, Le Nézet, and Jasseron 2005; LeLan 2006; Weinberg 2003). Consultation and reflection are a must.

In addition, given time pressures, many nurses are concerned that they cannot provide adequate care, much less the level of care they wish to deliver. They are unable to care for the patient as a total person as required by most codes of ethics. They are forced to overlook the personal contacts with patients that make a difference in the quality of care. Such contacts are also significant in terms of communication of information to patients and families, especially since consumers are now more knowledgeable than in the past and have a greater role in decisions related to their care. It is more difficult to nurture provider–patient relationships with the present "assembly line" approach to care. The National Health Service Institute for Improvement and Innovation in the United Kingdom claims that nurses spend less than 40 percent of their time on direct patient care. Other studies report a far lower percentage (*Front Line Care* 2010).

In many Member States, nurses have felt overwhelmed by organizational and bureaucratic requirements. Having accepted the necessity for increased administrative tasks in the interests of risk assessment and health and safety programs, they still are of the opinion that their basic purpose has been endangered by management's needs to the detriment of those of the patient (*Création d'une instance professionnelle infirmière* 2007; Meadows, Levenson, and Baeza n.d.). In short, they believe they are unable to devote their full energies to nursing per se and thus, the delivery and quality of care for many of these professionals is compromised. As one American nurse has rightly commented: "The things that aren't being done aren't things that you can catch up on later" (Weinberg 2003, p. 9). Moreover, work intensification is significant because of its potential to impact the transmission and acquisition of knowledge and skills. Furthermore, in spite of the significance of organizational socialization, efforts to meet efficiency requirements often deprive staff of the time necessary to induct new members of the profession and properly orient newcomers to the nursing staff (De Troyer 2000; Furlan 2006).

Nursing involves much more than technical competence and instrumental caring. Another dimension is involved. It is affective in nature and mirrors respect for the patient. The notion has been elegantly stated by Dame Christine Beasley, England's former Chief Nursing Officer. She posits:

> Nursing is more than the sum of its parts. Any health system needs nurses who are intellectually able and emotionally aware and who can

159

combine technical clinical skills with a deep understanding and ability to care, as one human to another. . . . This is a constant of nursing. It is the value base, on which public trust rests and the profession is grounded. As a profession it is our promise to society (cited in *Front Line Care* 2010, p. 63).

Unfortunately, a study of Belgian nurses (Siebens et al. 2006) reported that they did not have adequate time and support to integrate their medical-technical competence into a caring relationship. Moreover, time constraints have prevented the delivery of important aspects of nursing and, as a result, some needs have not been met. In the same vein, research in Sweden (Hallin and Danielson 2007), has evidenced similar consequences of work intensification. A less than satisfactory work situation related to themes, such as being unable to meet all demands, being insufficient, being unsure of oneself, and too little contact with patients due to time factors.

In the future, will nursing be limited to the delivery of medical-technical care or will there be movement in the direction of the skilled companionship that views nursing care as encompassing a harmonious integration of competences and caring (Siebens et al. 2006)? This is the question that remains to be answered. The response is important to the direction of the profession. It is evident that the focus on productivity, efficiency, cost-effectiveness, and performance within contemporary health-care systems has negatively impinged on the time nurses have for those special activities related to caring. Work conditions, in general, and particularly, the augment in the number of patients have decreased nurses' ability for management, prioritizing, and planning of team work and executing documentation with precision. Diverse values often separate administrators from nurses and other health-care professionals. There can be a conflict between a patient-oriented work ethos and one whose organization and structures stress the more technical, instrumental, administrative, or coordinating tasks. There is proof that the latter approach can augment institutional costs as a result of staff dissatisfaction, turnover, and adverse patient events (Kirpal 2003; Weinberg 2003). It can backfire.

In Scotland, the National Health Service has launched a workload project aimed at the recommendation of tools to be employed on a national basis for the measurement, comparison, and benchmarking of the workload of all nursing staff across a wide spectrum of sectors to include primary and acute care, mental health and pediatric nursing, as well as others. Efforts, such as this one, aimed at reducing work intensity would help achieve the objective of guideline number 18 of Council Decision 2008/618/EC entitled Guidelines for the Employment Policies of the Member States. It envisions the promotion of a lifecycle approach to work through "support for active ageing, including appropriate working conditions, improved (occupational) health status and adequate incentives to work and discouragement of early retirement." High work intensity is expensive in terms of occupational health and safety and it decreases the probability of viewing work as something to be endured (European Foundation for the Improvement of Living and Working Conditions 2009a; Peña-Casas and Pochet 2009).

The top of the list of nurses' work-related risks is occupied by physical strains or musculoskeletal injury to the back and extremities. These ergonomic hazards can be caused by frequent assumption of tiring or painful positions, due to the handling of heavy loads; moving, repositioning, and lifting patients; or by repetitive hand or arm movements or standing for long periods. Also, the recent obesity epidemic is important in this context. Nurses, in performing their duties, are involved in many bending and lifting activities and thus, they are susceptible to musculoskeletal disorders. These physical strains tend to be more visible in intensive, geriatric, and surgical care, as well as in nursing homes. In these settings, many patients are bedridden and unable to move. In most European health-care facilities, the availability of lifting mechanisms is limited. And, even if they are available, often, they are not used, although international benchmarking demonstrates that availability tends to promote usage. In most Member States, given the extensive need to perform physical tasks, the availability and use of lifting aids have been found to be unsatisfactory. Moreover, in Poland and Slovakia, availability is extremely inadequate in nursing homes and virtually nonexistent in hospitals.

It is noteworthy that there is also a strong correlation between stress and musculoskeletal conditions (Hasselhorn, Müller, and Tackenberg 2005; "Working" 2001). A path-finding study of nurses in seven Member States (Simon et al. 2008) confirmed this relationship, especially in the case of effort–reward imbalance and it concluded that psychosocial factors were more significant to these conditions than physical ones. Furthermore, the research did not find a meaningful identification with musculoskeletal disorders of lifting, bending, or the availability of or usage of technical lifting equipment. The major cause of health-related absenteeism is linked to these problems in Germany, the United Kingdom, and the Netherlands. Also, head nurses, having held positions at the bedside, have suffered as much as their younger cohorts from these ailments. Other investigations into these conditions have reported that 48 percent of French nurses complained of such maladies, as did 26 percent of their British counterparts and 68 percent of Slovakian colleagues (Bach n.d.-b; Estryn-Behar, Le Nézet, and Jasseron 2005; Hubačová et al. 2000). The proportion of nursing personnel free of musculoskeletal difficulties was the highest in home care, followed, in turn, by hospitals and nursing homes. Given that in the European countries studied, it was found that the type of institution as well as the nation determined the risk factor pattern affiliated with these disorders, the authors rightfully recommend that institutional typology should be viewed as an important ecological variable. With this knowledge, prevention becomes that much easier.

Another major hazard faced by nurses results from their exposure to biological agents. In fact, nurses' work sites, especially emergency departments and hospital wards, possess the potential to become venues for the spread of epidemics. Sources of infection abound, including contact with patients, microorganisms, body fluid samples, and infected blood. Also, with the reemergence and spread of infectious diseases, nursing personnel are exposed to enhanced risk. Bacteria, viruses, fungi, or parasites may be transmitted by contact with infected patients or contaminated body fluids (Cherry and Jacob 2005). It is for this reason that many health-care institutions have staff inoculation programs.

A major problem for nurses is injuries caused by needles and other sharp medical devices that can transmit potentially fatal diseases. Syringes, suture needles, scalpels, and glass instruments used regularly by nurses in the delivery of care are especially dangerous, if in contact with contaminated substances. Of all health-care workers, nurses are the target for a majority of these sharps injuries which are quite common. EFN (2008) has reported that in the Member States six million nurses have been subjected to more than two million unnecessary needle injuries. At a national level, in the United Kingdom, more than one hundred thousand needle sticks happen annually and in Germany, five hundred thousand sharps injuries have been recorded yearly (Wiskow, Albreht, and de Pietro 2010).

These are a definite professional hazard for nurses. In a study of more than one thousand five hundred nurses working in forty units of twenty hospitals, poor organizational conditions and heavy workloads accounted for 50 percent to 200 percent increases in the probability of needle stick injuries and near-misses among these practitioners and an augment in their exposure to infection as well (Stone et al. 2004). These injuries, needle stick and others due to sharp objects, as in other cases, are costly. Having the potential to lead to distress, sickness, and absenteeism, they place an extra burden on already strained human resources. They are also costly in terms of the diagnostic procedures required to determine if a serious illness has been contracted. And then, one must not forget the cost to the professional involved in terms of mental anguish (EFN 2007). Exposure to infection can also negatively reverberate into the area of recruitment and retention.

Chemical hazards complement the ergonomic and biological ones. Nurses can be exposed to a host of chemical agents, including medications, solutions, gases, cycotoxic agents, pentamidine, latex, PVC plastics and di-ethylhexyl phthalate (DEHP). In addition, hazards presented by radiation and lasers must not be forgotten. Some substances used in health-care facilities are carcinogenic and others harmful to one's skin or respiratory system. In fact, in a European sample, 28 percent of the nurses reported skin diseases. They were more prevalent in France, Italy, Germany, and Belgium. Many chemical agents constitute a health hazard. Exposure is related to site of practice. Skin disorders are more evident in medical and surgical departments and in intensive care than in home care, pediatric, or geriatric units. In the former units, the work rhythm leads to less hand washing, a major cause of these ailments. Then, women who do more work at home involving water are more at risk than men. It is interesting to note that studies have demonstrated that nurses working in operating rooms have experienced a higher rate of miscarriages than their colleagues working elsewhere (Bach n.d. b; Cherry and Jacob 2005; De Troyer 2000; Estryn-Behar, Le Nézet, and Jasseron 2005).

In terms of their physical health, it appears that among European nurses, the Dutch enjoy the best. On the other hand, the Polish and Slovaks seem to have the worst. On a European basis, 53 percent of nurses responding to a survey experienced musculoskeletal disease followed in descending order by skin disease (28 percent), digestive diseases (22 percent), neurological issues, including vision and hearing problems (19 percent), and mental ailments (19 percent). There were no differences based on site of employment in terms of their physical health. More specifically, when age and qualification level were taken into consideration, important variations did not emerge between nurses practicing in hospitals, nursing homes, and home care (Hasselhorn, Müller, and Tackenberg 2005).

Psychosocial Conditions

Not only must nurses contend with a stressful physical work environment, but the same label may be affixed to their psychosocial climate as well. With expansion of the service sector, given the multiple changes in working conditions, it has become more relevant to cite the psychosocial aspects of work along with the physical factors. The former, accounting for much of the work-related mental and emotional stressors, were late in being recognized because of difficulties concerning their measurement. In fact, having their origin in the workplace, they have been referred to as a disease of the twenty-first century (Hristov et al. 2003). Psychosocial working demands for nurses have been judged as elevated and they continue to increase throughout the Member States.

Stress

Stress, one of a group of psychosocial risks, according to the European Risk Observatory, is a most prominent health and safety challenge resulting from interaction between an individual and the environment. Basically, this condition is caused by a mismatch between people and their work. It is "a state which is accompanied by physical, psychological or social complaints or dysfunctions and which results from individuals feeling unable to bridge a gap with the requirements or expectations placed on them" (European Commission 2011, p. 90). The causes and consequences of this condition are many. Determinants relate to various areas of work which, if not managed in appropriate fashion, develop into sources of workplace stress. More specifically, these factors concern work organization and processes, work schedules, task design, individual control, autonomy and decision-making latitude, the congruence of workers' skills and job requirements, understanding of role, workload, work patterns, work conditions, and general environment (exposure to violence, abuse, biological and chemical agents, staffing levels, noise, etc.), changes in the workplace, current and future; communications concerning what is expected at work, change, employment security, the relationship between home and the workplace, inter- and intraprofessional relations, and certain subjective factors, such as emotional and social demands, being unable to cope, perceived level of support from the organization, managers, and colleagues; and value and ethical conflicts (European Commission 2011; Royal College of Nursing 2007).

Given the fast pace of the nursing workplace, job demand and control factors or decision latitude have become important contributors to stress. Practitioners, burdened by a high level of job demand and having limited control over the manner in which they perform, are definitely eligible for mental strain (European Working Conditions Observatory 2014; Karasek 1979). Actual changes in the work environment or threats of the same, such as new colleagues, supervisors, schedules, work patterns etc., are also an important source of stress among nurses who experience many changes in their work environment, including those related to the evolution of medical technology, new medical developments, and the structure and organization of services. All of these affect their relationships with patients and colleagues. Changes create uncertainty in the atmosphere and reactions can stir distress or eustress. In a sense, reforms introducing changes in work conditions have the potential to destroy the psychological contract between health-care institutions and their staff. It appears that a large number of Estonian and German nurses, favoring their traditional work modes, have been reticent to consider innovation in their routines. A survey of nurses' response to change indicated that those who had experienced reform, held more negative views of the patient care climate than their colleagues who did not have to deal with it. Moreover, it has been found that physicians and nurses are more prone to react to systemic changes, whereas other health-care staff tends to respond to layoffs and wage freezes (Kirpal 2003; Rigoli and Dussault 2003).

Often, nurses' evaluations of the effects of changes on their psychological well-being have been dismissed. However, research (Verhaeghe et al. 2006) on the subject undertaken in Belgium has confirmed these professionals' appraisal. Nurses, having had to deal with change, scored statistically significantly higher for distress. Furthermore, changes perceived as threatening had a negative impact on job satisfaction and a positive relationship with distress and absences due to illness. On the other hand, changes perceived as representing a challenge were positively related to job satisfaction and eustress. These had no impact on distress or absence. It is quite clear that changes in nurses' work environment, depending on their nature, can represent an occupation-specific work stressor.

The problem of change is much more complex in many of the newer Member States. In addition to the above-mentioned stressors, other psychosocial risk factors have been and some still are present. The work environment, hazards at the workplace, work organization, financial issues, public criticism, the professional environment, shift work, professional and intellectual demands and the general microclimate have had a role in generating a share of work stress. Research

165

(Golubic et al. 2009) has indicated that the importance of these occupational stressors relates to education. In Croatia, nurses with a vocational training perceived hazards at the workplace and shift work as statistically significantly more stressful than colleagues with a college degree. However, a most prominent determinant that preconditioned an elevated level of stress was the challenging transition to a market economy and a democratic system of government (Hristov et al. 2003). This penetrated all social structures down to the microlevel. Economic, political, and social transformation reinforced existing stress catalysts and created new ones. Transition for many nurses in the Central and East European Member States reaped job insecurity or even unemployment, a combination of work and other types of stress, decreased and often delayed wages, uncertainties, confusion, tension and conflicts regarding new arrangements in the health-care sector; the strains of tending a population in distress, a decline in living standards, and a host of other negative elements. According to Hristov et al. (2003), these stressors tend to be more virulent during transition periods. The multiplicity of these elements presents a serious challenge to nurses in societies in transition.

As noted, nurses just entering the world of work are especially subject to role stress. Very often, their professional socialization in educational institutions is not congruent with their work environment. Their self-expectations might not mesh with those of nursing management and the clinical staff. The situation can be intensified by fear of failure, making mistakes, and assuming total responsibility. Evidently, philosophical divisions between the norms and values of the health-care institution and those of the new graduate nurse present problems as well and lead to stress. Consequently, job stress can be quite severe. At one point in time, eight of ten English graduate nurses responded to these stressors by abandoning hospital nursing (Kelly 1996). The talents of these young professionals were lost along with any leadership potential. Young people are not the only ones worried about making mistakes. This fear relates to a 71 percent increase in mental disorders among nurses, in general. Stress is generated by uncertainties concerning equipment, lack of necessary information, constant interruptions in the rhythm of work, and dissatisfaction about the quality of care.

Effort–Reward Balance

An important element in the psychosocial environment is the effort–reward equilibrium. This is a measure of the balance between an employee's effort and the reward received. Effort relates to high emotional, physical, and quantitative demands and the reward factor to wages; recognition and respect, career development, and job security. These two forces should be equilibrated. To a large extent, however, the scale tends to tilt in the direction of imbalance and this signals increased risk of poor physical and mental health as well as possible exit from the profession.

There are substantial differences among the various Member States in nurses' effort–reward ratio. An extremely high ratio, indicating an especially undesirable situation, has been identified in Poland, Germany, Slovakia, and Italy, meaning that efforts are not matched with appropriate rewards. Nurses in these countries have felt slighted in terms of their compensation, financial and otherwise. In Poland and Slovakia, this high ratio may result from the aforementioned economic transition. In Germany and Italy, it could reflect change in the health-care delivery system itself. In either case, it is a warning signal. In general, nurses in transition societies have experienced the highest effort–reward imbalance (Hasselhorn, Tackenberg, and Peter 2004). On the other hand, as opposed to these scenarios, the ratio is the lowest in the Netherlands, indicating advantageous circumstances in which the scores for effort were low and reward scores higher. Effort scores were the highest in Germany and lowest among Dutch nurses. The difference between countries is significant, except between Finland, Poland, and Italy. With the exception of the latter nation, in all countries, females had higher scores than males. This was significant in Finland, France, Poland, and Slovakia.

Not only has the effort–reward imbalance differed among nations, but in some of these, substantial differences have been found between different types of health-care institutions. For example, in Germany, the imbalance was especially pronounced in hospitals as was true of Italy and Slovakia. In France, the imbalance was particularly high in nursing homes and in Poland, high visibility was found in hospitals, nursing homes, and home care (Hasselhorn et al. 2003, 2008; Hasselhorn, Müller, and Tackenberg 2005; Hasselhorn, Widerszal-Bazyl, and Radkiewicz 2003). Institutions enjoying low effort–reward imbalances can reap the advantages of a higher commitment on the part of nurses to their place of employment and their profession. On the other hand, nurses, who experience an intense effort–reward imbalance, have been shown to be more susceptible to burnout (Bakker et al. 2000). Given the research results cited here and nurses' evaluation of their wages mentioned elsewhere, one can appreciate the importance of supreme effort and inadequate reward to the nursing profession's agenda.

Work–Family Balance

A problem mentioned in another context that is also concerned with the psychosocial work environment is the impact of the demands of nurses' work on their personal life. Often, as noted, there is a gap between education and reality. Nurses discover discrepancies between their education, particularly, at the graduate level, and what is expected of them on the floor. Practitioners in Northern Ireland have experienced extreme stress related to confidence and competency in their role. This is not uncommon. Reflecting the complexity of care, this stressor can infringe on a professional's personal life. Both of these problems, considered major stressors, have been known to inspire nurses in many Member States to leave or consider leaving the profession (Chan and Lai 2010; Hughes and Claney 2009). Of all the variables related to job satisfaction and good physical and mental health for nurses, the work–life balance or work–home conflict, a significant indicator of the quality of life, has the most important gender dimension, given women's share of unrewarded work in the household.

This conflict, which is dependent on societal and family contexts as well as the individual's characteristics, represents one based on roles. Obligations in one domain cannot be attended to because of those in the other. The lack of congruence in roles relates to diverse types of work–home conflicts. A time-based work–family conflict results from problems related to the devotion of adequate time to both sectors. A strain-based work–family conflict revolves around stress originating in one site that transfers to the other, causing a failure to fulfill responsibilities in both camps. A behavior-based work–home conflict concerns difficulties in changing behavior between the two sites. High quantitative demands serve as a major predictor of this type of conflict, as revealed by studies of the European nursing profession. Pressures related to length and scheduling of work schedules, intensity of work, safety of conditions at the place of employment, and job security have been found to play a larger part in this conflict than family characteristics (Gallie and Russell 2009; Hasselhorn, Müller, and Tackenberg 2005; van der Heijden et al. 2008; Kasearu 2009; Simon et al. 2004). It has been determined that greater job demands lead to a higher level of work–home conflict, which, making a general deterioration in health more likely, in turn, generates increased job demands and work–home interference. The scenario represents a vicious circle.

Depending on where the conflict originates, it is referred to as a work-to-family conflict or a family-to-work conflict. The former has been found to be more prevalent among European nurses and it is the most prevalent among Slovakian and Italian nurses. Mean scores for this phenomenon were found to be the highest in Italy, medium high in France, Belgium, Germany, Slovakia, and Finland; and low in Poland and the Netherlands. Low scores have also been evidenced by nurses in the United Kingdom (Review Body for Nursing and Other Professions 2007). The problem has been of concern to a majority of Irish nurses as well (Adams and Kennedy 2006). Furthermore, among nurses, the work–family conflict is more visible in the early period of a career and between the ages of thirty and forty. Evidently, older professionals have fewer problems when attempting to integrate their work and private obligations. A major psychosocial stressor at work, this conflict impinges heavily on health, as well as attitudinal and behavioral outcomes. Thus, one can appreciate recent efforts to create flexibility in the workplace and a worker-friendly atmosphere. In fact, in most of the older Member States, support for family-friendly work provisions has been generally acknowledged and accepted. However, these efforts have been especially important to Central and East European Member States who have experienced a dramatic decrease in the birth rate creating consequences for pension funding, care of the elderly, and a host of other matters.

Job Insecurity

Job insecurity is another element that impinges on the psychosocial environment at nurses' place of work. There are two kinds of job insecurity. One is quantitative in nature and is attributed to perceived threat through imminent loss of a job. The second, qualitative job insecurity, results from the perception of a possible loss of quality within one's current position. An internal transfer or receipt of a less than desirable work schedule serves as an example of this second type. Quantitative work insecurity has been quite evident in many of the newly acceded Member States. It results from general problems related to the transition and particularly, from the restructuring of the health sector. Studies of European nurses (Hasselhorn et al. 2005; Laine and the NEXT Study Group 2003) revealed that in Poland and Slovenia, up to 90 percent of these practitioners were concerned about losing their jobs. Fear of job loss has also been found to be severe in Lithuania and Romania, and somewhat less in the Czech Republic. Thus, it becomes understandable why nurses show up for work, even when they are ill. The reality is that they are too insecure to take leave of absence when they are sick or entitled to annual leave. They fear their job might not be there when they return (*Health Care in Central and Eastern Europe* 2001; Rosskam and Leather 2006). In the older Member States, the percentage related to fear of job loss registered at ten or less with the exception of Finland where it was 17.3. Least concern was evident in the Netherlands (2 percent). In terms of locating another nursing position in the area, one out of four nurses interviewed in Italy, Germany, and Finland, thought this would be an arduous task. On the other hand, such was not perceived as a problem in the United Kingdom, Belgium, and the Netherlands. Results concerned with qualitative work insecurity were different. Nurses interviewed were primarily preoccupied with the possibility of an internal transfer and Italian nurses were the most worried. In Italy, France, and Belgium, but especially, in Poland and Slovakia, they worried about being assigned an undesirable work schedule.

Job insecurity also relates to gender and age. It seems that females in Germany, Finland, France, and elsewhere, are significantly more concerned than males about the possibilities of finding new employment should they become unemployed. The same has been found true for internal transfers in Italy and Finland and for receiving an unsuitable shift rota. In terms of age, preoccupation with losing one's job decreases with age in Finland, Poland, and Slovakia, but only slightly in France and Italy. Older nurses, it appears, are more secure in their employment. As one might expect, concern about finding a new nursing position increased with age in Germany, Belgium, France, Great Britain, and the Netherlands, whereas, strange as it might seem, in Poland and Slovakia, it decreased (Laine and the NEXT Study Group 2003).

Of the two types of job insecurity the quantitative variety has generally been the most prevalent. Circumstances identified with it are difficult for any nurse. Central and East European Member States have faced the most formidable challenges. Practitioners living in these nations, for the most part, have been less equipped than colleagues in other Member States to face labor market insecurity, primarily, because of the nature of this market prior to the transition and problems that appeared when and after transition took place. It must be recognized that attitudes transform as demands for the health-care workforce change.

Professional Relationships

In order to deliver efficient and effective care, nurses must interact with other health-care professionals. The nature of relations with colleagues, supervisors, and managers, or the organizational social infrastructure is central to career satisfaction, as well as a positive psychosocial environment at the workplace, and patient satisfaction and outcomes. Thus, group interaction assumes much significance along with leadership and management procedures. Moreover, the level of nurses' empowerment also relates to management practices, leadership styles, and work satisfaction. It is mirrored in the degree of nurses' participation in decision-making, where a larger amount of clinical freedom is identified with enhanced job satisfaction (Tovey and Adams 1999). Group relationships are especially important in the context of the nurse shortage, and the current focus on increased output and cost containment.

In the health-care world, the relationships between doctors and nurses reverberate into many quarters. In fact, nurses, in general, have believed that relations with medical staff exert a significant impact on their performance. Tension between the two groups has been most evident in the construction of a more holistic approach to health care and it has hindered nurses' professional ability to provide and improve care (Brown and Kirpal 2004; Institute of Medicine of the National Academies 2011). For an extended period of time, in the European setting, nurses, as noted, did not enjoy autonomy or discretion. Medical dominance, largely rooted in historically embedded values, was accepted. A nurse was a medical helper and nothing more. Moreover, this role was shaped by its familial affiliation within the configuration of health-care services. Given the feminized nature of nursing, the sexual division of labor concerning care giving within the paid labor force was congruent with that within the family (Dent 2003a, 2003b). Physicians dominated because of a hierarchical structure of authority, their social position, and monopoly of knowledge. It is noteworthy that Florence Nightingale, at one point in time, endorsed such a relationship. Even though she liberated females by giving them a profession and an opportunity to earn an income independently, she also limited them by affirming that only males should be physicians and that nurses should defer to their authority (Satterly 2004).

This command continues to exist, to a large extent, in the Central and East European Member States, such as Poland, Latvia, Slovenia, and Romania. Also, nurses are limited in Southern Europe as well (Dent

171

2003a; Sandin and Walldal 2002). They tend to be regarded as medical assistants with their role being determined by physicians. Moreover, the restricted duties of nurses do not allow them to be a threat to the medical profession. As for their status, it has been evaluated as lower than before transition. Not too long ago, it was revealed that in Slovenia, only 4 percent of nurses felt physicians respected their profession. The same attitude has prevailed in Romania (Filej et al. 2009; Vlădescu et al. 2008). It is interesting to note that in the latter nation before 1978, when nurse training was abolished for a period, nursing was a respected profession, but then the role developed into that of a medical assistant and in this part of the world, to a large extent, this role still prevails. These health-care providers are not viewed as members of an autonomous profession. There is no respect for the autonomy of nursing, little teamwork, and barely any understanding that the skills of a nurse and a physician are complementary.

The situation was appropriately exposed in reference to Slovenia. "[The] activity of nursing in everyday practice is still not a professionally and organizationally independent activity and not sufficiently comparable with other professionals employed in the healthcare system" (Filej et al. 2009, p. 167). Although written in reference to Slovenia, this judgment has a broader application. In Slovenia and environs, subordination of nurses has been attributed to the market culture, level of personal involvement, and amount of education. The professional development of nurses has been hindered by an organizational culture featuring hierarchical structures, a control orientation, a lack of collaboration and team building between doctors and nurses, as well as adequate participation of these professionals in change implementation activities (Skela and Pagon 2008).

In many instances, such as in Italy, where physicians and institutional organization generally fail to recognize the talents of new nurses with a university education, these professionals are still perceived in the traditional manner (Furlan 2006). However, in others, over the past few decades, physician-nurse relationships have been transformed, although not completely. French medical schools attempt to nurture greater understanding between the two professions with a unique program. In the second year of a six-year course, medical students are exposed to the hospital scene. At this time, they spend a month "shadowing" a nurse and an aide. Hopefully, they gain a true understanding of the role of this practitioner who is with the patient on a continuous basis. Moreover, in French hospitals, nurses, including those involved in direct patient care, participate in rounds with physicians (Gordon 2005). Activities of this sort have the potential to generate more productive professional relationships.

In many Member States, the medical world has been feminized and more males have entered the ranks of nursing. In addition to these gender changes, the social origins of nurses have experienced diversification, but not without a struggle. People with middle and upper class backgrounds joined the profession. Health-care institutions underwent change as well, as did nurses' educational preparation. New management tools have been invented. High technology has thrived. New methods of delivering care and work organization have been developed, disturbing professional boundaries. Nurses have become more autonomous and as they realize more autonomy in their practice, the potential to generate conflict with physicians becomes greater. Although autonomy has been enhanced in some Member States and nursing has become better defined, sometimes, as in Spain, distinctions between the professional functions of nursing and those of other professions lack clarity (López-Valcárcel, Quintana, and Socorro 2006). However, new social relations, not as stable as previous ones, have developed. Often, the outcome has been a fundamental reshaping of the traditional professional order.

It should be pointed out that Gordon (2005) presents the opposite side of the coin. She recognizes that there are more females in medicine and that nursing remains primarily a female profession. However, she argues that female physicians, reacting to the possibility of being mistaken for a nurse, do little to reduce the tension between the two professions. Claiming that gender and status politics must be considered, she continues to affirm: "The social distance between female doctors and nurses sometimes seems even more pronounced than that between male doctors and female nurses" (p. 47).

The result of these various developments has led to unstable relations between physicians and nurses, as identified in France (Picot 2005). The classical hierarchical structure of authority incorporating a completely powerless nursing workforce has become of limited utility. Nurses' line of action in many health-care institutions has changed. A new climate prevails. These professionals now perform a different role in defining the rules for interaction with others in health-care structures and patients' medical status. Their position has been fortified by their knowledge and understanding of patients, and the new team work organization. Nurse–physician relationships have been altered as the result of an enlargement of the arena for encounters between the two professions. A review of the literature concerning physician–nurse collaboration in the hospital setting (Tang et al. 2013) revealed that often physicians assigned it less importance than nurses and also, gave its quality a rating superior to that of their nursing colleagues.

Recognizing this scenario, Svensson (1996) has appropriately labeled the social order of health-care institutions, a negotiated order, the result of constant bargaining between nurses and physicians. This interaction determines power relationships in these structures. All participants have an active part in this process to preserve or modify the existing social order. Nurses' participation in institutional activities is of a different sort. Possessing now more command over decisions affecting patients, they can exert increased influence on norms for interaction and work performance. Their power and institutional role have changed for the better, but not completely. The RN4CAST project inquired into the nature of working relationships between the medical and nursing professions. The percentages of practitioners reporting an absence of positive ones indicate that more change must be realized. Results were as follows: Poland (44 percent), Germany (37 percent), Greece and Spain (34 percent), Belgium (30 percent), Ireland (23 percent), Finland (21 percent), the Netherlands (19 percent), and Sweden and England (11 percent) (Aiken 2011). Acknowledging that all social orders are negotiated orders, it is difficult to precisely define relationships between nurses and physicians. These depend on the people and settings involved. Power is distributed in diverse ways as is evident in the various situations found in Member States.

Nurses employed outside health-care institutions and those that are self-employed working with other professionals in the health-care and social sectors also have to negotiate their social order on a regular basis. Collaborative relationships involving several role partners from different organizational landscapes are complex and often frustrating. Scottish public health nurses, known as health visitors, have complained of a lack of recognition on the part of professionals in the field with whom they are expected to collaborate (Ellefsen 2002). Cooperation among various professionals and service agencies is at the foundation of community care. Each participant's competence merits recognition. Experiences (Vilbrod and Douguet 2007) indicate that, to a large degree, the interactions of nurses working in this capacity with general practitioners, service agencies, and other professionals, are difficult and often, they are pressed to "stand up and be counted" without direct confrontation. However, once again, knowledge of patients and their needs furnishes them an advantageous weapon, especially, when there are disparate points of view. With pharmacists, reference is made to engaging in a game of alliances and implicit understandings. In dealing with leaders and managers, defensive stakes are designed within their professional perimeters. It is noted that sometimes effective collaboration takes place as revealed in a recent study of community nurses in Lithuania (Zabarauskaite 2013) in which 63.1 percent of the respondents were satisfied with their relations with other providers of such care. On other occasions, as one might expect, such as in Bulgaria and Estonia (Index Foundation and Praxis Centre for Policy Studies 2007), relationships have been quite tense and marked by distrust, indicating again the social order is a negotiated order.

Nursing staff conflict, often referred to as horizontal violence, has been reported throughout the confines of the EU. A study of European nurses reported that in Italy 30.9 percent of nurses had a low interpersonal relations score, followed by Poland and France at 22.5 percent. On the other hand, the figure for Belgium was 8.4 percent and that for the Netherlands, 5.4 percent. Also, of interest, is the estimate that 43 percent of nurses' stress is related to poor relationships with colleagues (Dallender et al. 1999; Estryn-Behar, Le Nézet, and Jasseron 2005). Three levels of explanation for poor intrastaff relations have been offered. At the macrolevel, focus is on nurses' relations with dominant groups. Mesolevel explanations consider organizational structures, including workplace practices, many of which are controlled by nurses themselves. Microlevel analysis stresses the interactive nature of interpersonal conflict. Quite often, these explanations have underscored that nurses are at fault because they shackle and impede themselves (Farrell 2001). In other words, they are their own worst enemy. In nursing units, intragroup conflict has tended to be greater in smaller ones, featuring a higher ratio of nurses to total staff. Less than desirable interpersonal relations are not affiliated with anticipated turnover. Moreover, unit morale and the interpersonal relations aspect of team performance effectiveness are negatively associated with intragroup conflict and anticipated turnover, but positively associated with satisfaction with pay (Cox 2001).

Management style affects the general culture of an organization, job satisfaction, as well as the psychosocial environment at the workplace. Moreover, a style that facilitates and leads, rather than directs, and promotes and values staff contribution and multiple communication channels between management and personnel, especially enhances retention. It also nurtures trust. The quality of communication between staff and managers is a crucial issue in tempering stress at the workplace. In fact, a participatory management style, involving professional staff in the management process, is often assigned the highest grades. The Scottish National Health Service provides for such an arrangement. Known as Partnership Working, it represents an approach to employee relations and decision-making. At the apex of the structure is the Scottish Partnership Forum cochaired by the Chief Executive of the National Health Service and a trade unionist. Government is also involved at this level. Decentralized units include trade unionists, managers, and staff. The effort affords a triadic approach to decision-making concerning strategic human resource and operational matters. All structures must meet the Staff Governance Standard which indicates guidelines to assure that employees are well-informed, adequately trained, treated fairly and consistently, provided with a secure workplace, and afforded the opportunity to participate in decisions that affect them. To ensure that these conditions are met, a Staff Governance Committee in each unit oversees all activities (Steel and Cylus 2012).

Improvements in employees' well-being, competences, and productivity have been attributed to such managerial practices. Moreover, other performance benefits have resulted. These include lower levels of absences related to illness, patient mortality, and complaints, as well as stress and higher levels of job satisfaction and collaboration with colleagues. Equally as important, patients are more satisfied with care offered by a gratified staff. The culture generated by this management style nurtures institutions featuring teamwork that leads to a significantly higher safety climate. Moreover, all participants in the process are empowered (Ellins and Ham 2009; Hämäläinen and Lindström 2006; Speroff et al. 2010). In many sites, this management model was put into use to reduce tensions affiliated with augmented emphasis on management in health-care institutions, due to budgetary constraints and increased performance-related funding arrangements.

Western management principles and leadership styles in the form of participatory governance have been introduced into Estonian hospitals and their impact has been stellar (Kaarna et al. 2004). Obviously, this type of management was a new phenomenon for all health-care personnel. Känd and Rekor (2005) reported that it was immediately accepted by nurses who recognized they had an instrument for valuable input, not only into the decision-making process, but into total organizational development. They became acquainted with financial matters and thus, understood their low salaries, long hours, and poor working circumstances. They understood that institutional conditions left to be desired, but, at least, they could meaningfully contribute to their upgrade. Possessing the right to decide on the sequence of fulfilling professional responsibilities, they felt an integral part of the organization. In short, increased participation in institutional decision-making enriches loyalty, commitment, and retention, all affiliates of job satisfaction. When nurses are excluded from workplace management the importance of salary, security, and working conditions increases and grows out of proportion, often with disastrous consequences. The cost affiliated with participatory management arrangements is inexpensive compared to its benefits. It is of extensive value.

However, the same management model had a different experience in other parts of Europe, principally places in the United Kingdom and Sweden, where clinical participation in management structures has been the most developed. In these settings, staff was far from enthusiastic, believing involvement interfered with its principal interest— professional practice. In France, nurses demanded a greater say in management matters and the solution, manifesting a diverse scope, was somewhat different. The government established a nursing commission in all hospitals whose function is to address problems faced by these professionals, whether from a practice, training, or career point of view. These units have been able to deal with routine issues, but have met less success with matters related to general work organization and others of a complex nature (Bach n.d.-b). Problem solving in health care should not be unidimensional.

Although management received glowing evaluations by nurses in Estonia, the same did not occur in other Member States in the region. In Lithuania and Romania, leaders have been soundly criticized by a majority of staff and less so in the Czech Republic. Criticisms have asserted that health-care executives have become less concerned with the needs of personnel (*Health Care in Central and Eastern Europe* 2001). In the same region, leadership ability in nursing was censured. Evidently, it has been below par, due to a lack of educational facilities for the development of health-care management skills (Filej et al. 2009). Satisfaction with organizational leadership has been ranked as low in Malta, Finland, Poland, and Italy as well (Hasselhorn, Müller, and Tackenberg 2005; Muscat and Grech 2006). More positive evaluations have been forthcoming from Great Britain, Belgium, Germany, and

177

Slovakia. Even in these cases, nurses' evaluations of their organizational leaders were not sterling. They indicated they were only "more or less" satisfied with their superiors' efforts (Siebens et al. 2006; Stordeur et al. 2003b). It is important to note that evaluations of managerial quality vary according to work setting and level of education. They are important to the psychosocial environment.

In a more recent effort, the RN4CAST study reported on nurses' confidence in management's capacity to resolve problems in the workplace. In the Member States studied, a solid majority of practitioners lacked such confidence. The percentages range from 87 in Greece to 58 in Germany. No nation registered a favorable outlook. Attitudes related to questioning the decision or actions of those in authority were somewhat more favorable. Only in Poland (64 percent), Spain (55 percent), and Greece (53 percent) did a majority feel uncomfortable in doing so. Percentages in the cases of Finland (45 percent), Ireland (44 percent), and Belgium (43 percent), ranged in the 40s, whereas those for England (36 percent), Germany (35 percent), and Sweden (34 percent), placed in the 30s. The Netherlands was at the bottom of the scale at 12 percent, meaning the climate was more favorable to inquiry (Aiken 2011).

Leadership not only concerns what leaders do, but also, the way in which they do it. It seems that, in some cases, the methods utilized create tension and hostility, rather than harmony and fluid and open communications. In France, a large quantity of nurses (59 percent) has deplored hostile and tense relations with managers (LeLan 2004). Inadequate or nonexistent contacts with these leaders have been reported in other nations, including Belgium, Slovakia, and Finland (Siebens et al. 2006). As a result, dialogue is lacking and nursing personnel frequently feel they have no influence or input into organizational development. Poor communication often generates a lack of trust in administrators. In the Member States, nurses' involvement in organizational governance has varied, according to the hierarchical level of nursing within a facility. Shared governance models have ranged from nurses' informal and limited participation to those in which nurses' authority and accountability are formally recognized, allowing them to define and regulate not only nursing practice, but to have input into the general management of institutional resources (Page 2004).

A major criticism of leaders has focused on failing to create a supportive environment. Nurses have made reference to a lack of various types of support, including psychological support with particular respect to the emotional impact of the work situation, its ethical aspects, and violence at the work place. In France, psychological support has headed and still heads nurses' lists of criticisms of managers and needs. It is a matter that has required major attention in Belgium, where over 50 percent of hospital nurses have not felt supported by management (Siebens et al. 2006). In Italy, Germany, and Slovakia, this issue has been further down the list (Hasselhorn, Müller, and Tackenberg 2005; Muscat and Grech 2006). Comparative research has demonstrated the significance of organizational and managerial support to nurses. It is a major determinant of their dissatisfaction, burnout, evaluation of quality of care, and level of personal accomplishment (Aiken, Clarke, and Sloane 2002; Sundin et al. 2007). It is generally acknowledged that managerial support, as in Estonia, has the potential to reduce the negativities of a less than desirable work environment.

Given that lack of this support is perceived as a great stressor, it is imperative that access to it be enlarged. It can reap many benefits, not the least important of which is aiding the retention problem. Regular contact with other employees or colleagues can be an important part of organizational life. Such contact may be a source of support and provide a sense of belonging. It should also be underscored that in addition to support from management, that from colleagues, and even patients is just as important. This support has always been reported as higher than managerial support. The highest scores have resulted in the Netherlands and the United Kingdom and the lowest in Italy. With the exceptions of Poland and the United Kingdom, collegial support has universally decreased, as age increased (Hasselhorn et al. 2005; Sundin et al. 2007).

Florence Nightingale devoted attention to managerial problems in the workplace. Focusing on the relation of management to efficient nursing, she reasoned:

> Equal in importance to the provision of trained Nurses is the nature of the hospital authority under which these Nurses are to perform their duties. For unless an understanding is come to on this point, the very existence of good nursing is an impossibility (Nightingale 1954b, p. 285).

In the hospital realm, she proposed a triadic management scheme consisting of an administrative director, a medical director, and a nursing director. She was rightly concerned that only one trained as a nurse was qualified to govern other nurses. As it happened, not too long ago, this common triadic model assigning each director his/her own vertical hierarchy was introduced in most German public hospitals as part of a restructuring program. The theoretical equality of power within the management triumvirate was not translated into practice. Medical predominance prevailed. Nursing directors, ranked lower in terms of social prestige, enhanced the general lack of acceptance of an equal partnership. Moreover, nursing staff members tended to regard the medical director, rather than the nursing director, as their supervisor (Müller-Mundt 1997). Evidently, educational programs failed to erase traditional views. Times have changed and hopefully, further change will take place.

Burnout

There is no doubt that nurses' work world is marred by a galaxy of mental and emotional stressors. As noted, these are dependent on factors related to the nature and organization of work and job design. For example, empirical proof demonstrates that each additional patient assumed by a nurse adds a 23 percent increase to the odds of burnout and 15 percent to those of job dissatisfaction (Hayes et al. 2006). Moreover, stressors may result from interpersonal relationships with colleagues internal and external to the profession, with patients and their families as well as management. Effort–reward imbalances, work–family conflicts, lack of resources, staff shortages, and the technical aspects of nursing, especially the concern of nursing personnel in reference to their technical knowledge and skills or a moral conscience when they feel unable to provide the type of care they believe they should, play a role as well (Glasberg, Eriksson, and Norberg 2007). These are only some causes of stress that can result in burnout. There are many.

Stress has a detrimental impact on the individual's health when it is protracted over time, meaning it can lead to emotional exhaustion or burnout, a major risk and common problem for health-care professionals and particularly, nurses. The burnout syndrome, signifying the depletion of one's emotional resources, continues to increase within the ranks of nursing. It is generally acknowledged that the psychological well-being of nurses is constantly threatened. A British survey, undertaken by *Nursing Times*, revealed that these professionals felt the effects of workplace emotional stress as indicated by a greater consumption of alcohol, increased use of tobacco, and damaged sex lives ("British Nurses" 2007). Moreover, research efforts over time in the United Kingdom have noted a decrease in the psychological well-being of nurses. In fact, it has been evaluated as lower than that of the general population (Ball and Pike 2006a).

The most widely accepted definition of burnout is that offered by Maslach (1993). He refers to this condition as "a psychological syndrome of emotional exhaustion, depersonalization and reduced personal accomplishment that can occur among individuals who work with other people in some capacity" (p. 20). Burnout, which is now recognized as a significant social and individual problem, has major behavioral and health implications. Although it has been prevalent among health-care professionals, study of the phenomenon was limited, due to a lack of consensus as to its measurement. Maslach supplied an inventory for this purpose. Most recently, it was adopted in a large-scale, cross-national survey of nurses. It was concluded that the inventory was applicable to this type of research and could be utilized to determine the effectiveness of institutional and national policies aimed at reducing burnout among nurses (Poghosyan, Aiken, and Stone 2009). This is an important finding because burnout, according to one study (van der Schoot et al. 2003) of the nursing profession in Europe, in the past, has affected about 25 percent of its members. For nurses with high effective strain, the percentage registered at 64 and for those with high cognitive strain, it was 39.

Although they vary somewhat, burnout values have tended to be rather high in all nations, with the exception of the Netherlands. If the latter country has claimed the most favorable score, unfavorable ones have been allotted to Belgium and the United Kingdom and the most unfavorable to Slovakia and France (Gunnarsdóttir and Rafferty 2006; Hasselhorn, Tackenberg, and Peter 2004; van der Schoot et al. 2003). More recently, the RN4CAST study reported on nurse assessments of high burnout. Rates ranged from a high of 78 percent in Greece to a low of 10 percent in the Netherlands. England and Ireland registered 42 percent each and Poland 40 percent. Thirty percent was recorded for both Germany and Spain. In Sweden, 29 percent of nurses reported high burnout. The figure was 25 percent for Belgium and 22 percent for Finland (Aiken 2011; Schoonhoven, Heinen, and van Achterberg 2012). The picture is not positive. High burnout is a problem that requires attention, particularly in some Member States. Differences in burnout values have been identified on the basis of gender, in that males have consistently scored lower than females. In addition, personal burnout was found to be more prevalent among nurses employed in hospitals, outpatient care, and nursing homes than in home care settings. This is understandable, given the greater autonomy available in the latter and the diverse workplace climate. Intramural facilities revealed more occurrences of burnout. In fact, the mean score for burnout was highest among French hospital nurses. Interestingly enough, however, the same value was revealed in nursing homes and home care as well. The latter appears to be an outlier. However, within an institutional setting, it is generally accepted that the specific nursing unit does not have a significant effect on professional burnout. Also, problems concerning burnout vary considerably, depending on which patient care process has been adopted. Belgian nurses feeling at risk of burnout, have claimed their pressures resulted from conflicts related to the division of labor (Kalafati et al. 2005; Spitzer et al. 2006; Vandenbroeck et al. 2012; Vermandere 2014).

In a Croatian project personality traits were found to be weak, but significant predictors of burnout among nurses practicing in hospitals. Moreover, these traits only served as predictors of reduced professional efficacy. At the same time, organizational stress was found to relate positively to burnout. The importance of the interaction between personality and contextual variables in predicting burnout was revealed, given that the latter were found to be strong predictors of the phenomenon and personality weak ones (Hudek-Knezević, Maglica, and Krapić 2011).

Age is another variable that impacts on incidents of burnout. In general, nurses between the ages of thirty and thirty-five have reported the highest levels of the phenomenon, whereas their younger and older colleagues identified with the lowest. However, in reference to younger nurses, it is noteworthy that a recent Swedish study (Rudman and Gustavsson 2011) concluded that the newly qualified and inexperienced were especially vulnerable to burnout and particularly, during the second year after graduation. In general, however, it appears that within the ranks of the European nursing profession, there are no meaningful differences relating to burnout and seniority (Hasselhorn et al. 2005; van der Schoot et al. 2003). An earlier Hungarian study (Pikó 1999) found education to be a factor as well. Nurses with a baccalaureate degree suffered less from burnout than colleagues who had followed a diverse preparation for the profession.

Burnout appears to be a general phenomenon that is found in nations featuring diverse health-care delivery systems. It is costly from a variety of perspectives. The toll is great on the individual, members of the household involved, and colleagues, as well as others. Those afflicted suffer from poor health, are more prone to accidents and to committing errors at the workplace, in addition to experiencing low job satisfaction. Moreover, certain costs must be borne by the institution concerned. A survey of British nurses reported that about one-third of those polled indicated they had taken more sick days than usual. These were attributed to extreme pressures and in several cases, they accounted for thirty or more days in a given year ("British Nurses" 2007). Absenteeism obviously bears implications for staffing. In turn, medical costs reflect these situations that are also related to the individual professional's poor performance, lack of productivity, turnover, and a host of other factors. Society suffers in terms of the quality of care provided, health-care costs, loss of capacity for work, loss of social and intellectual capital, low levels of performance and loss of quality of life, to cite a few elements. Burnout is expensive and is something to be avoided.

Prevention has been related to the social environment at the workplace, organizational support and more precisely, a large amount forthcoming from colleagues; along with adequate demands, autonomy, and control over practice. An institutional culture manifesting these features has benefitted patient outcomes as well as those of nurses. It has been affiliated with more propitious patient outcomes and lower levels of nurse burnout. Health-care providers in larger workplaces tend to report a worse social environment than their colleagues in smaller ones (Aiken and Sloane 2002; European Working Conditions Observatory 2014; Gunnarsdóttir and Rafferty 2006). It appears that it is much easier to list the ingredients needed to avoid burnout than to actually obtain them. It seems to be easier said than done. However, the importance of the psychosocial work environment to health, perception, working ability, commitment, and productivity must be underscored

Work Ability

A significant individual and organizational resource closely affiliated with psychosocial workplace conditions is the work ability of employees, a notion that connects their resources and work characteristics. An individual's work ability consists of various elements that allow a person to perform a task in such a way that it results in a favorable outcome. In the first place, there are individual resources related to the mental, physical, and social capacities of the workers, in addition to their expertise. Thus, elements, such as education, training, and work experience, are important. In addition, aspects of the work environment,

183

such as the psychological, physical, and mental working demands and the social facet, must also be given consideration. The concept of work ability derives its importance from the fact that, as an organizational resource, it has the potential to increase output (Hasselhorn, Müller, and Tackenberg 2005; Hasselhorn et al. 2005). Moreover, a satisfactory work ability index has been found to be the significantly most important predictor for quality of life domains, such as the physical, psychological, environmental, and that concerned with social relationships. The highest odds ratio relates to the physical domain. Consequently, it is in the interests of all stakeholders for institutional managers to maintain or improve nurses' work ability scores (Milosevic et al. 2011).

Research on the work ability of nurses in European countries examined potential determinants of the phenomenon. Various factors, such as work schedule, sleep, multifaceted rewards, remuneration, work involvement, and motivation were taken into account. It was determined that work schedule was not related to modification of the Work Ability Index. However, responsibility for significant increases in this score was assigned to the quantity and quality of sleep and more favorable psychosocial factors. The other elements considered did not exert important effects on work ability (Camerino et al. 2008b). Croatian research has determined that statistically significant predictors related to low work ability are lower educational levels and older age. Thus, the availability of educational and career opportunities is an important ingredient of a decrease in occupational stress and an enhancement of work ability (Golubic et al. 2009). The Work Ability Index scores of Dutch and Finnish nurses have been found to be quite elevated, whereas those of their Danish, Polish, French, and German counterparts were the exact opposite. In fact, the Poles, especially older ones, had the lowest rankings. In Poland, personnel in the private sector have featured higher scores.

These indices are of importance because they are affiliated with work exposure, for example, to leadership positions, and with intent to abandon the profession. When work ability is low, nurses may have different turnover intentions or behaviors depending on their age. Relation of the index score to the professionals' age is telling. If younger nurses, as a group, have low work ability, it could mean a switch in profession. For senior nurses, it could signal early retirement. If all age groups manifest a low index, as in Germany, it could be a sign of hard times ahead. This could be dangerous in terms of the extensive shortage of nurses. To offset the departure of older workers from the workplace,

Member States have undertaken pension reforms, a reduction in early retirement pathways, and incentives to remain employed. Activities to enhance the Work Ability Index should accompany these efforts (Camerino et al. 2008a; Domagala et al. 1999; Hasselhorn, Müller, and Tackenberg 2005; Hasselhorn et al. 2005).

Research focusing on the working atmosphere in European nations (Widerszal-Bazyl et al. 2003a) has concluded that in terms of the psychosocial climate, nurses have been better off in Belgium and the Netherlands than in Finland, France, Germany, Italy, Poland, Sweden, or Slovakia. In the first two nations, job strain was found to be the lowest. Italy and Poland, featuring high work demands and low levels of control and support, represented the most difficult psychosocial work environment. As opposed to nurses' physical health, there are differences based on the site of employment in terms of their psychosocial health. It is noteworthy that a high degree of variance in psychosocial working conditions has been attributed to the nature of ownership, that is, public, private, or cooperative ownership, and type of operation. In Sweden, those employed in cooperative endeavors have considered their psychosocial climate superior to that found in the public sector. Those working in the latter are of the opinion that their psychosocial circumstances are significantly better than those in the private sector. Still, in all three ownership models, as they relate to the care sector, a sense of low control is evident (Höckertin and Härenstam 2006).

Violence: The Physical and Psychological Facets

Some workplace conditions, such as violence, have both physical and psychosocial facets. Nurses' workplaces are permeated by violence and although at the place of work, it is a global phenomenon, there is no agreement in the international arena as to its definition. This lack of consensus has been attributed to the fact that many different lines of conduct may be described as violent. Moreover, the dividing line between acceptable behaviors and violent or nonacceptable ones is not clear. Context and cultural interpretations complicate the matter as well. An act that is considered violent in one culture may not be considered so in another. Consequently, defining violence at work is a challenge (Chappell and Di Martino 2006; ICN 2008b; Tomev, Daskalova, and Ivanova 2003). A definition used in many quarters of the EU Member States is the one developed by the Commission. It describes workplace violence as "incidents where staff are abused, threatened or assaulted in circumstances related to their work, including commuting to and from work, involving an explicit or implicit challenge to their safety, well-being or health" (Cited in International Labour Office et al. 2002, p. 3). This statement is wide in scope. In terms of participants, violence in the health-care workplace is of a dual nature. When it involves solely health-care workers, including managers and supervisors, it is referred to as internal workplace violence. On the other hand, acts, involving these same workers and any other individual or individuals present at the site, fall under the rubric of external workplace violence. Groups at risk from external violence differ significantly from those at risk from the internal variety (Chappell and Di Martino 2006; Venema and van der Klauw 2012).

For a variety of reasons, but especially, the lack of consensus concerning a definition of workplace abuse and the fact that incidents are not always reported, it is difficult to specify its prevalence. However, there seems to be a general agreement that it is on the rampage and particularly, in the health-care sector. Kingma (2001) has labeled it "a problem of epidemic proportions" (p. 129) and in Italy, it has been said that the increase in violence in health-care facilities has triggered an alarm. Globally, it has affected on the average one of every two health-care workers. The EU Member States are no exception. Abuse in the health-care sector is more frequent than in any other field. In Sweden, 25 percent of the reported occurrences of workplace violence take place in health-care facilities, whereas those related to the retail, police, prison, and banking sectors represent only 5 percent each. Moreover, health-care personnel, in general, are eight times more likely to experience violence than people employed in manufacturing. Health-care providers' fear of violence is greater than ever before (Bartoloni 2007; ICN 2008b; International Labour Organization 2002; Wiskow, Albreht, and de Pietro 2010).

Of all health-care personnel, nurses are the most likely to experience violence in the workplace. In fact, they are at highest risk, it being three times that of other occupational groups. This is understandable in that they are in continuous direct contact with patients. Moreover, they frequently serve as a buffer between the patient and the physician (Daskalova et al. 2005; International Centre for Human Resources in Nursing 2007a). Within the nursing profession, females have usually been considered the most vulnerable. However, a study of violence risks in nursing in several Member States concluded that male nurses and younger nurses are more at risk (Estryn-Behar et al. 2008). The finding concerning younger nurses has been underscored in Sweden and Denmark. Being young and having a short employment tenure is a significant individual risk factor. In fact, the younger, the nurse, the more likely the exposure to violence. However, as the length of service in the work world increases, the risk of exposure to abuse lessens (Pedersen and Christiansen 2005; Sironi 2004).

ICN has also defined nursing students as "particularly at risk of workplace violence" (ICN 2006, p. 1). This affirmation has been confirmed in a recent study involving workplace violence and Italian nursing students. Thirty-four percent of the participants claimed to have experienced violence in various forms in the clinical setting. Moreover, these students reported being subjected to violence by colleagues, staff, and others, including teachers, physicians, and supervisors (Magnavita and Hepaniemi 2011).

Basically, there are two types of abuse at the workplace: physical violence and psychological violence. The former focuses on the patient and/or persons identified with this individual as the primary subjects. Also, in rare instances, health-care providers, including nurses, are the aggressors. Obviously, such behavior violates professional codes of conduct. However, it has been revealed that physical abuse by staff is especially high in Greece where 10 percent of the nurse participants in the RN4CAST study (Moreno-Casbas et al. 2011) reported the occurrence of such behavior a few or more times each month. In other Member States, the percentage registered at 3 and in the Netherlands at 0.

There has been an increase in incidents of physical violence in the health-care sector and in their severity. This type of abuse usually occurs along the line of conflict between patient/family and provider and it appears to be present in most countries. In some cases, such as Bulgaria, although it might not be typical for the health sector, it is not an exception. For example, a Bulgarian survey revealed that 7.5 percent of the respondents had been victims of physical violence in a given year. In addition, 10.2 percent had witnessed physical violence at the place of work in the same time period. As mentioned, any type of violence is experienced more by nurses than other members of the health-care team. This holds for physical violence as well.

An examination of physical violence in Bulgaria by professional group revealed that nurses have the highest relative share. The same holds true in Italy. A Royal College of Nursing poll carried out in the United Kingdom reported that more than one-quarter of the nurses surveyed had been physically attacked while at work. Although violence affects all health-care work settings, the risk of exposure to it depends

187

on one's sector of employment. Nurses in certain areas of practice are more prone to acts of physical violence. For example, in Sweden, psychiatric nurses are five times more exposed to this type of abuse than colleagues in other sectors. More specifically, in the United Kingdom, in acute care, 40 percent of nurses experienced violence on the part of patients or relatives. In the emergency department, the percentage climbed to 79. On hospital wards, the rate registered at 52 percent (Bartoloni 2007; Bennett, Davey, and Harris 2007; "British Nurses" 2007; Di Martino 2002; Ferrinho et al. 2003; *Informe* 1999; International Labour Office et al. 2003; Tomev, Daskalova, and Ivanova 2003).

An examination of the frequency of violence on the part of patients and/or relatives against nursing staff in some EU Member States ranked these nations from the highest number of incidents to the lowest in the following order: France, Germany, Belgium, Italy, Finland, Poland, Slovakia, the Netherlands (Camerino et al. 2008c). Another report (Vere-Jones 2008) has inserted the United Kingdom following France. A more recent ranking issued by the RN4CAST project (Moreno-Casbas et al. 2011) indicated the percentage of nurses experiencing occurrences of physical abuse on the part of patients a few times per month or more as follows: Finland (20 percent), Ireland and the United Kingdom (19 percent), Greece (11 percent), Poland (10 percent), Germany (8 percent), Belgium (6 percent), Sweden (5 percent), Spain (3 percent), and the Netherlands (1 percent). The more recent report includes some of the same Member States, but in different positions. Of note is the consistent low incidence of physical violence in the Netherlands.

Psychological violence, a form more subtle than physical abuse, encompasses a variety of behaviors and is more widespread throughout the health sector of the Member States. Moreover, its impact is as great, if not greater, than that of its physical counterpart. Verbal abuse, intimidation, bullying, mobbing, various types of discrimination, and harassment are some behaviors included under the rubric of psychological violence. It is noteworthy that the ICN (2006) cites excessive workloads, unsafe working conditions, and inadequate support as forms of violence as well. These types of aggression are not necessarily distinct. In fact, they frequently overlap (Chappell and Di Martino 2006; Wiskow, Albreht, and de Pietro 2010). Very often, the lines of confrontation are drawn between a superior and a subordinate.

Bullying, a form of harassment, is especially widespread and one of the fastest growing types of workplace abuse. It consists, according to the ILO, "of offensive behavior through vindictive, cruel, malicious, or humiliating attempts to undermine an individual or group of employees" (cited by International Centre for Human Resources in Nursing 2007c, p. 1). Colleagues, employers, supervisors, managers, patients or patients' friends and families, among others, serve as instigators of bullying. However, in nursing, bullying is, for the most part, intraprofessional, that is, between nurses. Moreover, research has concluded that it is a learned behavior within the workplace and not a psychological deficit within individual perpetrators and targets.

Mobbing is another common occurrence in health-care institutions. It too is on the increase. Colleagues or superiors isolate an employee via systematically directed hostile behavior. This type of conduct has been referred to as war at the workplace because the rules and strategies utilized are no different than those invoked in wartime. There are different types of mobbing: mobbing from below, mobbing from above, and horizontal mobbing. The first type involves an aggressor who is in a position inferior to that of the victim. The second kind relates to an aggressor occupying a rank above the victim's. Also, this term could be used to refer to an older attacker. The assailant and victim in the last sort are colleagues on an equal plane (Bromo and Bartolucci 2005).

There seems to be a consensus throughout the Member States that, in general, the most prevalent form of psychological violence is verbal abuse, as in Portugal, Bulgaria, and Italy. Nurses are subject to it on the part of patients and staff. Most of such abuse originates with patients as noted by the RN4CAST study (Moreno-Casbas et al. 2011). Nurses in Greece recorded the highest incidence (55 percent), followed by the United Kingdom and Ireland (49 percent each), Poland and Finland (41 percent each), Spain (37 percent), Germany (36 percent), Belgium (32 percent), Sweden (15 percent), and the Netherlands (9 percent). Verbal abuse on the part of staff is much more contained. Twenty-eight percent of Greek nurses reported occurrences of such behavior at least a few times monthly. Percentages then drop to 17 percent (Germany), 15 percent (Poland), 13 percent (the United Kingdom and Ireland), 10 percent (Belgium), 9 percent (Spain and Finland), 5 percent (Sweden), and 2 percent (the Netherlands). Of note, is the placement of Greece and the Netherlands in both categories.

Bullying and mobbing follow verbal abuse in terms of prominence. Incidents of these types of violence are not rare. For example, in Bulgaria, 38 percent of the nurses interviewed in one study reported experiencing bullying (International Centre for Human Resources in Nursing 2007c) and in Italy, at one time, almost 50 percent claimed they had been mobbed (Ban 2002). Of note, is the fact that not only is harassment on the part of management and superiors, such as immediate supervisors, on the increase, but this form seems to dominate in many instances. A study of workplace violence in some EU Member States revealed this phenomenon. In all cases, but one, that of the Netherlands, harassment by superiors was more frequent than that by colleagues. This type of violence was most pronounced in Poland, Germany, and France in rank order and once again, least pronounced in the Netherlands (Camerino et al. 2008c).

Psychological violence in the form of bullying and harassment in the United Kingdom has received much attention. In the National Health Service, 85 percent of the nurses have reported being targets of bullying (Lewis 2006). Results of studies carried out in this area are particularly interesting, given the conclusions related to black and minority ethnic nurses and those recruited internationally. Compared to white nurses qualifying in the United Kingdom, black and minority ethnic nurses and internationally recruited nurses are more likely to have been bullied and mobbed at the place of employment. Afro-Caribbeans have felt the most persecuted. One study indicated that one in six nurses reported experiencing such violence by a colleague. The frequency of such occurrences rose to three in ten for nurses with an ethnic minority background. In most surveys, white nurses qualifying in the United Kingdom report a lower incidence of bullying, mobbing, and related types of abuse. Ethnicity explains much of the variation. It is noteworthy that the abuse is related, in many instances, to minority issues. Over an extended period of time, surveys have repeatedly indicated that, as opposed to white nurses qualifying in the United Kingdom, greater proportions of black and minority ethnic nurses and those recruited internationally have considered these forms of psychological violence a major problem. Usually the perpetrators of this abuse have been nurse colleagues, but also medical and other coworkers, including managers. In reference to the latter, according to a Royal College of Nursing poll, it is noteworthy that almost 50 percent of the respondents claimed to have been bullied or harassed by a manager. Also, of note, is the fact that novice nurses are often the subjects of bullying which affects their productivity in negative fashion. More precisely, it impacts their cognitive demands and their ability to cope with their work responsibilities (Ball and Pike 2006a; Berry et al. 2012; "British Nurses" 2007; Pike and Ball 2007; Royal College of Nursing 2007).

Various facets of discrimination pose a problem for nurses in the Member States. This type of psychological violence can be direct or indirect. In the former case, prejudicial action is blatant, transparent, and outright. Indirect discrimination is quite subtle and cunning. It involves applying a rule or condition which, although applied equally to all groups, is such that larger proportions from favored groups meet its requisites than others. Moreover, this cannot be justified. There are several dimensions to discriminatory practices in nursing. These generally relate to gender, race, lifestyle, age, religion, social standing, nationality or geographic area, physical disability, and political convictions (Kingma 1999). Not all of these categories are prevalent in all Member States.

Since the largest part of the nursing profession consists of females, the gender dimension of discrimination is pertinent. In fact, it is of continuing concern to the predominantly female workforce. Sometimes, this discrimination has combined biases against females and nursing, as in the Central and Eastern European nations, where it has been assumed that managers should be physicians, meaning male, and attempts to create greater roles for nurse managers have encountered severe obstacles (Afford and Lessof 2006). In various health-care institutions in the Member States, preferential treatment has often been given to men. In terms of career development, a glass ceiling frequently exists for female nurses ensuring discrimination based on gender.

Not only are male nurses, in general, disproportionately represented in management and more responsible positions, as in Great Britain, Belgium, Germany, and France, but often, their career progresses at a faster pace than that of their female counterparts. They benefit more than women from available internal and external mobility. In Great Britain, there are a disproportionate number of men in more senior nursing positions and in Belgium, Germany, and France, the percentage of male head nurses greatly exceeds the overall percentage of men in the profession (Estryn-Behar, Le Nézet, and Jasseron 2005; *Front Line Care* 2010). In many instances, male nurses have moved directly into the higher salary brackets. Moreover, they have been known to earn more than females in the same position. Such has occurred in spite of the aforementioned norms concerning wages and the provisions of Article 141EC (Treaty of the European Union-ex Art 119 of the 1957 Treaty of Rome) which mandates equal pay without discrimination based on sex. It requires a policy of equal pay for equal work or work of equal value as between men and women. Moreover, this article has given a legal basis to a number of EU measures concerning equality between the sexes.

Hallmarks of positive practice environments include favorable strategies for continuing education and promotion that allow ample access to education and professional development opportunities, along with possibilities for the sharing of knowledge. In short, the climate should be one pervaded by a thirst for learning (Baumann 2007). Unfortunately, in the Member States, discrimination based on gender has also been identified in connection with access to career development instruments. Data reveal that more males are given the opportunity to pursue the training and specialization likely to lead to promotion and increased remuneration. In the United Kingdom, although at one time females constituted 93 percent of the nursing profession, males represented 45 percent of those involved in higher education courses and in senior management positions. Claiming that health-care job evaluations featured a gender bias, the Dutch Committee for Equal Treatment at one time ruled that the evaluation system used in the Netherlands discriminated against female employees (Kingma 1999). Obviously, such a finding had significant implications for nursing. Often, even when women have the appropriate qualifications, hidden gender assumptions in criteria are invoked in promotion and selection procedures. Over an extended period of time, it has been noted that the decision-making world in EU health-care institutions, for all practical purposes, has been one without women. The "glass ceiling" is almost shatterproof. The European Commission, in a report on equality between the sexes, concluded that, in the EU, sectoral and occupational segregation and gender pay differences have remained stable (European Commission: P.Vinay-Prospecta 1997; Vandenbrande et al. 2007; Weiler, Newell, and Carley 2007). In spite of many transnational and national policy initiatives, gender equality in career development is far from becoming a reality, as far as nursing is concerned. This discrimination against females in terms of career development is not based on differences in qualifications or skill levels.

One particular type of discrimination based on gender is sexual harassment. According to the European Commission, such acts of abuse consist, in part, of unsolicited and unreasonable behavior that is offensive to the recipient and conduct that places the person in intimidating, hostile, or humiliating work surroundings (European Commission 1991). This abuse may occur in the form of sexual jokes, comments and remarks of a sexual nature, inappropriate addressing of individuals, and inappropriate physical touching, among other ways. Given that most nurses are female and sexual harassment is, for the most part, directed against women, it has proven to be a significant thorn in the side of the profession. It is astonishing to read that in one study undertaken in the United Kingdom, 75 percent of the nurse respondents claimed they were subjected to sexual harassment at work. Surveys carried out in Bulgaria indicate such harassment has been a serious and extensive problem for female health-care workers, in general (Di Martino 2002; Kingma 1999). Interestingly enough, in Portugal, one report revealed that men working in health centers were more frequently victims of sexual harassment than women. This case is definitely an outlier. Also, of note, is the fact that, although in the Czech Republic, sexual harassment exists in significant proportions, public authorities and trade union officials, claiming the issue is overexaggerated, have chosen to overlook its significance (Vasková 2006).

In this context, culture is of importance. For example, in Bulgaria, the frequency of sexual harassment may be explained by the traditional social role of both sexes. Females are viewed as objects of sexual desire possessing a subordinate role in the family and society. Sexual harassment at the workplace is further bolstered by patriarchal stereotypes and behavioral models symbolizing male dominance and female emotional and economic dependence on men. These elements rationalize and legitimize this particular attitude toward women and make sexual harassment seem natural. Culture is also of significance in the case of Cyprus, where, given the Cypriot culture, society holds prejudices against victims of sexual abuse (Di Martino 2002; Stavrou 2007). Reference must be made to stereotypes and the images of nurses portrayed by the media that help nurture this type of psychological abuse. In many Member States, as in the United States, they have been presented as play things, sex objects, sex-obsessed human beings and romantic darlings (Stanley 2008).

Discrimination on the basis of race and nationality also presents a problem to the nursing profession in many Member States. It manifests several dimensions and nurses experiencing it face many of the same issues as those dealing with discrimination founded on gender. In the first place, immigrant and nonwhite nurses often find their work conditions less favorable than those of their native-born and/or white counterparts. A large number of the studies on this matter were undertaken in the United Kingdom. Problems illuminated in these extensive efforts serve as examples to document the situation in the United Kingdom and many practices found in other Member States.

Relations with patients and their family members have often proven stressful for the nursing constituency. In some cases, the discrimination has been direct as when patients or parents of children make it clear they do not want care by these health-care providers. In other instances, the discrimination has been more subtle. White patients treat white nurses in one way—favorably—and their minority colleagues in another—adversely. Studies have identified frequent examples of the first type of behavior, especially in the United Kingdom, but also elsewhere, as well. For example, in Portugal, in a survey of foreign nurses, 25 percent of the respondents reported discrimination on the part of patients who often became aggressive, racist, and xenophobic in their demands for a Portuguese nurse (Dhaliwal and McKay 2008; da Silva and Fernandes 2008). It appears that policies regarding zero tolerance toward discrimination from the public are the exception, rather than the rule, in most health-care institutions in the Member States.

Work schedules have also been of concern to nurses in minority communities. Among other things, shift patterns have created problems for these professionals who have had a significant role in providing continuity of care in several Member States. They have assumed a large part of night and weekend shifts. Twice as many of them have worked regularly at night and a disproportionate share has taken on Sunday work responsibilities (Dumont and Zurn 2007). More specifically, in reference to the United Kingdom, where rotating shifts have been used, it is noteworthy that a gigantic majority of these folks have regularly worked these shifts, making it difficult for them to organize their lives. Moreover, they have lodged complaints concerning the availability of alternate schedules, charging these and many other professional matters have been heavily dependent on social relationships with supervisors and managers, an element of the work culture that has excluded them. Most often, these nurses must accept their given schedules in light of financial obligations and tenuous employment status. This is especially true of those working in the private sector. In general, minority nurses are more likely to work extra hours, but they are less likely to be offered time off in lieu of salary. It has been established that there is a major variation, at least, in the United Kingdom's National Health Service, in work schedule by ethnicity and gender. Given this situation, some of these nurses have left acute care settings in favor of work in the community or elsewhere, where schedules tend to be more regular.

However, such a move impacts negatively on income as salary is at a lower level (Bach 2003; Dhaliwal and McKay 2008; Pike and Ball 2007; Royal College of Nursing 2007).

Career development in the United Kingdom has proceeded at a slower pace for minority nurses. These professionals have experienced difficulties at all stages of their careers. It has been established that, even though they possess the same qualifications as other colleagues, there is a difference of at least five years in career progression. South African nurses have been known to bitterly complain about the lack of promotion opportunities in hospitals. Research has revealed a stereotype of minority nurses in which they are portrayed as not possessing the necessary potential to become a supervisor or manager. Moreover, surveys have confirmed that ethnicity impacts on nurses' opportunity for promotion. In fact, in the past, this constituency was discouraged from pursuing it. Consequently, minority nurses have been heavily concentrated in lower professional rankings. To a large extent, most are staff nurses. Evidently, equal opportunity has been one thing, in theory and another, in practice. Formally, equal opportunity policies exist, but enforcement is another question. Minority nurses, given the realities of their career progression, have been skeptical of them (Bach 2003; Beishon, Satnam, and Hagell 1995; Dhaliwal and McKay 2008; Kingma 1999; Pike and Ball 2007; Royal College of Nursing 2007).

Another domain marred by discrimination based on race and nationality is that of training and development. Opportunities in this sector theoretically are supposed to be based on the needs of the health service involved and those of the individual professional. However, the literature indicates little systematic evaluation of needs and unequal access to these opportunities for minority nurses in the United Kingdom. In addition, given opportunities for time off and the nature of and availability of funding, participation in these programs has become a great challenge for them. Thus, it has been charged that this type of discrimination is also evident in the confines of the National Health Service. It is noteworthy that other groups completed more than double the number of continuing education activities than the minority nurse constituency. It could be that the inequitable manner in which training and development opportunities have been distributed accounts for the fact that most minority nurses are in the lower echelons of the professional rankings. Furthermore, the proportion of these nurses employed at this level has increased, whereas that for white nurses has decreased. In addition, the proportion of minority nurses at higher levels of the hierarchy has declined. Moreover, many of these professionals (53 percent) have stated their classification is inappropriate and they have reported they are carrying out responsibilities that should be paid at a higher grade (Bach 2003; Beishon, Satnam, and Hagell 1995; Kingma 1999; Meadows, Levenson, and Baeza n.d.; Pike and Ball 2007; Royal College of Nursing 2007).

Being identified with the lower grades of the nursing service, often full advantage is not taken of the technical skills of many minority nurses. Such has occurred in the United Kingdom, where a career path has developed that does not easily accommodate internationally recruited nurses, who usually possess an abundance of high-level technical skills and a lesser amount of practical skills. Unfortunately, the system these people enter expects them to assume a specific and subordinate position. The same occurs in Germany, Spain, and other Member States. Interviews conducted by this author in Italy with nurses recruited from overseas confirmed the same. The problem arises because very often nurses trained in a Member State acquire specific technical skills after registration and these techniques are often included in the preregistration curriculum of overseas-trained nurses. On the practical side, from the perspective of managers, it is to be noted that they want these so-called outside nurses to blend in with the other nursing professionals, their peers. Thus, their skill level is not always fully recognized (O'Brien 2007).

Even though it is less than that from patients, harassment and abuse from colleagues, due to race, color, or nationality, is another serious concern of minority nurses. A significant proportion of them in the United Kingdom, Ireland, and Portugal, have claimed that colleagues or their superiors manifested hostility toward them based on their race, nationality, or color. The same does not hold for members of the white national nursing staff. The Royal College of Nursing studied the experiences of internationally recruited nurses in the United Kingdom. It underscored the existence of institutional racism in that these professionals were touched by discrimination based on racial beliefs, skin color, ethnicity, and nationality. Furthermore, it concluded that this abuse is nurtured by personal, interpersonal, and structured social relationships that generate values and attitudes, not effectively addressed by policy statements (Adams and Kennedy 2006; Beishon, Satnam, and Hagell 1995; Royal College of Nursing 2007; da Silva and Fernandes 2008).

Given the discrimination experienced by minority nurses in several Member States, it is not surprising that they are not fervently positive about peer support and their relationships at work. They feel undervalued in the world of work. More specifically, many are of the opinion that colleagues, placing little trust in them, value them less than their counterparts as do patients and supervisors. This perception becomes more intense when coupled with often difficult experiences outside the workplace related to housing, bank credit, and even health care. These folks are under constant pressure to prove themselves. Still, in spite of negative experiences, it is interesting that many in this minority constituency appreciate the insights gained at the workplace. Collegial support and that of supervisors and managers are extremely important because of their significance to the quality of life within the workforce. They create trust, pride, loyalty, collaboration, and a spirit of willingness, among other important values. All of these are crucial to the performance of an institution and its employees. Moreover, such support is related to job satisfaction and thus, it becomes an important predictor of intention to leave the site of employment and/or the profession. Among the Member States, the Netherlands has reported the highest values of this type of support and the lowest has been traced to the Italian scene (Alexis, Vydelingum, and Robbins 2007; Gunnarsdóttir and Rafferty 2006; Royal College of Nursing 2007; da Silva and Fernandes 2008).

This discussion of discrimination has concentrated, to a large extent, on the experience of the United Kingdom's National Health Service. It so happens that it has been the focus of several major studies. Problems highlighted in this presentation are not limited to this particular Member State. Moreover, the bases for discrimination are multiple. In addition to the ones mentioned in this discussion, disability, religion, age, and, especially nowadays, sexual orientation should be recognized, among other elements. Unfortunately, all are alive and well as part of discrimination in nurses' workplace (Borg 2012). They are present in different proportions in most Member States.

Discrimination has been investigated in a study of different types of workplace violence in some Member States. The rank order of these nations for frequency of discriminatory violence is as follows from high to low: France, Germany, Slovakia, the Netherlands, Italy, Belgium, Poland, and Finland (Camerino et al. 2008c). It is noteworthy that certain types of violence are not typical in some Member States. For example, racial abuse is not typical in Bulgaria and the same holds for Poland. This type of harassment and violence in the workplace is not of primary concern. In part, this phenomenon is due to the significant homogeneity of the community in both nations (Domagala et al. 1999; International Labour Office et al. 2003; Tomev, Daskalova, and Ivanova 2003).

In a European sample, the most prevalent form of violence at the workplace for nursing personnel was that forthcoming from patients and/or relatives. This was followed by abuse from superiors and colleagues and discrimination in that order. Although nurses in France, Belgium, Germany, and the United Kingdom had the highest rate of violence from patients and/or relatives, France, Germany, and Poland had the most frequent occurrences of other kinds of violence (Camerino et al. 2008c). It is to be noted that the different types of physical and psychological abuse have not operated in a vacuum. At the workplace, they have been intertwined and frequently, they overlap. For example, it has been established that, in Portugal, verbal violence is closely affiliated with moral pressure, violence against property, and physical violence. The affiliation has been total as far as sexual harassment and verbal abuse are concerned. Moreover, all incidents of discrimination have also been identified with verbal violence and frequently, with moral pressure or bullying as well (Di Martino 2002).

It appears that violence at the workplace has been primarily experienced by nurses employed in the public sector. Abuse has been more widespread in public than in private health-care institutions. This seems a natural phenomenon due to the orientation of health-care delivery systems in the Member States. Moreover, it seems that, in most cases, violence is concentrated in hospitals, rather than in other establishments. This too is understandable, given the centrality of the hospital to the health-care sector, especially in the newly acceded Member States, and the nature of its clientele. Within this institution, violence is more widespread in the emergency, psychiatric, geriatric, and acute adult care arenas. Higher than the average number of incidents of abuse has also been reported in long-term care facilities and senior citizen residences. On the other hand, in several Member States, a relatively low rate of violence has been found in intensive care, surgical, pediatric, gynecologic, and obstetric settings, all of which feature a more specialized nursing staff (Ball and Pike 2006b; Estryn-Behar et al. 2008; Vere-Jones 2008).

As is often the case elsewhere, in the EU Member States, there is an underreporting of incidents related to the various types of violence. For example, many or, in fact, most incidents of racial harassment are not reported to the appropriate authorities. Very often, minority nurses accept such abuse, so to speak, as "part of the job." Moreover, they are not confident that their claims will be supported by management and dealt with in effective fashion. This perception holds true for most nursing staff members, not just minorities, and is found in a galaxy of Member States. Consequently, many nurses feel it is useless to file a formal grievance for such action would serve no purpose. Very often, those who report a grievance are not satisfied with the outcome. In a Royal College of Nursing survey carried out in the United Kingdom, almost 50 percent of the victims of abuse indicated they did not believe their employer appropriately handled their complaints (International Centre for Human Resources in Nursing 2007c; Royal College of Nursing 2007).

Frequently, it is difficult for the abused professional to complain. There is fear of dismissal, fear of revenge, fear of ramifications for future employment, and if one is not a citizen, fear of having to leave the country, among other barriers that impede pursuing a complaint. In addition, in a few instances, special reporting procedures and designated institutions have not been operative. This was the case in Portugal and Bulgaria until recently when the Joint Programme on Workplace Violence in the Health Sector, developed by the ILO, ICN, WHO, and the trade union entity Public Services International, became operative in these countries. Formal grievance procedures are now in place and compensation has been awarded for diverse types of violence experienced in health-care institutions.

In addition to the noted fears and the absence of organizational and institutional support of victims of abuse, underreporting of incidents of violence can also be attributed to cultural factors. For example, in Bulgaria, underreporting has been linked to the Bulgarian mentality and social factors, such as the tolerance of violence in the social fabric. In Cyprus, due to the taboos and prejudices that still pervade society, victims of violence have been discouraged from filing complaints. Also, especially in the past, professional associations did not make support mechanisms available to their members. Given these barriers and others, quite often victims of violence fail to take formal action. By far the most prevalent action, as in Slovenia, has been to tell family, coworkers, or friends, but not supervisors or trade union representatives. A small percentage of nurses has left their jobs, but more practitioners have requested a transfer in order to escape from the abuse (Ball and Pike 2006b; Di Martino 2002; International Labour Office et al. 2003; Tomev, Daskalova, and Ivanova 2003; Trbanc 2008).

ICN (2006), claiming underreporting has impeded the development and implementation of policies to deter violence in the workplace, has emphatically stated that every nurse has a personal responsibility to report incidents of abuse. For this responsibility to be translated into practice, there are major barriers that must be surmounted.

An understanding of why violence occurs is essential to its eradication. In the health-care sector, it is nurtured by a variety of complex factors, including the surrounding cultural, social, economic, and political elements. Also, certain structural and working conditions enhance the occurrence and frequency of violence at the workplace. Organizational factors and sociopsychological elements must be given consideration as well. Violence is not independent from the environment at work. In a discussion of its causes, one may begin with the individual who, in part, is responsible for that institutional environment. Individual factors have an important role in the explanation of violence in the health sector. Patients' individual characteristics, their personality, and behavior, in general, as well as the behavior of specific groups of patients impact the nature of violence in specific settings. The same holds true for nursing personnel. For example, it is well-established that stress and tension go hand in hand with the nursing profession. The relation between work stress and violence has been demonstrated (Di Martino 2003). Being able to cope with this situation is a key to survival for the professional care provider. Often, accumulation of stress and tension serve as a generator of some kind of violence. Fear, envy, burnout, and inadequacy nurture violence which has also been associated with uncertainty as to patient treatment, intent to leave the profession, and decisions to change workplace. As noted, younger nursing personnel with less professional experience are more open to aggressive behavior. Insufficient training and a lack of interpersonal skills to be employed in relations with colleagues as well as patients and dissatisfaction with professional life also nurture violence (Bromo and Bartolucci 2005; Camerino et al. 2008c; Estryn-Behar et al. 2008).

In addition, work-related violence relates to the way care activities are organized or to their organizational features. These play a key role. A study of a sample of EU Member States concluded that the prevalence of violence varies across countries, according to the existence of particular working conditions. It was indicated earlier that certain clinical areas are more prone to aggressive behavior than others. There are a host of work-related conditions affiliated with the existence of abuse. These include sudden reforms, shift work, especially working only the night shift; dissatisfaction with working time, inadequate staffing patterns, demanding workloads, including physical loads, coupled with pressures resulting from a lack of time and lack of recognition leading to a sense of injustice. Consideration must also be given to the physical design of the workplace, poor security measures, ward instability resulting, in part, from contentious nurse–physician relationships; less than desirable managerial and supervisory styles, the practice of interventions requiring close physical contact, worksites with little or no privacy, teamwork of low quality, and lack of appropriate organs and procedures to deal with abusive behavior (Camerino et al. 2008c; Estryn-Behar et al. 2008; ICN 2006; Roche et al. 2010). The list is long and, at the same time, incomplete. The importance of these working conditions is that they all have the potential to translate into internal and external violent interactions.

Environmental factors related to a nation's political, social, economic, and cultural arenas also influence the prevalence of abusive activities. The augment in physical violence may be explained by certain cultural developments. In most modern cultures, violence has received greater attention. It is more conspicuous and has grown in significance. Also, citizens have become more demanding. Their expectations and horizons have expanded as they have become more aware of their rights. However, these developments have not always been accompanied by a manifestation of civic responsibility (Ferrinho et al. 2003). Violence is embedded throughout the Bulgarian culture, as noted. It pervades all social classes, occupations, and ethnic communities. Psychologically, it has been based on people's dependence on a center of the power hierarchy where control has been exerted by a central force. When this ultimate source of authority is removed, as when Bulgaria turned to democracy, a vacuum is created along with an incapacity to cope with violence. Thus, many people look to it as a mechanism to regulate family, social, interpersonal, and institutional relations. There is a tolerance of violence in all its forms on the part of individual social groups, the public, and institutions (Di Martino 2002; International Labour Office et al. 2003; Tomev, Daskalova, and Ivanova 2003).

The Central and East European Member States recently liberated from Communism have been societies in political and economic transition. For these nations this transition has involved a difficult change from centralized state economies to market ones. The economies involved have been far from vibrant. Restructuring and reform in many sectors, including health care, have negatively affected work conditions and employment. Downsizing has been central to restructuring efforts in health care. A portion of the decrease in health sector posts has been absorbed by the private sector, but many of these laid-off workers failed to find other employment. As noted, the transition has shown resources are scarce, jobs are no longer secure, hospitals and other elements have a high level of indebtedness, pay levels are unsatisfactory, and wages are often not paid on time. In addition, many nurses have taken a cut in salary as a result of the transition. Fear, insecurity, and uncertainty related to reforms are a major threat to all health-care providers. Owing to these elements, those categories of personnel most affected by the transition in the health sector, physicians and nurses, have accepted violence as part of it. Nurses' ability and desire to address this situation is important to an abatement of the phenomenon. Moreover, these societies are penetrated by poverty, marginalization, and high unemployment. The situation is ripe for violence among health-care personnel and their patients and/or families (Afford and Lessof 2006; Daskalova et al. 2005; Di Martino 2002; Tomev, Michailova, and Daskalova 2003).

In summary, certain individual, structural, physical, and psychosocial work-related conditions account for the occurrence and frequency of violence. For example, Poland has featured a less than desirable social environment, plus many low-qualified nurses with an elevated uncertainty concerning patients' treatment, who have been ill-equipped to assume roles similar to their West European counterparts and a fast-paced rhythm of work, all of which have contributed to the high frequency of abusive behavior in nursing. Also, German and French nurses have experienced frequent violence accounted for by the high prevalence of risk factors, several of which have been cited here. On the other hand, given the low prevalence of these factors in Finland and the Netherlands, nurses have experienced violence less often than colleagues in other Member States. Organizational, societal, and individual factors are all important in an analysis of risks of violence, with multifaceted organizational matters assuming a key role. The frequency of the different types of violence in various nations depends on the presence and nature of these elements (Camerino et al. 2008c; Dubois, Nolte, and McKee 2006; ILO n.d.).

Violence committed at the workplace carries a high price. Its consequences are wide in scope and costly from several points of view. Perhaps the highest cost is borne by nurses involved in these incidents in terms of their individual health. Abusive activities can take a heavy toll on individuals experiencing them. First and foremost, they impinge on both one's physical and emotional health in negative fashion. It has been established that there is a correlation between violence and stress. A recent study confirms that abuse in the workplace leads to sleep problems and symptoms of severe stress among victims' physiological and mental health effects (Christiansen and Nielsen 2010). More specifically, psychological consequences relate to, among other things, posttraumatic stress disorders, anxiety, loss of self-confidence, and decreased motivation and job satisfaction. In addition, affected practitioners are more likely to terminate their employment or plan to do so. Moreover, these problems not only affect the individual, but very often, they are transferred to the victim's family, colleagues, friends, the institution where they work, and society as a whole. Moreover, the impact of such abuse on observers must not be forgotten (Bjorn 2012; Camerino et al. 2008c; Di Martino 2002; International Labour Office et al. 2003; Johnson 2009; Venema and van der Klauw 2012).

Health-care institutions pay a high price as well. The psychological consequences experienced by nurses reverberate throughout their confines. Very often, violent experiences lead to an increase in sick leave and absenteeism on the part of the victims which, in turn, in part, decreases potential productivity and availability of staff, while it can augment the workload for personnel on duty. In addition, employee attrition has been known to grow as a result of abusive activities and more nurses have exited from or consider leaving the profession, two serious matters in light of the extensive nurse shortage and the need to recruit new members to the profession. Retention and recruitment, problems of great magnitude, are impacted in negative fashion.

The workplace environment has been known to deteriorate as well as a result of violence. In part, the change is often caused by a decrease in staff morale and job satisfaction. In addition, there are greater costs related to security, litigation, and compensation, among other things. In short, in the end, performance, quality of care, efficiency, and productivity are dramatically affected. The impact on the practitioner, the institution, and, above all, the patient is great. Violence is related to adverse patient outcomes (Roche et al. 2010). Moreover, the internal and external image of the establishment is tarnished. Violence at the workplace negatively impacts observers, victims, family members, friends, patients, the specific institution involved, and eventually, all facets of and actors in the entire health-care delivery system. The cited and other psychological and organizational costs are not limited to the specific institution in which

203

violence occurred. The effects ripple throughout the health-care delivery system and society as a whole.

The EU and Member States have acted to control abusive behavior at the workplace, but evidently not enough. In addition, this type of violence is definitely not on the public agenda in the individual Member States in spite of efforts from multiple sources. Surveys have identified a considerable difference in awareness of the issue in the context of health and safety across Europe (Chappell and Di Martino 2006; Nystrom 2009). Many responses to the problem have been developed and/or supported by national, European, and international units. One source that has not been fully tapped is that of nursing educational institutions. Even though nurses are at the highest risk for violence in the health-care sector, many programs that prepare them professionally and many nursing orientation offerings have not furnished participants with adequate tools to cope with abusive behavior (Estryn-Behar et al. 2008; ICN 2006). Considerable energy has been spent on public education concerning the matter. For instance, ICN has repeatedly underscored the widespread violence experienced by nurses as has the European Federation of Public Service Unions, the ILO, the trade union organization Public Services International, individual nurses' associations, and national trade unions, among other units. ICN has taken an activist role and offers assistance in the development of different types of policy documents related to zero tolerance of violence. In addition, in a similar vein, it has developed a list of activities that could be undertaken by national nursing associations. Collaborative efforts are also evident as well. The aforementioned framework guidelines for addressing workplace violence in the health sector that became operative in Portugal, Bulgaria, and the Czech Republic, among other nations, were developed, as noted, by several international associations. These guidelines were issued as a stimulus to the development of policies to control violence appropriate to specific circumstances in various nations.

Individual employers have developed equal opportunity policies that are extensive in scope. Health-care institutions have featured training projects directed at discrimination. Also, sometimes, in the individual Member States, there is a specific office responsible for tackling workplace abuse, like the Swedish Work Environment Authority, the Irish Health and Safety Authority, the Cypriot Equality Authority, the Greek Gender Equality Unit, or the Office of the Estonian Equality Commissioner, to cite a few. Collective agreements in several Member

States provide for employers and trade unions to undertake measures to combat physical and psychological violence at the workplace. For example, in Bulgaria, the agreement, a national one, is applicable to all health-care facilities. In this manner, it has furnished a framework for confronting various types of workplace violence within institutions (Daskalova 2006). Similar types of agreements exist in other Member States, such as Denmark, France, and the United Kingdom.

Trade unions have been active in this sphere in many Member States. Unfortunately, many have avoided sensitive issues, such as sexual orientation, and have focused on traditional matters, such as age. Also, several have failed to develop specific strategies related to particular issues. Once again, there is a division between the older and newer Member States. The former have undertaken more initiatives than the latter and their focus has been wider in scope. Frequently, trade unions have not monitored their activities or evaluated them. Even though they have been active, it has been concluded that there is much room for improvement (European Commission: Directorate-General for Employment, Social Affairs and Equal Opportunities--Unit G-4 2010).

The many facets of violence at the workplace have received considerable attention in several Member States. Legislative initiatives concerning the different brands of abuse have been undertaken with diverse results. For example, in the Netherlands, the Working Conditions Act contains provisions related to abuse and aggression and the promotion of humane working conditions. Evaluations of this important measure are positive because workplace violence has stabilized, even though it has not decreased. Furthermore, there is greater awareness of the problem and employers are more inclined to confront it. Elsewhere, outcomes have not been as favorable. In Spain, Law 55/2003 (Spain 2003) refers to discrimination and other workplace issues related to violence in the health sector. In terms of meeting its requisites, employers, public institutions, and social organizations have been criticized in that their efforts concerning prevention and elimination of harassment have been labeled limited. In Germany, the same report card has been issued because the law for protection against abuse has had restricted influence on personnel policies and in the courts (van den Bossche 2005; Corral and de Munain 2006; von Wahl 2005).

With the exception of the Netherlands, the legislative approach has assumed that violence at work falls under the rubric of the framework type of health and safety regulations and the civil and criminal codes. Moreover, implementation of legislation usually happens in reference to these legal doctrines. It is noteworthy that the implementation phase of the legislative process encounters prominent obstacles, which include a lack of awareness, difficulties found in smaller units of employment, and a scarcity of resources for enforcement (Chappell and Di Martino 2006). It is no wonder that the guidelines to deal with violent behavior at the workplace are not uniform throughout the Member States. Very often, excellent initiatives are taken. Unfortunately, frequently, they are not followed up or they suffer from a lack of coordination and cooperation, two significant activities (Nystrom 2009). Long-term, multifaceted, and multipartner strategies are warranted because violence at the workplace is not only a professional risk, but, in addition, a public health problem and a violation of human and workers' rights.

Job Satisfaction and the Meaning of Work

Nurses' physical and psychosocial work conditions impact on their views concerning various aspects of their relationship to their place of work and their profession. Even though there is a large quantity of literature concerned with job satisfaction or with how nurses feel about their work, there appears to be no consensus as to a standard definition. However, it is generally agreed that it depends on many factors. Gunnarsdóttir and Rafferty (2006) refer to the phenomenon as "a pleasurable or positive emotional state resulting from the appraisal of one's job or job experience" (p. 167). Much research has been carried out on this topic as it relates to nurses, in general, and to those in disparate work and geographical settings. Many elements that contribute to this state have been identified in these efforts. The ingredients are many and the recipe is complicated.

The importance of job satisfaction cannot be overlooked for the simple reason its significance reverberates in many quarters. For the individual practitioner, it relates to motivation and performance. Elevated job satisfaction produces augmented motivation in work performance and, at the same time, it means the nurse is less likely to resign or change jobs frequently. Job satisfaction impinges on retention and continuity in staff, providing many benefits. Moreover, it is significantly related to intent to abandon the profession. Also, it has been designated the principal determinant of patient satisfaction and outcomes. A decline in patient satisfaction and poorer patient outcomes result, in part, from a decrease in job gratification. Nurses' relations with patients and their families are also tainted along with the quality of care provided. Having an impact on work performance, nurses' job satisfaction relates to productivity, organizational profit, and cost containment as well (Busse and Schlette 2004; Curtis 2007; Duddle and Boughton 2007; Hinno, Partanen, and Vehviläinen-Julkunsen 2011; ICN 2008a, 2008b). The recipe for this condition has a galaxy of possible ingredients, some of which change over time. Work prospects, the physical work environment, work setting characteristics, such as leadership, opportunities to use one's talents, and to provide patients the services they require; recognition and support from the institution, superiors, and colleagues; organizational communication patterns, nurse–patient relationships as well as those with coworkers, career development possibilities, organizational pride, status, role definition, task requirements and outcomes, amount of responsibility, organizational policies, feeling valued, employment security, perceived participation in decision-making, resource issues, and external pressures are some of the many determinants of nurses' job satisfaction. These various factors can be related to general rubrics, such as work characteristics and organization, work environment, organizational culture, and human resource management practices. Each element has a different significance for the individual practitioner and different combinations result, as if they were part of a kaleidoscope. Within the context of this change, the one stable ingredient is the amount of professional autonomy (Basso and Salmaso 2004; Baumann 2007; Gunnarsdóttir and Rafferty 2006; ICN 2008a, 2008b; Review Body for Nursing and Other Health Professions 2007; Tovey and Adams 1999; Widerszal-Bazyl et al. 2003b).

Of the various research efforts on the subject, some are comparative in nature and others are case studies. These projects (Gunnarsdóttir and Rafferty 2006; Hasselhorn, Müller, and Tackenberg 2005; Hinno, Partanen, and Vehviläinen-Julkunsen 2011; Hubačová, et al. 2000; Kaarna et al. 2004) have assigned labels to the countries involved in terms of the levels of work gratification. Throughout the Member States, there are significant variations in nurses' job satisfaction. Sweden and the Netherlands merit a rating of high, whereas Estonia receives a grade of moderately high. Then, there are a group of countries with low levels of job satisfaction that include Slovakia, Belgium, Germany, Italy, Poland, Ireland, and the United Kingdom. In the case of the latter nation, it is noteworthy that there might not be a consensus as to the level of gratification. An official report (Review Body for Nursing and Other Health Professions 2007) claimed that 50 percent of the sample was satisfied and the other 50 percent was neither satisfied nor dissatisfied. Also, of interest is a study (Ruzafa-Martinez et al. 2008) of

Spanish nurses working in England whose overall work satisfaction was termed medium.

Some of the variables accounting for job gratification have a stronger identification with that state than others. Various elements of human resource management practices have been designated by nurses as of prime importance. For example, in Estonia, management protocols concerning supervisory relationships with staff, planning policies, feeling part of the organization, and perceived involvement in decision-making were singled out for special attention by practitioners. The latter two elements are of particular significance because not only do they enhance satisfaction, but they reinforce links with other factors that fashion job gratification (Kaarna et al. 2004; Känd and Rekor 2005). Organizational policies and leadership were also found to be an important dimension of satisfaction in Belgium, Ireland, and the United Kingdom. In fact, nurses in Belgium, Slovakia, Germany, and the United Kingdom have claimed a quality of leadership superior to that of their Italian and Polish colleagues. Patient contacts and especially, those with persons who acknowledged their work and the value of the care they were provided, were also identified by nurses in several nations as significant contributors to job satisfaction, along with professional status and organizational pride. For Czech and Slovakian nurses, control over work activities, responsibilities, and scheduling was of importance (Ball and Pike 2003; *Création d'une instance professionnelle infirmière* 2007; Curtis 2007; Gunnarsdóttir and Rafferty 2006; Gurková et al. 2013; Stordeur et al. 2003b; Willem, Buelens, and De Jonghe 2007). Of interest, is the fact that the ingredients nurses believe to be important to their job gratification are not always the same ones to which they attribute their present state of satisfaction. Evidently, once again, theory is one thing and practice is another. According to the literature, organizational factors seem to exert more influence than individual ones.

As one might imagine, individual characteristics as well as those relating to the workplace correlate with the nature of job satisfaction. Emotional reactions to nursing are important and obviously, these are determined, in part, on the basis of the individual practitioner's physical and mental health. A study of Slovakian nurses (Gurková et al. 2012) identified a positive correlation between positive emotions and job satisfaction. Age and years of experience are other variables that have impacted nurses' levels of job satisfaction. According to the literature, younger nurses reflect lower job satisfaction than their senior colleagues. However, it has been affirmed that, as a general rule in Europe, younger nurses and their senior colleagues identify with a higher level of gratification than middle-aged practitioners. In the case of the younger set, this outlook has been attributed to the assignment of fewer responsibilities to these people, less pressure, fewer demands from colleagues, and less identification with the work–family conflict. Senior nurses, having, in general, fewer demands external to the profession, benefits linked to seniority, better knowledge of nursing, more practical experience, and being able to say "older and wiser" are more susceptible to higher satisfaction levels. Evidently, superior gratification begins to decline when the nurse reaches thirty years of age. This rule, however, does not apply to Belgium, where job satisfaction is low for older practitioners or to Italy, where it is low for both younger and older members of the profession (Flinkman et al. 2008; Gurková et al. 2013; Hasselhorn, Müller, and Tackenberg 2005; Stordeur et al. 2003b).

In addition, nurses, based on their age, often place different weights on ingredients of job satisfaction. They have different priorities. For example, a study of nurses in Belgium revealed that younger practitioners, as seems logical, assigned more importance to promotion and career development than older and more senior ones. On the other hand, the latter were more interested in job security and status of their employer (De Gieter et al. 2006). In Finland, well-being at work for senior nurses was founded solely on reciprocity in reference to colleagues and patients, nurse to nurse interactions, and nurse–patient relationships. In short, the communal aspects of patient care served as the basis for job gratification (Utriainen, Kyngäs, and Nikkilä 2009).

From the perspective of gender, there are also differences concerning job satisfaction that have been related to diversity in professional ambitions. The lower expectations of females have been explained on the basis of their inferior position in the labor market and greater commitment to the domestic realm. Perhaps, as a consequence of being skeptical of the traditional image of nurses and reflecting a conflict between what males do as nurses and what they think they should be doing in terms of career development, male practitioners tend to be less satisfied with the ways in which their talents are used. In some cases, they feel they are discriminated against. They claim that they have to tolerate higher performance standards than their female colleagues and, in addition, endure resentment for having selected a traditional female profession (Stordeur et al. 2003b). Consequently, their level of job satisfaction can be inferior to that of their female coworkers.

Education is another variable that has been used to account for diversity in satisfaction ratings. In general, nurses with higher educational achievements tend to produce lower scores. Usually, these professionals are ambitious and possess higher expectations than colleagues who have less education. Often, they find themselves in organizations that are unable to or do not make full use of their talents. Career development encounters obstacles and job satisfaction declines. On the other hand, in Belgium, it was found that hospitals with more specialization and formalization have more gratified nurses (Willem, Belens, and De Jonghe 2007). Evidently, these facilities are able to take advantage of the nursing staff's talents. However, even though Coomber and Barriball (2007) affirm that the level of education achieved is affiliated with job satisfaction, they caution that outcomes for this factor are not consistent. It is noteworthy that demographic characteristics, such as age, education, and years of experience, according to a recent study (Gurková et al. 2012), are not related to nurses' job satisfaction, at least, in Slovakia.

Nurses' evaluation of their work situation has been found to be significantly different between one health-care facility and another. One of the determinants of this situation relates to institutional structure and the distribution of power within. Thus, it is a question of centralization versus decentralization. Research (Willem, Buelens, and De Jonghe 2007) has determined that centralized institutions have a less satisfied nursing staff. Thus, given the negative effect of centralization, executives can enhance gratification by restructuring and the implementation of devolution. Such occurred in Estonia. Moreover, within a specific institution, job satisfaction is increasingly fashioned by the professional's position within the organization. It tends to rise with occupational level. Usually, those with higher professional grades register more elevated scores than rank and file nurses. These have been attributed to the exertion of more control over their work situation, their position vis-à-vis other health-care professionals and within the nursing hierarchy, plus greater social recognition (Estryn-Behar et al. 2003b; Ruzafa-Martinez et al. 2008; Stordeur et al. 2003b; Tovey and Adams 1999).

In addition, work gratification also varies according to the area of nursing. For example, a study of European nurses (Stordeur et al. 2003b) revealed that those working in home care, rather than in nursing homes or hospitals, were more satisfied with their work situation. This is understandable in light of their work conditions. As mentioned, they experience greater autonomy, more control over work requirements, and more close-knit relationships with chronic patients. In addition, their work pressures and administrative tasks are reduced. The same results were issued in Italian and French case studies on the subject. On the other hand, nurses affiliated with acute care settings tend to generate lower ratings (Basso and Salmaso 2004; Estryn-Behar et al. 2002; "Preserving the Nursing Workforce" 2008).

Moreover, variations in job satisfaction have been identified between nurses employed in the public and private sectors. For example, in the United Kingdom, professionals in the independent sector have displayed greater satisfaction and pride than their counterparts in the National Health Service. They have also valued different elements of job gratification. For those in the private sector, good job security, pay, respect at work, appropriate management practices, and harmonious management–employee relationships have been considered of prime importance. For nurses in the National Health Service, contact with patients, accomplishing a worthwhile job, and feeling valued by the organization have been singled out for special attention. These factors were the least important for those nurses employed in the independent sector. Similar differences between the two spheres have been found in Poland and other nations. Diversity in satisfaction levels has also been identified on the basis of union membership. It seems that union members are less satisfied with their work than their nonunionized colleagues (Ball and Pike 2003; Domagala et al. 1999; Seago, Spetz, and Others 2011). The lower level of satisfaction could be the reason for affiliation with a trade union.

Job satisfaction is of import, but dissatisfaction is as well. In some countries, work dissatisfaction in the health-care sector is much higher among nurses than other employees. Such is the case, for example, in Ireland and Italy, where there is substantial dissatisfaction within the ranks of nursing. The RN4CAST project (Aiken 2011) in an examination of job dissatisfaction among nurses identified distinct variations, ranging from 56 percent in Greece to 11 percent in the Netherlands. The following dissatisfaction rates were generated: Ireland (42 percent), England (39 percent), Spain (38 percent), Germany (37 percent), Finland (27 percent), Poland (26 percent), and Belgium and Sweden (22 percent). The average for the EU was 28 percent (Schoonhoven, Heinen, and van Achterberg 2012). Of note, once again, is the most favorable situation in the Netherlands and the least favorable in Greece. Job dissatisfaction relates to site of practice. It has been determined that nurses involved in direct care in hospitals and nursing homes experience greater job dissatisfaction than colleagues in other roles (McHugh et al. 2011). Obviously, this state carries consequences for the individual involved, the patient, and the health-care institution, especially, if the dissatisfied nurse remains in the workplace for a long time. Negative factors arise. These, among others, include decreased productivity, inferior patient relationships, lowered quality of patient care, an increase in the potential for errors, a decline in patient satisfaction, health and mental well-being; increased absences, conflict, and further dissatisfaction. It is a vicious circle. There are economic considerations as well, such as continued rising costs, due to inefficiencies and a decline in output. Moreover, organizational objectives are compromised (Basso and Salmaso 2004; Chan and Lai 2010; Curtis 2007; Duddle and Boughton 2007). The price is high and not only in economic terms. Job satisfaction is essential to the overall well-being of nurses, health-care institutions, and patients.

Closely related to job satisfaction is the meaning of work which is of importance because it provides individuals their perception of the significance of their undertaking. It is generally acknowledged that many health-care professionals assign high values to their endeavors because as a group, they include highly motivated persons. However, as in the case of job gratification, within the European nursing profession, research demonstrates that there are great differences related to the meaning of work. Of note are the low values reported in the Netherlands, Poland, and Italy. The Dutch result was unexpected because in terms of other facets of the profession, the Netherlands has produced superior grades. Extremely low stipends and the discrepancy between nurses' loyalty to their work and the sparse recognition they receive explain Polish circumstances. In Europe, except for Poland, Slovakia, Italy, and the Netherlands, there is a continuous decrease in the meaning of work after one year of employment.

Differences in perspective also relate to institutional types. Values were especially elevated in home care as opposed to hospitals. As in other instances, the difference may be due to a greater amount of autonomy in practice and fewer administrative encounters. Overall, scores tended to be significantly higher than in hospitals. Gender also relates to reported values. Male nurses, with the exception of Italian ones, assigned less meaning to their work than their female colleagues. This could result from the fact that, as mentioned earlier, nursing has traditionally been viewed as women's work and many female nurses perceive their profession as a calling. In Italy, where there are a large number of male practitioners, the values were equal for both sexes. Age was reflected in the scores in that younger and older nurses, especially in Italy and France, reported higher scores in the meaning of work. It could be that the younger professionals were reflecting the enthusiasm of youth and thinking in the long-term with hope for the future. Elder colleagues could be mirroring the notion of having participated in a calling. In the case of the newly acceded Member States, it is the middle-aged practitioners who have borne the largest brunt of poor economic conditions and extreme work and extraprofessional demands, due to child rearing and other domestic obligations (Pokorski et al. 2003).

Job and Organizational Commitment

Commitment to a specific organization and to a job is closely related to job satisfaction. For the most part, European nurses appear to be a solidly committed group. There is a general tendency for them not to develop a strong commitment to an employer. Their strongest attachment has been toward their field of specialization, their team, the broader professional community, and the patient (Kirpal 2003; Stordeur et al. 2003b). It seems that professional commitment tends to be much higher than organizational commitment. This tendency has been attributed to the fact that nurses often change employers without exiting the profession. Given the extensive nurse shortage, in general, they do not encounter grave difficulties in switching jobs, with the exception of those in the newly acceded Member States. Loyalty to a specific organization often is not fully nurtured, given the time required for orientation and socialization processes. Even though the Slovak nursing profession has been referred to as in crisis, it has been found to be committed. The same holds true for nurses in Poland and Germany, in spite of their lesser degree of job satisfaction. Nurses in Belgium and Finland may lay claim to high commitment (Hasselhorn, Müller, and Tackenberg 2005; Kovarova et al. 2003).

Professional commitment has been highest in France and low in Great Britain, Germany, and the Netherlands. Organizational commitment has been highest in Finland. In Italy, professional commitment has been labeled moderate and institutional commitment very low. Even though, in general, nurses have been highly committed to their profession and less so to their organization, strenuous working conditions have correlated with reduced commitment (Miettinen 2005;

213

Stordeur et al. 2003b). In the discussion of job satisfaction, it was noted that certain variables exerted influence on outcomes. The same holds for nurses' commitment. In terms of institutional affiliation, their professional commitment has been found to be highest in nursing homes and outpatient care and organizational commitment higher in nursing homes and home care as opposed to hospitals. From the professional perspective, in nursing homes, the nurse has more opportunities in terms of provision of services. Higher commitment to institutions, such as nursing homes and residences, is understandable, given the bureaucracy and hierarchy identified with larger structures. Gender also enters the picture in that scores for both types of commitment tend to be lower for males. In terms of seniority, nurses, having some, have demonstrated more professional and institutional commitment. Age also correlates with commitment. In Belgium and the United Kingdom, commitment of older nurses was found to be lower and the opposite trend was identified in Finland. Younger nurses tend to exhibit lower organizational commitment than their senior colleagues and a Finnish study demonstrated that among graduate nurses their professional commitment, as noted, decreases during their first year of employment (Flinkman et al. 2008; Hasselhorn, Müller, and Tackenberg 2005; Stordeur et al. 2003b).

Factors that have related to strength of commitment on the part of European nurses include a favorable view of one's own physical health, mental health, and work ability, along with the possession of a sound socioeconomic situation and a supervisory position affiliated with strong organizational commitment. Then, there are the elements that reduce commitment, such as a negative evaluation of the value of work, few opportunities for career development, little influence in organizational policies, less than optimal use of one's talents, poor work environment, and leadership of low quality. In particular, sparse organizational commitment has been identified with poor promotion prospects and lack of possibilities to provide patients with necessary services. Low commitment to nursing resulted from having to work a high proportion of night shifts and disapproval of physical working conditions (Miettinen 2005). Human resource management policies can be used to rectify these situations. In the United States, Magnet Hospitals, those characterized, in part, by low staff turnover, excellent patient outcomes, and nurses' job satisfaction and commitment are heavily conditioned by stellar, decentralized, participatory, managerial practices and a healthy workplace environment.

Intent to Leave the Place of Employment and/or the Profession

A cloud that persistently hangs over the heads of health-care executives is the possibility that nurses intend to leave their place of employment or, even worse, the profession. The rationale for exiting the profession is complex. Many elements, individual ones and those related to work, enter the picture. Research (Pokorski et al. 2003) has indicated that many of the aforementioned factors, such as the meaning of work and job commitment, are clearly important to European nurses' decisions on this matter.

In general, it is working conditions, rather than individual factors, that play a prime role in the choice to leave a nursing position or the profession. As noted, there are significant variations in these conditions throughout the Member States. A prime reason for the intent to leave, as in Finland, has been dissatisfaction with salary. Financial rewards have been viewed as incompatible with work demands, both physical and mental. Research on the quitting decision of nurses in the British National Health Service found that while the effect of salaries is statistically significant, the predicted impact of an increase in nurses' wages on retention rates is miniscule. Thus, in some cases, pay raises might not be the answer to halt exits (Frijters, Shields, and Price 2007). Moreover, work patterns, shift work, and schedules have received negative evaluations, along with opportunities for career development. Lack of status, respect, and support have soured many practitioners as well. In Belgium and the United Kingdom, withdrawal has been enhanced by poor organizational leadership and clinical management (Estryn-Behar et al. 2002; Flinkman et al. 2008; Gunnarsdóttir and Rafferty 2006).

Nurse-to-patient staffing ratios and the work environment have been found to be significantly associated with intent to leave (Van den Heede et al. 2011). Other work issues related to the matter include increased work load, work schedules, a perceived decline in the standard of care, violence at the workplace, lack of autonomy, and poor career development opportunities. These last factors have been of importance to Irish and Swedish nurses, in particular (Adams and Kennedy 2006; Sjögren et al. 2005). An element most strongly linked with intention to leave, especially in the United Kingdom, has been relationships at work (Ball and Pike 2006a, 2006b). Occupational health risks, low work ability, the work–family conflict, personal burnout, and low institutional commitment are other elements taken into consideration in decision-making, along with poor health, both physical and emotional, as exemplified in Belgium, the

Netherlands, and Denmark. These are some of the reasons cited by European nurses for their intention to leave a job or exit the profession. Any one of these elements or combinations of them can impinge negatively on job satisfaction. Low job satisfaction, as noted, is found among nurses in many Member States and it is affiliated with a more sincere or higher intention to leave the profession (Flinkman et al. 2008). Also, it accounts for the widespread demoralization in the ranks of nursing staff, as in the United Kingdom. Here the extreme number of practitioners claiming to leave the profession has been attributed to a low level of morale. There is definitely a linkage between exposure to these various stressors and the probability of nurses being satisfied with their work situation or whether they consider leaving it. In addition, institutional culture and intent to leave the profession are closely related. Both structural and contextual elements impinge on the decision-making process (Ball and Pike 2006a, 2006b; Gould et al. 2003; Hasselhorn et al. 2005).

Throughout the EU, the proportion of nurses who express interest in leaving the profession varies greatly. It has been determined that almost 50 percent of Finnish and Greek nurses display this intention and in the United Kingdom, one out of three practitioners surveyed wanted to leave. Italy, identified with the lowest sense of professional accomplishment, follows with its percentage registering at 20.5. Many Italian nurses wish to exit, but this does not necessarily augment the risk of actual departure. In descending order, places are assigned to Germany (18.5 percent), Slovakia (12.4 percent), Poland (11.2 percent), the Netherlands (10.6 percent), and France (7.3 percent). Also, in Belgium, the proportion desiring to leave is very low. The intent to exit in Italy, the United Kingdom, and Germany contrasts sharply with that in the Netherlands, France, and Belgium. This could be due to the fact that nurses in the latter group of nations often assign higher grades to work environment and health outcomes. Moreover, in the Netherlands, as in Belgium, in terms of job demands and influence in the workplace, the situation seems to be more favorable than in other countries (Estryn-Behar et al. 2003a; Hasselhorn, Müller, and Tackenberg 2005; Hasselhorn, Tackenberg, and Müller 2003; Hasselhorn et al. 2005, 2008; OECD 2012).

Also, it must be remembered that very often, the decision to leave is dependent on the existence of optional paths. For example, in Poland and Slovakia, in spite of harsh working conditions, few nurses actually think of leaving. One study (Hasselhorn, Tackenberg, and Müller 2003) reports over 80 percent of the Polish and Slovak nurse participants expressed fear of encountering major difficulties in having to find new employment. It is for this reason that these practitioners do not often leave. Job insecurity, as noted, is prevalent. Also, the same applies to nurses with poor work ability. Very often, they too fail to leave the profession, primarily because of sparse alternatives. In addition, to a certain extent, some institutions actually tolerate practitioners of this type (Hasselhorn, Müller, and Tackenberg 2005).

Variations in the intent to exit the profession have been identified in major comparative research efforts focusing on European nurses. Intent has been found to vary with respect to several variables: age, gender, type of institution, level of qualification, seniority, health, work ability, and burnout, to cite some. In terms of age, it appears that, in general, younger and older practitioners more often express an interest in leaving. In most Member States, it is the younger that are the most intent. In Germany, nurses between the ages of twenty-five and thirty-nine have considered leaving most frequently, whereas in France, the group with the highest intent was in the thirty-five to thirty-nine age bracket. The same intensity was found in younger practitioners in Finland and Poland in age groups under thirty and in Slovakia, in those only up to twenty-four. The situation in the United Kingdom is somewhat different in that nurses between forty and forty-nine years of age registered the highest desire to leave. This is interesting because, at one time, over half of the deserters were under thirty.

In most nations, with the exception of Slovakia, where those practitioners over fifty-five considered leaving the least, it is the older nurses, like the younger, who register the highest intent to exit. However, the literature indicates that more mature and experienced practitioners will continue to practice when certain conditions are met. These include flexible work arrangements, participatory governance, autonomy in practice, the availability of appropriate continuing education opportunities, a safe, secure, and friendly workplace climate; and a communicative management style (International Centre for Human Resources in Nursing 2007a). In the case of the young, their intent is understandable in that these employees are the most likely to have lower wages than their colleagues, more routine in their work, and sparse participation in organizational decision-making. There is a definite identification between age and intent to leave the profession (Estryn-Behar et al. 2003a; Flinkman et al. 2008; Gould et al. 2003; Hasselhorn et al. 2003, 2005; Kovarova et al. 2003; McCarthy, Tyrrell, and Cronin 2002; Widerszal-Bazyl et al. 2003a, 2003b).

217

In terms of gender, comparative research has found that among European nurses the proportion of those desiring to exit their professional world is higher for males than females. Exceptions, however, are provided by Slovak and Italian practitioners. Also, in France, men displayed no significant difference with women (Estryn-Behar et al. 2003a; Hasselhorn et al. 2005; Kovarova et al. 2003). If consideration is given to the qualifications of those expressing interest in resignation, in general, it is the more qualified nurses, and especially, those with a specialization, that voice such a desire. This is the case in France, Finland, and Germany, to cite a few examples. Interestingly enough, in Slovakia, qualification was found not to influence decision-making (Estryn-Behar et al. 2003a; Flinkman et al. 2008; Hasselhorn, Müller, and Tackenberg 2005; Hasselhorn et al. 2003; Kovarova et al. 2003). This trend related to the well-educated, combined with that concerning young age, raises a warning signal. Young practitioners with solid qualifications, frequently at the university level, are a high-risk group.

Among European nurses, as noted, there are large diversities in turnover rates. These often vary according to type of institution and sector. To a large extent, nurses employed in hospitals are more prone to consider leaving their positions, as in Germany, Belgium, Poland, and Ireland. However, in Poland, the relationship between intent to leave and type of institution has been found to be insignificant. Frequently, the most highly qualified nurses abandon the hospital for other types of nursing. They react negatively to what they consider relationships that are restrictive and authoritarian in character. The intent to desert these hospital positions ranges from 19 percent in the Netherlands to 49 percent in Finland and Greece (European Commission 2012a). Primarily, these nurses work in general medical and surgical units. Turnover has been significantly less in critical care. The same holds for care of the elderly in nursing homes and home care institutions. On the other hand, in Finland, it has been nursing staff working in long-term care institutions that most often gave thought to departure. Frequently, these professionals have desired to switch to hospital or outpatient care positions. For them, the least attractive option has been the health center ward. In Germany, an interesting pattern has been identified when differentiating between institutional types in terms of the age of professionals thinking of leaving. In nursing homes and home care, younger nurses have considered the intent to leave much less frequently and the older practitioners much more frequently than those associated with hospitals. Diversities have also been identified between the public and private sectors. For example, in the United Kingdom, nurses in the private sector are a little more anxious to exit than those in the National Health Service. In France, nursing personnel in private clinics and noncommercial hospitals give more thought to the intent to leave than colleagues affiliated with psychiatric hospitals (Ball and Pike 2003; Estryn-Behar et al. 2003a; Hasselhorn, Müller, and Tackenberg 2005; Hasselhorn et al. 2003; Van den Heede et al. 2011; Widerszal-Bazyl et al. 2003b).

Professional seniority is another variable relevant to intent to leave and again, there is variety among European nurses on this matter as well. In many Member States, such as France, Germany, Finland, the Netherlands, and Slovakia, intent, as mentioned, is higher at the very beginning of one's nursing career. It has often been fully nurtured at this stage. Then, at a certain point, it reaches a summit and declines. Timing of the climax is not fixed. For example, in Germany, it is reached by males and females in the second and fourth year of a professional career, respectively. In Ireland, decline commences after the third year. Dutch and Finnish nurses find themselves at the other end of the continuum. The former peak after six to ten years of seniority and then their thoughts concerning departure decrease. The latter become less eager to depart only after fifteen years of experience. Practitioners in the United Kingdom portray a different cycle. Intent is the lowest among nurses with two to four years of experience and it peaks among those into their professional career for eleven or more years (Flinkman et al. 2008; Gould et al. 2003; McCarthy, Tyrrell, and Cronin 2002; van der Schoot and van der Heijden 2003).

The length of time one has been employed in a facility or institutional seniority is also important to one's career outlook. For example, in Slovakia, nurses, having a shorter period of employment with a specific employer, were more preoccupied with intent to leave. In similar fashion, in Germany, those with more institutional seniority gave less thought to the matter. In France, after six to twelve months with an employer, nurses consider leaving less often. Although in Poland, professional seniority registered no significance for intent to exit, institutional seniority was significantly related (Estryn-Behar et al. 2003a; Hasselhorn et al. 2003; Kovarova et al. 2003; Widerszal-Bazyl et al. 2003b).

Practitioners' physical and psychological health also play a role in decision-making concerned with intent to leave. It has been found that younger nurses with low perceived health exhibit a greater tendency to give frequent consideration to exit than older colleagues in the same state. It could be that younger practitioners are seeking other employment, whereas the senior professionals perceive a greater threat of unemployment and are, therefore, complacent in their present position. Musculoskeletal disorders and burnout correlate with intent to leave as well. In regard to burnout, it is definitely affiliated with intent in many Member States, but not in Slovakia, where the relationship has been recorded as weak (Kovarova et al. 2003).

Research on European nurses has also focused on the aforementioned work–family conflict and its relationship to the intent to leave. Results underscore a definite link between the two elements. The interdependence was found to be especially strong in Germany, Belgium, France, and Italy. On the other hand, in Slovakia, it was exceptionally weak. There is a clear association between these two variables in West European nations, but the affiliation is less firm in the newly acceded Member States. This is understandable in light of the nature of their labor market (Simon et al. 2004).This conflict is a significant predictor of giving thought to the intent to leave. For example, in France, nurses bearing the burden of a work–family conflict have been twice as likely to do so. Also, it is important to note that, within the EU, the meaning of work and work ability perform prominent roles in decision-making as well. The latter for younger and older nurses, especially in Poland, France, and Germany, is affiliated with the wish to prematurely exit the profession (Estryn-Behar et al. 2002; Hasselhorn et al. 2005).

It has also been affirmed that the intensity of intent to depart the profession is closely related to the aforementioned effort–reward imbalance. Nurses experiencing this imbalance more often desire to leave their jobs. In fact, those with an especially intense imbalance, as found in Germany, Poland, Italy, and Slovakia, are approximately three to six times more likely to entertain such thoughts (Hasselhorn, Tackenberg, and Peter 2004). A more recent study (Li et al. 2011) has reconfirmed the effect of this imbalance and its critical nature.

Changes in a common characteristic of nurses' work environment, job strain, have been deemed important to fluctuations in their reasoning on departure from the profession. Longitudinal inquiry has indicated that European nurses, not originally exposed to job strain, but who encountered it within a year, demonstrated higher risk of giving thought to departure from the workplace than colleagues that never experienced it. As one might expect, those practitioners exhibiting continuous job strain over time have manifested an even higher likelihood of considering exit from the profession. Continuous exposure to job strain was found to be the highest predictor for Finnish, Dutch, French, and Slovak nurses to develop interest in intent to leave. An encounter with job strain among previously untainted nurses, in Germany, Belgium, Italy, and Poland, was deemed more predictive of entertaining thoughts on departure from professional ranks (Hasselhorn et al. 2008). There is a definite identification between job strain and nurses' decision-making concerning their relationship with their profession.

A notion of the intensity of the intent to leave is disclosed by nurses' responses to the following question: How often during the course of the past year have you thought about giving up nursing completely? Responses were surprising, given the amount of attention focused on possibilities of departure from the profession. Never was the response for 63.8 percent of Slovak participants. In decreasing order the "never" responses registered 63.3 percent in Poland, 55.5 percent in France, and 47.3 percent in Germany. In terms of giving thought to the subject sometimes in a given year, results were as follows: 34.2 percent in Germany, 29.1 percent in France, 24.9 percent in Poland, and 24.5 percent in Slovakia. Percentages then drop to single digits for the options of sometimes in a month, sometimes in a week and every day, except for German nurses' response to the month category which was 10 percent. Germany, Italy, and Finland are the nations with the highest proportions of nurses who frequently consider turnover. The Netherlands, Poland, Slovakia, and Belgium exhibit lower proportions (Estryn-Behar et al. 2003a; Hasselhorn, Tackenberg, and Peter 2004; Hasselhorn et al. 2003; Kovarova et al. 2003; Widerszal-Bazyl et al. 2003b).

It would seem that practitioners in these nations are attached to their profession. Very often, as in Belgium, the intent to leave an organization is greater than the intent to leave the profession. A large proportion of European nurses want to remain in its ranks. Sometimes, as noted, no or few other options are available, as in Poland and Slovakia.

Reasons for remaining in the profession include: loyalty and commitment, flexible work patterns, a family-friendly work environment, control over work, autonomy in practice, and opportunities for training and development (Hasselhorn, Müller, and Tackenberg 2005; Hasselhorn et al. 2003; Meadows, Levenson, and Baeza n.d.). Unfortunately, these elements do not prevail throughout the Member States. It is crucial to avoid nursing unit turnover as well as exit from the profession. Both are costly from many perspectives. From the economic perspective, the replacement, training, and other costs related to a nurse's departure are significant, possibly adding up to double or triple of the salary involved. These phenomena also leave their marks on key workgroup processes, such as group cohesion, relational coordination, and workgroup learning, as well as on patient outcome measures and satisfaction (Bae, Mark, and Fried 2010; Gordon 2005).

Research has indicated that nurses' expressed intentions are stronger predictors of working as a nurse than job satisfaction. Thus, these practitioners tend to act in accordance with their intentions and perceptions of control over behavior. According to this theory of planned behavior, people's actions can be quite accurately predicted from intentions when control is not excessively restricted. Up-to-date evidence related to the percentage of nurses who intend to leave their job in the next year was made available by the RN4CAST study (Scott, Matthews, and Kirwan 2012). It reveals that in several of the Member States such intentions are held by a noteworthy quantity of practitioners as exemplified by the following data: Greece and Finland (49 percent each), Poland, England, and Ireland (44 percent each), Germany (36 percent), Sweden (34 percent), Belgium (30 percent), Spain (29 percent), and the Netherlands (19 percent). Once again, the consistency in the positions of Greece and the Netherlands is of note. The average for the EU registered at 34 percent. Given these figures, health-care executives should identify any early signs of exit and implement strategies to abolish them (Murrells, Robins, and Griffiths 2008; Schoonhoven, Heinen, and van Achterberg 2012).

Conclusion

As in the United States, European nurses, like other health-care professionals, continue to report dissatisfaction with their working conditions. A multitude is calling for improved work environments and sufficient and suitable human resources, leading to an improvement in the quality of health care. In articulating their demands, these practitioners are making reference to many of the subjects cited in this volume. Many of these issues have been acknowledged for decades. However, they have become compounded, due to the enhanced pace of social, economic, and political changes that have called forth modifications in health care and thus, in nurses' work conditions. An historic inability to take action on many of these interrelated areas is found throughout the Member States. Challenges lie ahead in regard to the workplace environment. Although these workforce matters occupy a prominent position on nurses' agendas, they are not necessarily a priority for health-care managers, who instead, often, are preoccupied with other financial matters, waiting lists and times, emergency room admissions, and the like.

The importance of environmental and organizational factors, rather than individual or demographic ones, to the configuration of a healthy workplace is generally acknowledged. It has been demonstrated that negative elements are found in all four of the components of institutions: organizational management practices, workforce deployment practices, work design, and organizational culture (Page 2004). The result is work environments that lack several positive features and thus, nurture obstacles to nurses' health, appropriate behavior, and quality of care. The signal focuses on human resources management which, according to Buchan (2004), for the most part, until recently, has been overlooked. The literature has provided an indicator of the management styles and workplace factors that nurture a healthy physical and psychosocial climate in the workplace and nurses' job satisfaction. These elements have proven to be relatively consistent across various specialties and jurisdictions, highlighting a common predisposing climate. Moreover, it is nurses' perceptions of management features and work climate that are critical to their job orientations (Hayes et al. 2006; Stordeur, D'Hoore, and the NEXT Study Group 2007).

The reasons for the nursing crisis are complicated and varied, but a critical one relates to unhealthy work environments that carry consequences felt throughout the health-care sector. As management endeavors to construct positive practice environments, it is imperative that nurses be involved. These surroundings have been defined as "settings that support excellence and decent work. In particular, they strive to ensure the health, safety and personal well-being of staff, support quality patient care and improve the motivation, productivity and performance of individuals and organizations" (International Centre for Human Resources in Nursing 2007b, p. 1). Nurses' participation in the development of this model is essential. It affords an opportunity to influence the general clinical environment and aspects of practice that matter, in addition to administrative and organizational issues.

A distinguishing mark of European industrial relations is employee representation at the workplace. A Communication (COM (2001)313 final) released by the Commission dated 20 June 2001, affirmed its belief that all employees should be informed of elements important to their working life and they should be involved in its development. A Directive (2002/14/EC) followed that set forth in broad terms the regulatory framework for a system that would allow for the realization of these beliefs and thus, informing and consulting workers. Minimum requirements were established for the institutionalization of mandatory workplace representation, without harmonizing it. As a result, such representation, usually based on statutory regulation, voluntary agreement, or collective agreements, has been realized in the Member States in a wide variety of forms, reflecting diverse national definitions and regulatory mechanisms as well as the nature of the particular environment involved.

In terms of the operationalization of these units, the directive specified what information and consultation should cover and how and where consultation should occur. More specifically, employers are obliged to inform these bodies on a regular basis of issues concerning the work site and the specific sector of employment. These units oversee the implementation of labor laws, health and safety regulations, conditions of work, and the like. In some Member States, they act in a capacity that exceeds information and consultation and extends into codetermination. These structures are important as participatory mechanisms that have the potential to strengthen dialogue and aid in the development of mutual trust. Also, of significance is the fact that nurses can use these instruments as a vehicle for work place advocacy and making their voice heard on a series of related matters. There is a divide among the Member States in terms of their impact. For the most part, it appears that they have only moderately influenced work conditions. They have been judged as less influential in the Member States of Central and Eastern Europe and in the South. In still others, such as the United Kingdom, their importance has diminished, indicating the perception of the National Health Service staff that they exert little control over events at the work place and that their voice is not fully considered (Bach 2004; European Commission: Directorate-General for Employment, Social Affairs and Equal Opportunities--Unit F-1 2006). Hopefully, this arrangement will be fine-tuned so that it will become more functional and be able to realize its objective.

5

Industrial Action

Introduction

The term "industrial action" refers to any noncooperation with management for the purpose of reducing productivity in the workplace. It may occur in the context of a labor dispute or it may be meant to impact social, economic, or political change. Measures that may be undertaken are varied and wide in scope. They range from participation in certain demonstrative activities, such as picketing or petitioning and the refusal of certain duties, on the one hand, to the complete withdrawal of labor or striking, on the other. The latter activity has been a controversial form of collective action. It has presented particular problems for all health-care providers in terms of professional ethics and the impact on patients' well-being. Obviously, its ethical standing depends on its ends and the nature of the organization of the means.

In some Member States, nurses traditionally could not or would not undertake industrial action. Being doubly defined as caring, because the majority of the providers are women and due to the nature of their work, industrial action for many members of the nursing profession was deemed inappropriate. Moreover, it was considered immoral for females to disrupt the workplace (Chadwick and Thompson 2000). However, most recently, as in the United States, throughout the EU, many nurses have cast aside traditional restrictions on collective activities. For example, in Great Britain, nurse disenchantment with National Health Service reforms resulted in a rule change, in the mid-1990s, that authorized certain types of collective action. Italian nurses were not prone to industrial activities, especially strikes, because being imbued with idealism and dedication, they viewed their profession as a mission. However, given dramatic changes in many facets of their professional life, they too came to recognize the need to protect themselves via industrial activities. The same occurred in many other Member States. Collective actions are undertaken to create better conditions for the profession and for patients. Nurses' role as patient advocates justifies industrial action related to the quality of care (Sala and Usa 1997).

Moreover, in the most recently acceded Member States, strikes, which were once considered taboo under Communist rule, are no longer perceived as such. Before the transition to a democratic order, the traditional trade union role of organizing and coordinating industrial action was not significant. However, there has been an increase in the use of various industrial activities, especially strikes, which are now considered a powerful resource for trade unions in their efforts to protect workers. In many Member States, nurses have come to hold a new view of collective action and strikes, in particular. No strike clauses have been eliminated from the rule books of many national nurses' associations as they underwent a change in style and philosophy. In fact, ICN, in underscoring the importance of collective action to these organizations, has forcefully suggested that they put in place proactive policies and contingency processes and structures to guide members in their industrial activities (ICN 1999; Trif 2007).

At the transnational level, according to the Charter of Fundamental Rights of the European Union, all workers in Member States, regardless of the nature of their employer and whether they are engaged in the public or private sector, possess the right to undertake collective action. Article 28 of this document reads: "Workers and employers, or their respective organizations, have, in accordance with Community law and national laws and practices, the right . . . to take collective action to defend their interests, including strike action." In addition, the Community Charter of the Fundamental Social Rights of Workers promulgates the right to resort to collective action, and the right to strike. Moreover, the latter is also confirmed in the European Social Charter and the International Covenant on Economic, Social and Cultural Rights.

Collective action, a fundamental element of all industrial relations systems, is closely related to specific national contexts. In a majority of the Member States, its legal basis is embedded in the constitution. In others, such as Belgium, Finland, Germany, and Luxembourg, it is derived from the constitutional freedom of association. It is generally understood that this freedom embraces the right to participate in all facets of an association's life, including collective action. Moreover, industrial action is regulated by national legislation, collective agreements, and case law. In some states, such as the United Kingdom and Malta, legislation provides the legal basis for industrial activities, whereas in others, for example, Ireland, this basis is founded on a combination of legislation, collective agreements, and case law. In the Netherlands, collective action is based on case law. Austria is atypical because the legal basis for such activities is not codified (Federation of European Employers 2004, 2011; Warneck 2007; Welz and Kauppinen 2004). The spectrum of permissible industrial action ranges from the narrow to the extremely broad.

Unfortunately, as in other instances, there are difficulties related to accurate discussion of these activities, especially, on a comparative basis, due to severe problems with availability of data and its nature (Vandenbrande et al. 2007). In Greece, the Czech Republic, and Slovenia, data related to labor disputes is no longer collected and in Croatia, there are no official statistics concerned with any type of collective action. In other nations, statistics only concern certain forms of industrial action. Moreover, as in other matters, coverage and the methodology utilized tend to vary from country to country. Often, they depend on the number of workers involved, the duration of the action, the sector in which it occurs, public or private; the activities' relationship to the political arena, and the inclusion of indirectly affected workers. In addition, some nations do not report statistics related to the effects of collective action in certain sectors. For example, Portugal excludes public sector and general strikes. Thus, given the diversity in coverage, methodology, and even definition of terms, cross-national comparisons of collective action are tenuous at best (Carley 2008; Eurofound 2012; Hale 2007; Vandenbrande et al. 2007; Weiler, Newell, and Carley 2007).

Issues Spurring Collective Action

In the Member States, nurses and health-care workers, in general, on many occasions have responded to specific threats to their working conditions as well as more universal issues with collective activities. Reform arrangements, their focus, their basis, and the method utilized for their preparation have served as causes for action. For example, the potential effects of privatization and deregulation were challenged with collective action in Slovakia, the Czech Republic, and Lithuania (Dragu 2006; Lethbridge 2004). The same holds for the Polish government's reform effort entitled "Let's save Polish hospitals" which was committed to turning these facilities into commercial endeavors with considerable financial help and tax advantages (Mrozowicki 2013; "Nurses Fired" 2009). Similar challenges to liberalization have come forth in other

Central and East European nations. Also, in Portugal, nurses protested in the public health-care sector where there was experimentation with new forms of governance. From their perspective, this activity caused concern because it was perceived as privatization of essential services. Thus, it was believed that consumers possibly might not receive the same quality of services as previously. Moreover, nurses were of the opinion that a curative approach to public health threatens prevention and that the resultant recruitment system would not enhance job security. In addition, they worried that with the new governance formula they might lose their civil service status (Cristovam 2001; Quintas and Cristovam 2002).

And, at one time, fifty thousand Italian nurses marched through the streets of Rome claiming that not enough attention was being focused on the public nature of the health-care system and better education for health-care professionals (Martellotti 2005). In France, nurses, challenged the government's enactment of the thirty-five-hour work week for purposes of containing costs. The national nurses' association, the Fédération Nationale des Infirmiers claimed that such a policy only made a bad situation worse. In addition to living with a shortage of nurses, nurses would have to accomplish in thirty-five hours what they could not do in thirty-nine (Silvestro 2002).

Action has also been directed against EU reforms as well. Named after the former European Commissioner for the Internal Market, Fritz Bolkestein, the so-called Bolkestein Directive applied the country of origin principle to the service sector. Its objective was to abolish legal and administrative impediments that might impede enterprises from offering their services in another nation and to stimulate cross border competition. More specifically, it provided that an institution in a Member State could recruit employees in other Member States, using the law of its home country. In other words, service providers are only obliged to meet the rules and regulations of the country of establishment and not the nation in which services are provided. Under the rubric of "Stop Bolkestein," in 2004, Italian nurses and others demonstrated for the preservation of social and labor rights and the defense of the public good and public services.

The reference points used in reform efforts have also encouraged nurses' collective action. In Ireland, these professionals have been heavily involved in a dispute focusing on the defense and improvement of public health services. It was their contention that management was concentrating too much on the internal organization of the health-care delivery system to the detriment of improvements for consumers of services (Sheehan 2008). For Maltese nurses, cost-effectiveness played too great a role in reform efforts and for them, not enough consideration was given to patients' needs, appropriate standards of clinical nursing practice, acceptable staffing levels, and patient classification. The same concern was held by British nurses who, in 2007, protested proposed reforms of hospital services which they deemed were driven purely by financial considerations with no recognition of nursing standards of care ("Maltese Nurses" 2001; Triggle 2007). Polish nurses have been of the same opinion. In 2012, they organized nationwide protests to demonstrate their opposition to the bypassing of minimum staffing ratios in hospitals, the requirement that nurses and others become self-employed practitioners so as to decrease costs, and the increase in the retirement age for nurses to sixty-seven (Mrozowicki 2013).

These standards, descriptions of desired quality, have a special significance because they are used to evaluate nursing care. Thus, they are utilized to measure its quality, decrease its cost, and determine nursing negligence. More specifically, they relate to nursing structure, nursing process, and nursing outcomes. Structural standards refer to the organizational framework in which nursing is implemented and the optimum relationships between the nursing unit and other elements. Therefore, they are institutional or group oriented. Referring to the criteria that detail desired methods for specific nursing interventions, process standards are nurse oriented. Outcome standards, being descriptive statements of desired patient care results, may be termed patient oriented. Moreover, in this era of cost containment, patient classification systems are of importance because they are used to gather data concerning the workload of nurses for purposes of case costing. Given the significance of these standards and patient-classification systems, protesting nurses have felt their challenges to a wide variety of reforms are justified.

Methods used in achieving reform have also been of such importance to nurses as to cause collective action. For example, in Bulgaria, doctors and nurses, discontent with the transformation efforts of the authorities, demanded a referendum on the subject as well as public discussion on the financing of health care in the public and private sectors. Both constituencies felt that such efforts would clarify the criteria for reform and enlarge the decision-making base (Savova 2008). Maltese nurses have also been concerned with the scope of decision-makers in health-care reform efforts. Opposing imposition from above or from external sources, their collective action has stressed the notion of social dialogue and underscored greater possibilities for success, if reforms were implemented in concertation with health-care workers' representatives ("Maltese Nurses" 2001).

In all Member States, there exists preoccupation with health-care spending. However, of special note, is the lack of investment in the health-care sector in Central and East European nations. These systems are extremely underfunded and, in addition, a lack of transparency is often detected as well. For example, Polish people recognize corruption in the health-care system as a serious problem as do the Greeks. Thus, it is not surprising that health-care providers in these countries have acted in reference to reform of the financial arrangements for health care. More specifically, Polish nurses and colleagues have demanded that the government inject more funds into the health-care delivery system by raising its rate of contribution from 3.7 percent to 6 percent of the Gross National Product. Such, they believed was necessary to counterbalance a financial system which was not only forcing health-care facilities to assume enormous debts, but was destroying services, threatening the release of workers, and the closing of many institutions (Sroka 2006; Sula 2004). Health-care trade unions in other nations have acted on the same issue with similar demands. Such has occurred in Romania and Latvia, where the percent of Gross National Product devoted to health care has consistently decreased and is significantly less than in the 1990s.

In addition, Hungarian nurses and others have demonstrated to underscore the disastrous financial condition of their health-care sector and to issue a warning to parliamentarians that a proposed budget could only lead to the collapse of patient care. And Greek nurses have issued a call for more funds for public health as well. Danish health-care trade unions have pressured the government for its failure to raise family allowances as promised ("Demi-victoire" 2007; Kleitsa 2003). Also, in a financial vein, Latvian nurses and others have advocated broader use of tax revenues to ameliorate the country's social situation and increase public sector employees' social guarantees (Karnite 2005).

Issues related to reforms that have sparked collective action by nurses have also focused on changes in the profession. Portuguese nurses sought earlier retirement. Instead of being able to retire after thirty-five years of service and at age fifty-seven, they demanded earlier retirement after thirty years of service, at age fifty-two. In Italy, nurses requested, via industrial activities, the creation of a professional governance chamber (*ordine professionale*). This, they considered extremely critical for enhancement of professional status, the recognition of professional autonomy, and the achievement of equality with other health-care professions, especially physicians. In many Member States, nurses' changing self-perceptions have generated dissatisfaction with restricted role definitions, dependency in the power hierarchy, and restricted opportunities for advancement.

Nurses in Slovakia also requested changes in the profession. They appealed to Members of Parliament to adopt legislation that would specify minimum personnel standards for nurses working in intensive care units and the same for other departments, so that they would be able to care for a patient for at least one working hour in a shift, while, at the same time, the number of patients per nurse would not exceed ten. In addition, they requested the opportunity to provide nursing care as standardized care in social service and retirement facilities and to be able to perform all nursing activities that a nurse should perform, meaning to have all the necessary instruments and the appropriate environment for doing so (Barošová 2005).

As one might imagine, collective agreements have served as a source of protest in a galaxy of Member States. It is noteworthy that in a majority of these nations, a peace obligation is in existence, meaning that signatories to a collective agreement during its lifetime are prohibited from taking industrial action directed against the accord in its entirety or any of its provisions. However, once the agreement has expired, collective activities may take place. In some nations, such as Finland, Germany, and Greece, matters unrelated to the accord may provide subjects for action. In others, the peace obligation is total. And, in some others, such as France, it is nonexistent. Renewal of accords has stimulated nurses' action and sometimes, as in the case of Ireland, some collective agreements have not been fully implemented, requiring third party settlements be put in place after industrial action (Sheehan 2008).

Nurses and health-care workers have also responded collectively to matters of business in different stages of the legislative process and on disparate topics. In Hungary, health-care trade unions' industrial action was directed against new rules that imposed litigation costs on employees, in addition to expenses incurred by the opposing party. Bulgarian nurses were involved in advancing a law that was to provide state subsidies to hospitals to cover uninsured persons. In Germany, in the interests of health-care quality, nurses took industrial action against government plans to pass a law regulating workload (*Informe* 1999; Mihailova 2007).

An important public policy issue for nurses in all Member States, but especially, in Bulgaria and Romania, is the exodus of medical workers. In both cases, nurses and their trade unions have protested to seek governmental response to the problem. The issue has been especially sensitive since these countries joined the EU in 2007. As noted, free circulation of health-care personnel in search of better pay has exacerbated grave staff shortages (Beekman 2007; Luminita 2007) which are of prime importance not only in these countries, but in others as well.

Various facets of remuneration serve as the most common cause of industrial action for health-care workers, and especially, nurses, in practically all Member States. Nurses have a lot of company in their protests related to this issue which is often coupled with social benefits. Most recently, Croatian practitioners held a strike against governmental austerity measures. They protested reduced benefits and cuts embodied in a public sector wage bill (Carley 2008; "Nurses Strike" 2012). Nursing professionals have requested recognition for the value of their work in the form of higher wages. Pay and professional status are supposed to be at a level considered commensurate with their education and job demands. French nurses, including those in private practice, have been especially quick to forge links with wage-earning and skills recognition. For Swedish nurses, gender enters into the picture. Their salaries are relatively low and the situation becomes more complicated, due to the high number of part-time workers and the gender segregation identified with the so-called caring professions. Thus, their protests have stressed not only better wages, but more equal pay between the sexes. It is noteworthy that the gender pay gap in Sweden has registered at 17.9 percent and is now at 15.4 percent (European Commission 2013; Lovén 2009). Nurses have forcefully argued that employment sectors dominated by females should reach the same pay levels as those dominated by males. Increase in stipends has become a gender equality issue (Bach n.d.-b; Swedish Association of Health Professionals 2008) and not only in Sweden.

Parity related to pay also has another dimension as far as nurses' protests are concerned. In Spain, collective action has been taken on behalf of equality of pay in the public and private sectors. Nurse employees in the latter have claimed that public sector health-care workers earn 50 percent more and work an average of one hundred eighty-five hours less per year. According to them, this situation warranted industrial action because workers in both sectors are required to have the same qualifications and skills (Gancedo 2006).

The process for determination of wages has nurtured industrial action as well. For example, in Portugal, nurses unhappy with salary scales were concerned that in terms of their profession, pay indexing was lower than that of other professional employees and that the criteria for overtime pay were not uniform (Cristovam 2001; De Troyer 2000). Polish nurses also have had concerns with the rules for assessing additional remuneration (Sroka 2006). In addition, process has also irritated British nurses enough to vote industrial action as a warning to the Chancellor of the Exchequer, the head of the governmental department responsible for public revenues in Great Britain, to remain aloof from their independent pay review process (Carvel 2007; Mulholland 2006). For nurses in all Member States, salary increases provide the major subject for collective action under the pay rubric. It must be remembered that, in some of these countries, as noted, nurses' wages have been decreased in order to manage budgets. Also, as noted, public sector pay freezes or cuts were typical responses to the impact of the recent economic crisis on public finances. For example, such was the case most recently in Ireland, Greece, and in the Central and East European Member States, specifically, Slovakia, the Czech Republic, Estonia, Latvia, Lithuania, Romania, and Bulgaria (Carley et al. 2010; Cziria 2006; "Nurses Vote" 2009). In the latter countries, average wages in health care have grown less than in other sectors. These occurrences explain, in part, the flood of protests for pay increments. While wage increase demands are a significant issue, it must also be remembered that wage arrears are just as important in many of the Central and East European nations, especially Bulgaria and Slovenia. In fact, the 2009 Croatian Labour Act provides that salaries must be paid at regular intervals and at least once a month. Arrears are to be forthcoming by the fifteenth of the following month (Article 84).

Nurse protests have also related to professional changes and career development initiatives. An issue known to American nurses involving the introduction of new, less qualified, and less paid nursing categories has received the same negative reaction and encouraged industrial activities in Germany and elsewhere throughout the EU, as in the United States. At the same time, collective operations in Portugal and Ireland have been related to improvements in professional status and career development. More specifically, with their actions, nurses have highlighted the fact that they lack access to senior posts and that there is a gap between their career paths and those of other public employees. Nurses, they claimed, are systematically excluded from management positions in the hospital sector in favor of physicians. Thus, they have issued a call for the establishment of career ladders, career paths, and promotional posts that recognize their seniority and professional capacities (Cristovam 2001; De Troyer 2000; Swedish Association of Health Professionals 2008). There is also a facet of this issue that relates to gender. In this regard, it is to be noted that the European Commission has recognized that nurses are not the only people to face this problem and that, in general, regardless of field, there exists a glass ceiling for women that obstructs their entry into senior positions. Thus, it created the EU level network of women in positions of power to deal with this issue.

Career ladders, consisting of successively higher titles and job categories tied to salary increases, higher status, and often, greater autonomy and/or more responsibility, have served as mechanisms for recruiting and maintaining staff nurses and more recently, as instruments to motivate personnel and increase productivity. Obviously, they have consequences for the quality of services delivered and patient satisfaction. They are important for any profession. Selective socialization of employees is ensured via promotion of internal staff members. Moreover, promotions based on merit stimulate coworkers who see that superior performance and productivity enhance possibilities for career development. In addition, successful career ladders protect an institution from employees seeking advancement opportunities elsewhere (Gillies 1994). Given the nurse shortage that exists in many nations, this is a particularly cogent argument. Educators, employers, and nurses' professional organizations should assume responsibility for fostering career ladders.

Throughout the EU, many efforts relate to the shortage of nursing personnel. For instance, in Bulgaria, with the scope of combating the shortage, protests by health-care professionals' trade unions underscored the need to reduce the length of university studies from four to three years (Beekman 2007). Irish and Maltese nurses have also been concerned with education as it relates to the need for additional nurses. The former undertook collective action to increase the number of nursing students and the latter, with a similar scope, wanted changes in the nursing curriculum in order to attract more students ("Maltese Nurses" 2001). Given that the supply of nurses has failed to keep pace with increasing demand, and thus, improvements in care outcomes are threatened, these efforts are not to be overlooked.

Working conditions have been almost as important as pay issues in terms of stimulating industrial action. Nurses in most Member

States have related to this issue with protest activities. Staff reductions, recruitment restrictions, and shortages, in general, have been of critical importance to health-care personnel. They have rallied around these matters in a variety of ways in Hungary, Belgium, Bulgaria, Greece, Ireland, Malta, Poland, Portugal, Romania, Spain, and other Member States. The list of nations is long. The focus of protests was not necessarily money, but rather maintenance of minimum standards and protection of the quality of services. In fact, in the case of Spain, it was noted that the staff shortage in the private sector was so severe that, in some instances, it was greater than the number of workers. Obviously, such situations impact on the working time of health-care providers, as in Poland, where nurses and other health-care professionals have been known to work up to eighty hours per week (Dunin 2007; Gancedo 2006).

Working time which has been coupled with increased workload and resulting pressures is another issue that has generated collective action. It has been a significant subject for debate over the years. In fact, Germany experienced its longest strike ever in the public sector over this matter (Vandenbrande et al. 2007; Weiler, Newell, and Carley 2007). In general, unlike their French colleagues, nurses, with their actions, have sought reduced working hours. These efforts have been evident in Belgium, Greece, Ireland, Poland, Portugal, Slovakia, and Spain to indicate only a few of the Member States. In many instances, specific reference has been made to the need for more humane hours and the reduction of the excessive amount of overtime, as in Greece and Slovakia.

The principal dimension of working time that determines the work–life balance is the number of hours worked. It has been demonstrated time and again that long working hours have a negative impact on the quality of working life. The longer the hours worked, the greater the likelihood that employees will deem their schedules incompatible with family and other commitments. More specifically, the detrimental effect sets in with work weeks that are longer than forty-eight hours. Although scheduling is merely one facet of the staffing function, it is crucial to productivity, the morale of the workforce, and the overall work environment (Cziria 2006; European Foundation for the Improvement of Living and Working Conditions 2009c; Gillies 1994; Kleitsa 2003). Supplies and equipment have been at the heart of many a protest by nurses and others. Reference has been made to a lack of investment in the health sector in Central and East European countries.

A deterioration of working conditions in many facilities outfitted with outdated technical equipment, often in a poor state, has been attributed to this fact. Not only does this situation impact on the provision of good clinical practice, but it affects health and safety conditions as well (Lethbridge 2004; Mihailova 2007). Human resource shortages and those related to supplies, along with poor equipment maintenance, lead to not only a progressive deterioration of services, but also to employee dissatisfaction (ICN 2008b). In Greece, the lack of supplies (medications, compresses, syringes, etc.), due to the state's failure to pay hospital suppliers over a period of four years, brought the healthcare system to a point of collapse. This situation, reflecting corruption in the system, triggered protest reactions in many sectors. Needless to say, productivity is not only related to motivation, but its quantity and quality depend on an appropriate supply of materials, human and otherwise, to meet demand.

There are other issues that might be noted, but the ones cited are those that have surfaced on a regular basis. Relative deprivation, in one sense or another, is important to a discussion of these issues which have encouraged nurses' collective action. It signifies the perceived difference between what one believes to be one's just deserts and what one actually receives, the perceived difference between justice and achievement. In other words, it represents the difference between actual attainment as perceived by the individual or group and the best possible level. Obviously, such perceived differences breed dissatisfaction and various theories have designated dissatisfaction as a main source of unrest and cause for action (Barnes, Farah, and Heunks 1979).

Collective Action Tactics

Although it exhibits a preference for social dialogue to resolve professional and workplace problems, ICN justifies collective action in situations in which negotiations between employees and employers have been refused, unsuccessful, or unsatisfactory. In addition, industrial activities are considered appropriate when problems with the remuneration of nurses' wages and deficiencies in the quality of their working environment have become so severe as to impinge negatively on high standards of nursing care well into the future (ICN 1999). Throughout the Member States, nurses have engaged in a galaxy of diverse types of collective action. They have been imaginative and often surprising in their choice of tactics which obviously are dependent on available resources, both human and material. These means are of significance.

236

Institutional resources are important to groups, especially, in terms of their behavior and outcomes of their actions. Opportunity and mobilization are important variables between dissatisfaction and action. It is to be noted that in the various Member States, very often, a different label is assigned to the same collective activity. Moreover, some types of industrial action are legal in some nations and prohibited in others.

Health-care systems, in part, are shaped and guided by what providers of services believe and the way they learn their beliefs, change them, and articulate them. Persons affiliated with organizations are more likely to engage in collective action. Organizational involvement serves as a stimulant. Of the various dimensions of affiliation, it is the commitment of time and money to the association that links members to protest activities (Somma 2010). Nurses have a broad range of available options to make their issues known. To highlight specific problems, many practitioners and their organizations have utilized methods well-known to the American scene. Petitioning is a most familiar tactic, Most recently, Swedish nurses initiated a nationwide petition campaign, entitled Mission 24K, in favor of establishing a basic level for nurses' starting salaries (Irish Nurses and Midwives Organisation 2013). Practitioners have used other familiar activities, such as the release of expert communications and results of research endeavors, press conferences, legal challenges, picketing, the holding of workshops and public meetings, distribution of leaflets to the local population, and lobbying politicians, professional organizations, and other interest groups.

As in the United States, trade unions in many Member States have traditionally commented on draft laws or implications of specific public policies. However, in the Central and East European Member States, given historical circumstances, they were not used to such activities. They had little training or experience in this area and, given the economic situation, funds have not been readily available to compensate specialists or attorneys on a regular basis. Thus, this has been a relatively new practice in the region. It has been used in Bulgaria to challenge health-care reform efforts. Trade unions, being excluded from discussions concerned with health-care reform, were forced to "take the bull by the horns" and send precise warnings concerning the decision-making framework and to propose alternative programs designed to alleviate what they perceived as the negative social effects of reforms. They organized many of the above-mentioned activities and, in addition, participated as experts in the proceedings of the parliamentary health commission to launch alternative legislative initiatives and to submit arguments in favor of amendments to the materials being discussed (Daskalova et al. 2005).

Dissatisfaction is often manifested through protest behavior which may be viewed as action, based on disagreement with policies, undertaken to reverse practices and realize benefits from a particular system, while operating within that system (Lipsky 1975).Very often, such action is characterized by showmanship. Formal protests have been lodged by nurses with public authorities on many an issue and on a regular basis throughout the Member States. In Portugal, health-care trade unions undertook this type of activity in connection with the aforementioned new management models. Moreover, Polish nurses and colleagues, in reference to a shortfall of funds, gained entry to the National Health Fund in Warsaw for purposes of protest to public authorities. Formal letters and declarations with demands and deadlines for action have been used in Bulgaria, where they were delivered with a certain fanfare to the Prime Minister, the Minister of Health, and members of parliament and the parliamentary health commission (Cristovam 2001; Mihailova 2007; Sula 2004). One of the most direct ways to convey a political message is to deliver it directly to a politician or governmental authority.

In most of the Member States, as in the United States, marches and demonstrations have a long standing tradition. They are usually staged to publicize unfair treatment of a group or groups and to oppose an unpopular practice. In Spain, the Czech Republic, Belgium, France, Latvia, Poland, Slovakia, Portugal, and Bulgaria, among other Member States, health-care trade unions have used demonstrations as a protest tactic. It has been suggested that the presence of trade unions makes it easier for dissatisfied individuals to relate their personal state of mind to what occurs in a given system, in this case, a health-care delivery system (Barnes, Farah, and Heunks 1979). Perhaps Polish trade union demonstrations have been the most interesting. Polish nurses have had numerous instances of national industrial activities. As part of wider collective action, they and twenty thousand other health-care workers have staged a long-term demonstration in front of the Prime Minister's office in the hope of forcing the government to increase spending for health care. In addition, they have also displayed their displeasure with the Polish health-care delivery system in front of the Parliament, desiring that such action would guarantee legislative approval of more spending on the public health sector, including a pay raise for them.

Previously, they had spent two weeks protesting without break in front of other government buildings. As part of the demonstrations in front of the Prime Minister's office, nurses inaugurated and operated a street hospital for patients that were refused admission to institutions because of health-care workers' long-term absences. Nurses labeled these activities the "Protest of White Slaves" (Dunin 2007).

Demonstrations vary in terms of their duration. In Latvia, those of the public sector trade union confederations, carried out under the banner "We are against poverty," and those of the categories employed in private health centers in Spain have been relatively short in comparison to the cited Polish case, or the Bulgarian one in which daily demonstrations by all hospital workers have lasted more than forty consecutive days (Gancedo 2006; Karnite 2005, 2008; Mihailova 2007). Although Latvian protest actions are relatively short, it is to be noted that they quickly reoccur. No one is satisfied with these efforts. The government's response is to create divisions among health-care providers. It blatantly asks protesters to identify the category of health-care workers whose stipends should be decreased in order to meet requests. Thus, the government responds positively to one set of workers' requests and reduces pressure by realizing a separate agreement with a trade union. In this way, temporary "fixes" and peace are achieved, but the discontent only returns (Karnite 2005, 2008).

Picketing is another common tactic utilized by nurses in their protests. It is used extensively in Western Europe, with the exception of France, where it is illegal. In the Central and East European region, it is allowed in some Member States (Latvia, Lithuania, Slovakia) and, in others, it is not regulated or, as in the case of Hungary, it has not been used in practice (Warneck 2007; Welz and Kauppinen 2004).

The boycott is an important tool of protest that has been attractive to nurses. ICN has sanctioned the boycott of elective interventions and certain services involving nonnursing duties, for example, domestic, clerical, portering, and catering tasks. In the above-referenced dispute with the Chancellor of the Exchequer in Great Britain, 95 percent of the members of the Royal College of Nursing voted for the first nationwide action since its founding in 1916. Boycott actions were a part of the decision. More specifically, collective activities were to include boycotting completion of forms that the National Health Service trusts use to satisfy government targets (Carvel 2007). According to the Royal College of Nursing code of practice on industrial action, any measures undertaken by nurses must not work to the detriment of patients' or clients' well-being or interests. The code then identifies several activities which might meet this requirement. Essentially, they involve use of the boycott in reference to various matters. Illustrative of the list are refusal to work overtime, refusal to attend nonpatient related meetings, refusal to participate in meetings called outside of working hours, refusal to change work time on short notice, and refusal to attend training sessions outside of working hours, to cite a few elements.

More recently, Irish nurses and other health-care workers launched collective action against a recruitment freeze in the public health service. Tactics included some of the aforementioned boycotts. They involved refusal of all nonemergency overtime and out-of-hours work as well as certain types of activities, such as covering posts left vacant by recruitment restrictions and cooperation with specific Health Services Executive advisors (Sheehan 2008). On another occasion, the Irish Nurses Organisation proclaimed a hospital-wide boycott on all unpaid acting-up, that is, assuming responsibility for the performance of tasks affiliated with personnel of a superior grade. Swedish nurses have banned overtime work as have the Finnish along with rota changes. Greek and Maltese nurses have boycotted the performance of particular duties as well. More specifically, the Maltese declined all nonnursing duties in addition to the taking of nonemergency blood samples (Jokivuori 2007; Kritsantonis 1998; Warneck 2007).

Another obstructive measure designed to interrupt ordinary activities that has been used by nurses is the blockade. For the most part, this tactic has been utilized in reference to traffic. For example, in Bulgaria, trade unions and physicians' and nurses' associations organized protests advocating better working conditions that blockaded traffic on Sofia's main streets for a half hour each morning over an extended period of time. Polish nurses have also on a regular basis brought traffic to a standstill in the streets of Warsaw (Fawcett-Henesy 2000/01; Mihailova 2007). Another type of blockade was threatened by Maltese nurses in 2007. They proclaimed that if the university did not come forth with appropriate resources, there would be no alternative, but to block the opening of any new health services planned by the government.

Go-slow is another form of collective action used by nurses in many Member States. Essentially, as is evident from the name, it involves a reduction in the pace of work. It is a form of workplace activity in which employees seeming to be routinely engaged, deliberately ration their productivity in order to exert pressure for the achievement of a desired objective (Hammett, Seidman, and London 1957). Rules in the workplace are applied widely, literally, and carefully, even those that are normally overlooked in the interests of efficiency.

Closely related to go-slow is work-to-rule, another labor practice invoked by nurses to lodge a particular dissatisfaction. Using this technique, employees meticulously perform each and every task explicitly associated with one's position. However, ancillary duties related to core responsibilities are overlooked. For example, nurses, declining to perform tasks they are not contracted to do, might refuse to answer the telephone. Only the minimum requirements of a position are met. Very often, the two terms, go-slow and work-to-rule, are used synonymously. Both tactics are illegal in certain Member States, namely Belgium, Denmark, and France, and could be considered inappropriate forms of action in the Netherlands, where all collective activities must be reasonably proportioned to the demands presented. If not, the action is termed "out of proportion" (Warneck 2007). Both of these techniques have been used by nurses throughout the Member States where they are allowed. It is interesting to note that, in Ireland, trade unions evaluated work-to-rule in a positive vein, claiming it improved the time nurses spent with patients and, in turn, the overall quality of patient care (Irish Nurses Organisation 2007).

Challenging the issue agenda, in some nations, involves utilizing additional forms of behavior not necessarily sanctioned by the established order. To articulate their demands, some forces step outside the regularized channels of action. Although unlawful in France and Spain (Warneck 2007), sit-ins or occupation of public buildings have been a favorite of nurses in Greece and Poland. In Greece, nurses in a protest involving reform took over the health ministry and even invited the minister to go with them to do the same at the Ministry for Economic Affairs (Kritsantonis 1998; "Tensions Rise" 2008). Having occupied government buildings in the past, in 2007, some disillusioned Polish nurses, as part of an enormous health-care workers' collective action, entered the Prime Minister's office and waited for a meeting with him which only took place seven days later. In the meantime, they also occupied another office in the Prime Minister's chancellery. In addition, as part of these takeovers, nurses and hundreds of colleagues undertook a hunger strike.

A nontraditional collective action that made its debut in California, in 1966, and in Europe, in Sweden, in 1998, has become fashionable and is used in other Member States as well. This is the weapon of mass resignations. In its first European use, 150 Swedish nurses employed in

241

the same intensive care unit advertised for new employers. It was their method to exert pressure to maintain flexible work schedules. The idea spread fast and resignation became contagious mass action. The following year, nurses across the country by the hundreds threatened to or actually did resign. Even though at the time, national unemployment figures were high in most fields, the same did not hold for the nursing profession. Employment opportunities were plentiful, either at home or in Norway and Denmark where salaries were higher. The purpose of the resignations was to focus public attention on the spotlights of the profession: underpaid, overworked, and understaffed (Berg 1999; De Troyer 2000).

Finnish nurses have also used resignation as an industrial weapon. They turned to this technique because of the government's response to their strike action. It was ignored. Also, given that the government can legally force striking nurses to return to work, they were convinced that this fact undermined their power position. So they undertook mass resignations. However, in retaliation, the parliament passed emergency legislation forcing nurses to work, even though they had resigned and were formally unemployed. This was an historic measure in that it was the first time a European legislative body passed a law nullifying and voiding an employee's resignation. Moreover, perhaps in anticipation of the mass resignations, the Finnish Labour Court had ruled such action unlawful (Carley 2008; Ibison 2007). Those who resigned did not enjoy the same type of job security as employees participating in strike activities. However, as in the case of Sweden, the labor market for nurses worked to their advantage and acted as a security measure along with the fact that all participants in the action agreed not to return to work until everyone was reinstated (Jokivuori 2007).

In the newly acceded countries of Central and Eastern Europe, resignation has been relied on in Bulgaria and Poland. As noted above, Polish nurses have staged numerous industrial activities on a national basis. Disliking the government's response or rather lack of same, they and their colleagues undertook massive group resignations that in some facilities amounted to 90 percent of the personnel. There were political implications to these actions as well in that health-care personnel were hoping to weaken the government in a major way and possibly even realize its collapse (Dunin 2007).

Threats have also been a part of collective action in the Member States. Perhaps the threat to strike is the most common, but actually, threats may relate to a galaxy of possible activities. They may relate to a single action or several, as happened in Malta, in 2008. The Malta

Union of Midwives and Nurses, while in the midst of industrial activities over continued staff shortages, threatened to stop treating patients when understaffing was evident, to refuse to admit patients to hospitals and homes for the elderly, to shut down district health centers, to not change dressings of patients not in their units, and to operate on a work-to-rule basis. Threats can represent an efficiency and economy of means. Depending on the particular situation, very often, utterance of a threat serves to resolve the conflict.

Solidarity or sympathy activities provide support to colleagues or others in their primary actions. With some exceptions, such as Latvia, Austria, Luxembourg, the Netherlands, and the United Kingdom, such efforts are legal. In Germany, Italy, and Spain, legality depends on the circumstances involved. In Poland, secondary action is only permitted on behalf of those workers who do not enjoy the right to undertake collective action. Fire workers, the police, and the military would be in this category. However, in Poland, nurses have enjoyed solidarity support. To engage in international secondary action, in most Member States, some conditions must be met. For example, the primary activity abroad must be lawful in nature or there must be some community of interest between the workers of the two countries involved. Belgium may be singled out for the fact that there are very few restrictions on trade union support of workers abroad. In some instances, there are also time limits placed on sympathy actions. These range from half a day in Poland to three days in Estonia (Warneck 2007).

In terms of industrial action, the strike is the most extreme means available to nurses and their organizations for advocacy of social and economic interests. Although these professionals use the strike, it must be remembered that it is formally regulated by national legislation, case law, collective agreements, and other legal instruments. Thus, there is much variance in its use throughout the Member States. When a general definition of the public function is adopted, as usually happens, it is most probable that there are restrictions on health-care workers' right to strike and especially, on those professionals employed in the hospital sector. Interruption or complete cessation of services could endanger life, security, or health of the total population, or part of it. Thus, limitations are necessary. Strikes in essential services are regulated by several mechanisms. Often, restrictions are placed on certain categories of workers' right to strike. Given the nature of the nursing profession and its role in the health-care delivery system, one might expect to find controls on its use of this right.

Such is the case in Romania, Finland, Lithuania, Luxembourg, Cyprus, the Czech Republic, and Slovakia, to cite a few examples. Often, as in Slovakia and the Czech Republic, strikes are prohibited in certain professions and work places. Another approach is represented by Latvia, where employees in essential services are required to balance their limited right to strike with public interests. Sweden is unique in that legislation restricting strikes in these services is nonexistent. Industrial action involving these services and nearly all of the public sector is lawful. However, trade unions and employers' organizations in the public and private sectors have concluded accords of indefinite duration not to undertake industrial action that threatens the public interest. Austrians are required to adhere to the principle of rationality in that action must be based on reasonable cause (Ahlberg and Bruun 2005; Warneck 2007).

Another regulatory mechanism involves enforcement of the obligation to continue work at a minimum level and to carry out any necessary emergency tasks. In many Member States, it is proclaimed that minimum services must be maintained. In fact, most Member States have opted for this mandate. Romanian legal instruments not only refer to the requirement of providing minimum services, as do most nations, but they specify the level at one-third of normal activity. Different models are utilized throughout the Member States to determine the nature of essential services. In the option that is most prevalent, employer and worker representatives agree on these services and the minimum number of personnel required. In Cyprus, a special committee, consisting of representatives of the parties to the dispute, exists in each workplace to monitor and implement the established services and to deal with any problems that may arise during a strike. Another process, utilized in Italy, provides for a neutral commission to make these determinations. It is also possible for governmental authorities to designate the appropriate conditions, as happens in Spain. Or, if the strike is in the public sector, the employer makes the decision, and if in the private sector, the union involved decides. This is the practice in Greece. There are several different options.

Within essential services strikes are also often regulated by placing constraints on methods utilized. This is another general phenomenon applicable to a galaxy of Member States. For example, in the United Kingdom, nurses are not to behave in ways that could be detrimental to the well-being of patients. A similar restriction holds for Hungary where health and human life are not to be endangered. Obviously, physical violence is covered by a universal ban.

In addition, there are other constraints placed on the use of collective action. Reference has already been made to the peace obligation. In several Member States, the strike is considered *ultima ratio* or an act of last resort, the last possible solution. Originally, this phrase referred to the final arguments of kings. In this context, it means that other efforts to resolve a conflict must precede strike action. In fact, in a majority of the Member States and for ICN, alternate dispute resolution is obligatory before the advent of collective action. Actually, this mandate offers legitimacy to strikes in that efforts to resolve a conflict have taken place before the calling of a strike. According to ICN's policy, the only restriction on the right to industrial action is the establishment of independent and impartial mechanisms for extra-judicial dispute resolution (ICN 1999).

Strikes have achieved positive results for nurses and have also indicated why their general use is problematic. Although they are undertaken with optimistic visions, they can be divisive, humiliating, and destructive in a variety of ways to those who participate in them and to others as well. Decisions to call a strike are not to be taken lightly for they bear consequences for all sectors. For example, in the United Kingdom, a nurse participating in industrial action could theoretically face disciplinary proceedings before the employer, criminal proceedings, civil proceedings for negligence, and professional conduct proceedings. There are also possibilities of loss of earnings and loss of employment rights, among other things (*Code of Practice* n.d.; Dimond 1997). Potential risks are great. Involving many uncertainties, use of the strike must be given careful consideration. Thus, in most nations, there are established procedures to ensure that special and appropriate attention is focused on the strike. Certain conditions must be satisfied for a strike to be considered legal. These procedures principally contain requirements related to the formal vote to authorize a strike and the requisite notices related to action.

In the Member States, there are two methods to sanction a strike. In some nations, only trade union members may take the decision to initiate such action. This is the situation in Germany, where a strike cannot be other than a trade union strike. In other countries, both union members and nonmembers decide whether to strike or not. Such is the case in Poland and Latvia where union membership has no relevance in the matter (Dimitriv 2007; Warneck 2007). Usually, in such situations, the right to strike is considered an individual as opposed to solely a trade union right.

Often, it is mandated that a secret ballot be utilized to ratify strike action, that there be a specific number of participants in the decision-making, and an established threshold for the portion of affirmative votes. The secret ballot is used in many Member States, including Ireland, Slovakia, Cyprus, and Portugal, but in others, such as Greece, the vote is taken in the general assembly of the trade union involved. The quorum required to take legal action varies throughout the Member States. For example, in Poland, the Czech Republic, and Slovakia, it is established at 50 percent of the constituency involved and in Latvia, at 75 percent. Also, the threshold of affirmative votes fluctuates in the same fashion. A simple majority is required in many nations, such as the Netherlands, Bulgaria, and Slovenia, whereas nurses in the Royal College of Nursing in the United Kingdom need a two-thirds majority to make application to the Council, the governing body, for authorization to engage in industrial action. The threshold is even higher in Denmark, where it is set at 75 percent. Regardless of the particulars, these votes are of importance. Furnishing authorization to the workers involved in strike action, they legitimate it.

These ballots are especially significant when decisions for militant action result from pressure by members of a union disillusioned with the actions of management and the trade union leadership. Such has happened with the Federation of Hospital Workers in Greece. Members took decisions opposed to the leaders' wishes. In France, the trade union rank and file with their vote has been known to challenge leaders' practices in reference to nurses' industrial action. Then, attempting to bridge the gap between the official trade union authorities and the membership, "coordination groups" have been established by the rank and file to organize strike action in opposition to the official trade union channels. Such behavior served as a lesson to the labor organizations involved. They were quick to consult workers more frequently and on a regular basis (Greenwood 1998; Kleitsa 2003).

In addition to ballot requirements, there are usually other procedures that have to be followed before strike action may be undertaken. For the most part, these relate to the time frames for serving notice of a strike and the type of information that has to be supplied and to whom. The time frames for announcing strike action vary a great deal throughout the Member States. Notice periods range from twenty-four hours in Greece to fourteen days in Finland and Estonia. The timing of the announcement can also be related to the nature of the collective action and its stage. For example, in Estonia, solidarity actions require less notice than other types. In Spain, there is one time frame for strikes taking place in the public service and a shorter one for those in other settings. Lithuania makes the distinction between essential and other services. And, in Slovenia, action of special importance requires more advance notice. The Netherlands seems to be the most flexible of all Member States. There are no specific times for the issuance of strike notices. However, it is expected that management will be given a list of demands and a deadline for response before action is undertaken. And, in the case of nurses in the United Kingdom, industrial activities must commence within four weeks from the date of the ballot. Diversity is evident (Federation of European Employers 2011; Warneck 2007). These notice periods are important to the preparation of programs to be relied on during strike action.

Variance also relates to the type of information that must be furnished and the proper authorities to be contacted, such as governmental figures, employers, health service administrators, trade union officials, and the public. Required information often relates to the exact nature of the action to be taken, participants, etc. And, in the case of essential services, such as health care, written agreement between the parties providing for the maintenance of a minimum level of services is often requested or, as in Greece, a list containing the names of employees who will remain on duty during an eventual strike is expected to be on file and updated annually (Federation of European Employers 2011; Warneck 2007).

There are various types of strikes. Some are temporary walkouts and this technique has been adopted by nurses in Ireland using a rota system throughout the country's hospitals. On the other hand, rotating strikes are not allowed in France. It has been claimed that these selective strikes provide less effective action because the number of nurses withdrawing from the provision of services is not sufficient. In most Member States, political strikes are theoretically prohibited. Exceptions are provided by Finland, Ireland, Italy, and Denmark, if the strike is short and for a reasonable matter. In nations where political strikes and sympathy or secondary actions are allowed, the trade union movement possesses excellent means to exert pressure against the government (Finland: Ministry of Labour 2003). Warning strikes serve notice of a forthcoming effective strike. Permissible in some Member States, they have been a favorite mechanism of hospital employees in Poland. Workers in more than one hundred public facilities throughout the country have staged warning strikes on many an occasion. In countries where they are allowed, the duration of such activities is usually restricted. For example, in Estonia, a warning strike is limited to one hour and in Poland, to two hours (Mihailova 2007; Sroka 2006; Warneck 2007).

When strikes are in effect, ICN's strike policy dictates that nursing personnel maintain minimum essential services and adhere to other principles. The latter include minimum disruption to the general public, crisis intervention for the preservation of life, continuous nursing care to those incapable of caring for themselves, provision of nursing processes critical to essential therapeutic services, and diagnostic procedures related to potentially life-threatening conditions, as well as observance of the provisions contained in national and subnational legislative instruments concerning strike action (ICN 1999).

It is noteworthy that, in some cases, certain governmental structures have the authority to postpone collective action for a certain period of time, ranging from fourteen days to two months, depending on the nation involved. Usually done on the basis of the existence of a threat to the public interest, such is possible in Estonia, Portugal, Finland, Spain, and Sweden. This power is broader in Cyprus, where the Council of Ministers, the executive branch of government, enjoys discretionary power to ban strikes in certain services that it considers essential. Also, in some nations, such as Slovakia and Denmark, the government can also end strike action. For example, in the latter country, parliament has intervened to terminate nurses' strikes. Arguing that such action effectively meant that these professionals had lost their right to strike, the Christian People's Party proposed a measure to formally abolish it. The proposal failed to elicit parliamentary support, principally because it was believed that the legislative body should not develop rules for Danish industrial relations. The general consensus of a majority of the parliamentarians was that such interference would represent a death measure for the so-called stellar Danish model. In addition, it was thought that the rights to take collective action and to strike are closely linked to the right to collective bargaining and thus, cannot be discussed in isolation.

The replacement of employees on strike by other workers recruited from outside the workplace, that is, strikebreakers, is generally prohibited throughout the EU. In some countries, for example, Italy, Portugal, Austria, and Slovenia, to cite some examples, employing new workers or replacing workers during a strike is not permitted. However, in Lithuania, it is possible to employ alternate people as replacements for striking employees when minimum services are not forthcoming.

In addition, there are instances in which employees may be used in strikers' positions. For instance, in Germany, management may use employees, if they volunteer to fulfill the responsibilities of strikers. And, in France, employers are free to assign nonstriking employees to the positions of strikers. They may even require them to work overtime. And, in Greece, public sector employees under civil mobilization may be replaced, but only on a temporary basis. The situation in Cyprus is most unique in that replacement workers may be hired, but only in the northern portion of the island, that part which, in 1974, was invaded and occupied by Turkey. It is noteworthy that ICN and national nursing associations vehemently oppose the use of strike breakers. They view this practice as a mechanism that stems the urgency for serious social dialogue (Federation of European Employers 2004, 2011; ICN 2011; Warneck 2007).

It is generally understood that persons participating in a lawful strike cannot be penalized. However, this understanding has not always been honored. In 2006, the first official strike in the health-care sector by hospital workers took place in Slovakia and some nurses participating in the activity were suspended by the hospital director. Also, in several cases, unfairly dismissed Latvian public sector workers have won court actions for employment law infringements. More recently, in Poland, nurse trade union leaders were fired for strike activities which hospital management claimed were illegal. The release of these employees from their nursing duties took place before the case could be heard in court where the chances of it being dropped were very high (Carley 2008; Karnite 2005; "Nurses Fired" 2009; Tragakes 2008).

It is noteworthy that legal protection from discrimination against trade union members is provided in most nations throughout the EU, with Cyprus, being one exception. However, in reference to Lithuania, it is remarked that there is little protection in practice and protection is judged limited in Romania. In Poland, it has been evaluated as not very effective and it is noted that union leaders may be dismissed without union authorization as happened with the incident involving nurses cited above (Federation of European Employers 2004).

An important facet of collective activities consists of activating other elements to participate in the action in a manner favorable to protest objectives. Thus, nurses frequently undertake collective action in the company of others for the simple reason that there is often greater security in numbers, an important resource. Also, as the old saying goes: "Misery loves company." On multiple occasions, in many or most of the Member States, nurses have joined forces with a wide range of other health-care workers. In other instances, they have limited their collaboration to physicians. In Bulgaria, the Czech Republic, Germany, Estonia, Poland, and Sweden, to cite a few nations, these two professions have organized joint protests on more than one occasion. However, the possibility of such efforts has been criticized. One nurse, presenting an argument for noncollaboration, has commented in typical fashion:

> I think if nurses don't speak up, nothing will change. Nobody is going to solve things for us. But to join in with the doctors would be stupid. I know we all work in health care, but if we joined them, the focus would be only on their demands. Their needs and our needs are two different things. A nurse's job is completely different from a doctor's, so we need separate strikes (Heitlinger and Trnka 1998, pp. 63–64).

In opposition to this opinion, it is generally believed that a broad front of health-care workers, including more than one profession, is needed for optimal articulation of demands. Moreover, engagement in separate battles within the health-care sector often puts members of the different professions in conflict with each other.

Intra- and extraprofessional strategic alliances are important for long-term success in realizing demands. When groups find common ground on which they can join forces, the probability of developing a correspondence between their desires and the underlying attitudes of proximate decision-makers to whom they must appeal is increased. Other things being equal, the more similar the goal orientations of the units involved, the greater the likelihood of realizing success. The involvement of multiple forces creates a process characterized by reciprocal relations in which strategies are developed based on the leaders' perception of the needs of many actors. It is also a very indirect process in which the media and reference publics of protest targets play critical roles.

Frequently, health-care providers' trade unions work in unison with other labor organizations. For example, in Slovakia, health-care workers have enjoyed support from other trade union representatives in their demands for higher wages and better working conditions (Cziria 2006). In Bulgaria, nurses and physicians have garnered assistance in their causes from disparate trade union organizations: the Trade Union of Transport Workers, the Union of Teachers and labor organizations affiliated with the forestry and timber industry plus taxi drivers (Mihailova 2007). Members of the European Federation of Public Service Unions, a federation of more than two hundred independent trade union organizations representing over eight million workers in public services in Europe, enjoy this organization's support in their activities at the national level. Moreover, this supranational association also undertakes efforts on their behalf at the European level. In addition, it operates on a European basis with mechanisms available to labor organizations. It also works in partnership with the European Trade Union Confederation, another pan-European trade union network. Together these two associations develop policy documents, many of which result from research efforts, seminars, conferences, and social dialogue.

Support for health-care workers and specifically, nurses, in the articulation of their needs has been forthcoming from a multitude of sources internal and external to the health sector. In many Member States, nurses rightly engage in broad cooperation with a wide variety of nongovernmental organizations, social movements, and social sectors. In the United Kingdom, in 2007, auxiliary hospital staff supported nurses' industrial action short of a strike. The same collaboration resulted from patients' organizations in Bulgaria and elsewhere. Most recently, Polish nurses and other health-care providers were joined in their opposition to public health-care policies by miners and workers from the automotive industry. Of note are the activities in the United Kingdom that unite trade unions and local community and faith groups, embracing both workers in the health-care sector and consumers of health services (Carvel 2007; Lethbridge 2004; Mrozowicki 2013; Savova 2008).

In reference to the aforementioned "Stop Bolkestein" protest, it is to be noted that demonstrators included not only nurses, but citizens, members and representatives of organizations advocating for consumers of health-care services, students, trade union members and supporters, adherents of a galaxy of social movements, supporters of various political parties, health-care providers, and spokespersons for their professional associations, among others. All joined ranks to oppose liberalization of the service market. Moreover, it is to be noted that this collaboration spilled over national borders. Protest marches occurred at the same time in Greece, Italy, Finland, Germany, France, and other Member States (Fusani 2005). Communal and group activities of which there are many different types are important to the articulation of demands. Involving communication and group efforts to confront problems, this mode of articulating demands requires much initiative. Participants must come to agreement on agenda, strategies, and timetable. This type of action places control of participation with the group and thus, enhances its influence.

Formal collaboration with politicians varies from country to country. In many cases, it has been in a positive vein. Parliamentarians in Slovakia, as noted above, were most cooperative with health-care professionals and the same holds for those from both political parties in England who committed support for nurses in their aforementioned pay dispute with the Chancellor of the Exchequer ("British Nurses" 2007). Viewing labor conflicts and industrial activities as the traditional responsibility of social partners, Swedish politicians do not customarily become involved. However, manifesting visible support to the low-paid women's struggle for higher wages, in the recent past, they have collaborated with Swedish nurses on strike. The dispute was primarily viewed as a gender issue. In the aforementioned long-lasting Polish protests, it is not surprising that strikers received support from opposition political parties in their effort to weaken the government.

In several instances, collaboration and support for collective activities have been forthcoming from important personages. Again, in Poland, Polish bishops, on behalf of protesting nurses, issued a call for dialogue, hoping that such a mechanism would lead to industrial peace. Well-known artists have also lent their support in many nations.

Material and other types of support from the public in general and different groups within it have been important to the outcomes of nurses' industrial action throughout the EU. In several instances, the citizenry has actually joined protests, as in Bulgaria and Slovakia. Material solidarity was forthcoming again in Poland in the form of food, tents, blankets, and funds. To reciprocate the protesting nurses, midwives, and physicians provided free physical examinations for Warsaw residents. In addition, these health-care providers were joined in their efforts by groups of miners, steelworkers, and teachers (Cziria 2006; Dunin 2007; Mihailova 2007).

Without public support, industrial action can be futile. For the most part, the public in various Member States has been sympathetic to nurses' collective activities. For example, public opinion denounced the corruption in a fragile health-care system and manifested complete understanding of the aforementioned Greek protest efforts (dsegretain 2009). The media, in addition to public opinion, has been positive in attitude toward nurses' endeavors, especially in Finland and Sweden. In fact, these two elements have always sided with Swedish nurses. And, the aforementioned mass resignations of Finnish nurses received media support and a public approval rating of 61 percent. A similar positive response was given to striking Polish nurses. On the other hand, the situation in the Netherlands is different. Although strikes are few in number, when they do occur, given cultural attitudes and the impact of the notions of consensus and evolution on which Dutch society is based, the general public is seldom very sympathetic (Berg 1999; Dunin 2007; Jacobs 2005; Jokivuori 2007).

Nurses must articulate their objectives and select strategies, so as to maximize their public exposure through the media. The latter has always been eager to cover the unusual. The protest-media-outcomes triad has significance. There is interplay between these three elements in creating and communicating issues and in affecting the final result. News coverage is critical to the success of industrial action. Thus, the nontraditional and unorthodox tactics, such as building takeovers, street clinics, and mass resignations, could be worthwhile. Catching the fancy of the media, protest forms and conflictive framing of demands promotes publicity of a particular cause and its message, exposes the public to issues it might not otherwise encounter, and influences the outcome. Furthermore, public opinion can be used as a source of information for the construction of dispute conclusions. The public, its temperament, and its reactions to conflict impact the result. However, public opinion alone does not solely determine outcome. There are, according to Chard, (2004) mediating influences on outcomes from various facets of public opinion and a multitude of other factors. In terms of public opinion, its two dimensions, direction and intensity, are of note. The first refers to its orientation, approval or disapproval of something. The second indicates the strength of this orientation, that is, very strong, less strong, etc. Intensity is an important dimension of identification with groups.

Moreover, direct actions, such as those cited above, can be very effective in transmitting preferences to authorities with the aid of the media. The triadic relationship between outcomes, protest, and the media is of significance. Without media attention, collective activities become like the tree falling unheard in the forest. Information is power. Nurses' organizations may well be capable of increasing the saliency of their issues by utilizing the communications media and successful appeals or threats to the public. Given the media's capacity to reach massive audiences fast, simultaneously, frequently, and conveniently, it is critical to nurses' endeavors. If an incident of collective action is not assigned importance or is overlooked by the media, protesters' chances for success are automatically reduced. It has been claimed that this powerful instrument of communication actually determines the agenda, civic and otherwise (Lipsky 1975). Collaboration with the media is imperative.

There is also an international facet to collaborative efforts. They are not as frequent as other types, but they are evident. In Maltese nurses' industrial action that included strikes, both ICN and ILO intervened. This international pressure resulted in the initiation of social dialogue. ICN also collaborates with national nurses' organizations addressing labor matters by providing technical support. In addition, it encourages ILO to influence national policy in each member country in a positive manner. In the aforementioned nurses' agitation in Poland, the Human Rights Commissioner for the Council of Europe gave support to these professionals on the basis of his understanding that the protest was based on social and economic rights which, according to him, are fundamental to human rights. Interestingly enough, international collaboration is not always accepted. Whereas Italian nurses supported French colleagues in their challenge to the thirty-five-hour work week, the Swedish Association of Health Professionals requested that sister organizations in the Nordic and Baltic regions remain neutral in its conflict with employers (Swedish Association of Health Professionals 2008). Nurses' collaborative stage is large in scope. There are many actors of various origins, but the ones for each scene involving a specific situation should be carefully selected.

In a discussion of the frequency of collective action, accuracy and comparisons are most difficult due to the aforementioned data problems in this sector. In most nations, official or semiofficial data on industrial activities are only available long after they have taken place, if at all. Among the Member States, some countries have experienced more frequent collective activities and are more strike prone than others. Belgium, Ireland, France, Bulgaria, Spain, Italy, Greece, Cyprus, Denmark, Poland, Portugal, Finland, and Malta may be included in the top ranks of the Member States' collective action league. It is to be noted that considerable industrial activities have taken place in the health-care sector in Sweden, Denmark, Estonia, Lithuania, Portugal, France, Ireland, Latvia, Malta, and Poland. In fact, Poland has experienced a sharp increase in strike action, and the most frequent strikers have been health-care workers, especially nurses. Also, Maltese nurses have had their share of industrial actions over the past few years. Moreover, the public sector has been involved in high-profile conflict in some

254

Member States, such as Ireland, Lithuania, Romania, Germany, and Italy. (Carley et al. 2010; Curtarelli et al. 2013; European Foundation for the Improvement of Living and Working Conditions 2009a). Empirical studies have shown that higher levels of protest potential are affiliated with extreme dissatisfaction and perceived deprivation. It is usually the least satisfied and the groups that feel most deprived that are high on protest. However, it must be remembered that, in addition to perceived deprivation and dissatisfaction, there are other variables that serve as important contributors to protest potential.

Denmark has manifested a special strike pattern of many small strikes. In fact, it has been singled out as the most strike prone of the Nordic countries. Short but irregular work stoppages related to organizational issues have been a common occurrence in Spain as well. Strikes have become more common in Finland in the last two decades, culminating in the worst outbreak of nurses' industrial unrest for a generation in 2007. Finland has had a high level of industrial conflict. This situation results from the fact that workers' organizations are firmly entrenched at the local level. In addition, the trade union movement is pervaded with intense political rivalries, leading to inflated demands that have not been able to be accommodated in the confines of a centralized bargaining system. Also, important interunion and interconfederation competition has been prevalent (Finland: Ministry of Labour 2003; Ibison 2007; Lilja 1998; Lucio 1998).

Among the older Member States, Germany, Luxembourg, the Netherlands, Sweden, and Austria have lower overall collective action records. Also, in these countries strikes are not frequently used as a strategic weapon. The German strike record has been, in general, among the lowest in Europe. Here, there are limitations on strike actions, but it is noteworthy that intersectoral bodies have settled most conflicts in a peaceful fashion. The major strike of nurses and physicians, in 2006, was unique in that it was the first of its kind in fourteen years. Although the 2008 national strike of ten thousand health-care workers in Sweden that lasted over five weeks was singular, it is to be noted that the number of strikes has decreased and their range is limited in comparison to other European countries. In the Netherlands, as opposed to other Member States, an environment of industrial peace has prevailed. Major long-term disputes have been rare and even though the nation is near the bottom of the transnational strike league with Austria and Germany, it has experienced most types of industrial activities. Also, the United Kingdom has had fewer industrial conflicts than many other

Member States (Blanke and Rose 2005; Curtarelli et al. 2013; European Foundation for the Improvement of Living and Working Conditions 2009b; Federation of European Employers 2004, 2011; Jacobs 2005; Lovén 2009; Vandenbrande et al. 2007).

The newer Member States jointly have displayed the least amount of collective action. The level of activity has approximated one-quarter that of the others. Industrial measures are rarely undertaken at the workplace level in Romania and Latvia and Lithuania have been essentially strike free. The latter phenomenon is interesting in light of the fact that Latvia features the lowest standard of living in the area, the longest working hours, and the lowest salaries along with many other negative trends. Recently, in Lithuania, a court decision has impeded the right to strike (Carley 2008; Curtarelli et al. 2013; Karnite 2005; Tragakes 2008).

For the most part, throughout the EU, there is more collective action in the public than in the private sector. In the newer Member States, industry and manufacturing have been the areas most prone to conflict. They are followed by transportation and communications which, in turn, are followed by the broad public sector, including health care. Over an extended period of time, it has been health care or the health and social work sectors grouped together that have been most affected by industrial action in Belgium, Italy, Hungary, Poland, Ireland, and Slovakia (Carley 2008; European Foundation for the Improvement of Living and Working Conditions 2009a).

Moreover, physicians and nurses have responded in different fashion to strikes, according to some scholars (Chadwick and Thompson 2000), because of their diverse histories. On the one hand, physicians belong to a liberal profession with a long history. On the other, nurses are part of a new or neo-profession linked to both social status and gender questions and others concerning whether theirs is a profession or not. Lacking the power of medicine, the dominant health-care profession, industrial action has been selected by nurses for this reason. The power differential between the two groups, in part, can be explained by gender. The family serves as a model to illustrate relations between service providers and patients. In family terms, the father is equated with the physician, the mother with the nurse, and the patient with the child. Power differentials are evident in the economics of health care, as well as in its politics. The differential between the wages paid to physicians and nurses reflects a gender bias. Moreover, nurses have had to invoke industrial action more frequently than physicians because of gender and the power image affiliated with the profession. Having lacked the type of professional autonomy and influence that garners the respect of those in the managerial and governmental worlds, nurses have been forced to undertake collective action more often than their medical counterparts. Physicians, being more autonomous professionally and enjoying greater prestige, have been more fortunate in achieving their demands, most frequently, without resorting to strikes.

Alternate Dispute Resolution

As mentioned previously, in many Member States, collective action may only be taken after attempts have been made to resolve the dispute in question by other means. These efforts involve extra-judicial or alternate dispute resolution: conciliation, mediation, and arbitration. The scope of these procedures is to aid industrial partners, management, and labor, in their search for a viable solution to their disagreement without resorting to traditional legal structures. This objective has been sanctioned by the EU in its 1989 Community Charter of Fundamental Social Rights for Workers. Article 13 of this document reads: "In order to facilitate the statement of industrial disputes the establishment and utilization at the appropriate levels of conciliation, mediation and arbitration procedures should be encouraged in accordance with national practice."

Almost all countries in the EU have mechanisms, provided either by the state or the social partners themselves, for the resolution of industrial disputes that rely on these processes. A common feature of these procedures is intervention by an independent third party. The three techniques are distinguished on the nature and degree of this intervention. The most modest involvement of a third party is represented by conciliation. In seeking resolution of the disagreement, in this process, the third party acts as a facilitator to render certain dialogue and exchange of information between the conflicting parties. The role of the conciliator is to create a favorable climate for resolving the conflict and to encourage the parties to develop their own solutions. When mediation is used the third party has a more active role in that this person may actually suggest possible remedies to the problem and articulate opinions. The dividing line between conciliation and mediation is very fine. In fact, in some Member States, such as Malta, there is no recognition of the nuances between the two procedures and in others, principally, Estonia, Slovakia, and Slovenia, the boundaries between the two overlap.

In arbitration, the third party has the most active role. This person designs the solution to the dispute which is final. Conciliation and mediation are common features on the EU stage, whereas arbitration has a much more restricted role in the resolution of industrial disputes. Although alternate dispute resolution systems exist throughout the Member States, like other structures, they have been operationalized in diverse fashion in the various countries. All Member States adopt some, if not all, of these mechanisms. In the older ones, the seeds for these instruments have been nurtured by an industrial culture marked by concertation and cooperation over conflict. In the nations that have joined the EU most recently, alternate dispute resolution instruments only came into being in the last decade of the last century and the early years of the present one. Most of the extra-judicial systems in these countries are, for the most part, regulated by national legislation, whereas in the other Member States, they principally originated in and are governed by collective agreements. Greater heterogeneity, fragmentation, and fragility among the social partners in the newly acceded countries account for the diversity in the source of extra-judicial conflict resolution (Düvel et al. 2004; Welz and Kauppinen 2004).

Throughout the EU, one finds a wide range of extra-judicial institutions and procedures available for solving disputes. Welz and Kauppinen (2004) have classified these services in a useful manner. In many nations, the mechanisms are internal to public institutions. For example, the Maltese may turn to the Department of Industrial and Employment Relations, the Romanians to the Ministry of Labor, Equality of Chances and Family; the Portuguese to the Ministry of Employment, the Luxembourgish to the National Conciliation Office, and the Bulgarians to the National Institute for Reconciliation and Arbitration in the Ministry of Labor. Moreover, very often there are specific officials within the labor administration charged with conflict resolution responsibilities as in Belgium, Denmark, Finland, and Estonia.

In addition, there are independent public dispute resolution agencies. The Labor Relations Commission in Ireland, the National Mediation Office in Sweden, and the Labour Mediation and Arbitration Services Office in Hungary can be included in this category. In general, there is not a large population of these entities in the newest Member States. Another type of organization limited to Spain, Malta, and Greece is the private conflict resolution agency. Such obviously serves as an alternative to similar services offered by government. A practice that is not prevalent throughout the EU is the designation of a person to deal with the dispute that is independent of the official labor world. Where utilized, this being is selected from a list usually maintained by the Minister of Labor. Such a procedure has been adopted in the Czech Republic and Slovakia.

Voluntary, autonomous structures established by the social partners are also utilized in extra-judicial dispute resolution. This is the practice in Germany and many of the Central and East European Member States. As strange as it might seem, it is possible to speak of circumstances in which conflict resolution procedures and institutions are nonexistent, as in the Netherlands. Such has resulted from the significant influence of the social partners in the development of a highly functional system of collective bargaining and tripartite concertation. As previously mentioned, the incidence of industrial action is extremely low. It is interesting to note that when health-care workers experienced difficulty in reaching a collective agreement in 1998, it was the Prime Minister who served as the mediator. In situations such as this, methods for resolution of disputes are realized as needed.

Two relatively new developments related to alternate dispute resolution should be singled out for special attention. One concerns the new Irish health forum created, in 2007, for purposes of dealing with critical industrial relations issues related to reform of the health-care delivery system. More specifically, this body focuses on work practice issues and new work processes across the health sector, as well as the broad spectrum of nonpay matters. It brings together employers, trade union representatives, and a wide range of health-care workers, including physicians, nurses, those in clerical and administrative grades, therapists, and laboratory staff, as well as employees in various support grades. Its scope is notable. Another new method of alternate dispute resolution was introduced in Poland, in 2003. It relates to the so-called good-will missions. Essentially, the procedure allows a social dialogue commission to examine conflicts between management and labor and to determine if it is necessary for the maintenance of social peace to appoint someone to help resolve the dispute. The unique objective is to reduce the number of conflicts and to enlarge the territory of discussion by going beyond the legal realm and tackling social and economic matters as well (Sheehan 2008; Welz and Kauppinen 2004).

In spite of the diversity that pervades the various extra-judicial dispute resolution systems in the Member States, they do share common features. In the first place, utilization of these procedures does not preclude recourse to legal structures. Second, for the most part, these processes are completely separate from each other and use of one is not dependent on use of a specific other. Parties to disputes are free to choose one arrangement or another. Generally, not being standardized, but rather, more or less, formalized, the parties enjoy significant latitude for self-regulation. Third, all of these techniques are optional or compulsory depending on the type of dispute involved. Last, as far as the role of the third party is concerned, regardless of its form, whether an individual or a collegial unit, independence and impartiality are taken for granted. In addition, disputants are autonomous in selection of the third party and they can issue a challenge, if confidence fades (Düvel et al. 2004).

Alternate dispute resolution is a manifestation of an industrial culture based on social dialogue and it has performed an important role in the Member States. ICN has deemed this role to be of such significance that it urges national nursing associations to develop programs to familiarize and train nurses in their catchment area in the various techniques of extra-judicial dispute resolution (ICN 1999). Not only has this process strengthened social dialogue, but it is suitable for different types of conflicts, meaning it can be applied to individual or collective disputes as well as conflicts of rights and conflicts of interest. The first two types are self-explanatory. The latter two need definition. Rights disputes arise when employers and employees have differences of opinion on matters related to the conclusion, alteration, termination, or fulfillment of an agreement, as well as the application or interpretation of provisions of a collective agreement or work procedure regulations. Interest disputes are different in that they refer to diverse opinions concerning collective negotiation procedures and accord contents. These matters arise when a collective agreement is not in force. These extra-judicial mechanisms, in comparison to others, allow for flexibility and acceleration of decision-making time. Moreover, given the expertise and experience manifested by the third parties involved, the resultant solutions might be more appropriate. Also, in terms of cost, alternate dispute resolution is definitely less expensive and more cost effective than procedures within traditional legal structures (Düvel et al. 2004).

Dispute Resolution and the Courts

In addition to the extra-judicial processes, throughout the Member States, tribunals also play a large part in the settlement of industrial relations disputes. From the perspective of specialization, certain models are detected in the EU framework. In some instances, there is a completely separate court system specialized in labor law, as in Germany, where the system operates at the local, regional, and federal levels. Sentences issuing from the Federal Labour Court have been deemed as important as legislation as far as regulations in the realm of labor are concerned (de Silva 1998). It is interesting to note that at the local level, the judicial panel includes a judge by profession and two honorary nonpaid judges possessing equivalent legal powers, one appointed from the ranks of employers and one from those of employees. Although the systemic framework is different, the principle of the judicial panel is the same in Luxembourg, where it consists of a judge an employer, and union assessors (Jung 2001; Tunsch 1998).

In many Member States, such as Malta and Finland, there are special industrial tribunals with exclusive jurisdiction over employment and industrial relations conflicts, but not a separate system. In others, such as Hungary, the special labor courts enforce employment laws and agreements, but the affected parties may appeal the labor court's decision in a civil court. This latter procedure represents another model featuring courts specialized in labor law only at the first level of jurisdiction. Another situation is represented by the Swedish case. The Labour Court deals with disputes between social partners. However, parties not subject to collective agreements lodge their complaints with the civil court system and the Labour Court serves only as a last resort.

In addition, in the EU framework, there are specialized panels or departments within the common law court system that deal with industrial relations conflicts. And, in some cases, labor disputes are adjusted by common law courts. The legal patterns are multiple. As far as costs are concerned, here again, there is no uniformity. They are shared equally, sometimes they are paid by the government, or they are borne by a party to the dispute, usually the defeated one (Dimitriv 2007; Federation of European Employers 2004; Finland: Ministry of Labour 2003).

Summary and Conclusion

Nurses' industrial action throughout the EU has been generated by multiple issues. Some of the collective activities discussed in this chapter have only recently come to the newly acceded Member States, primarily because of their previous political orientation. Most of the actions undertaken by European nurses are familiar to their American counterparts. As in other instances, this discussion has highlighted variation in practice from one Member State to another. Not all activities are sanctioned throughout the EU. However, there is some communality in the guidelines related to nurses' collective action and to the vital role of alternate dispute resolution in the various nations. Given its development and composition, the variety of collective pursuits has been important to the profession and its agenda. Olzak and Ryo (2007) appropriately affirm: "Protest ensures continued public attention on issues that concern the movement's constituents, and thus it constitutes an important indicator of movement strength" (p. 1566). Many or most of these issues also affect the public in one manner or another. Collective instruments have been used in diverse ways, but public support and that of other workers and the media have been particularly helpful to the nursing profession. Moreover, even though it has been more active in other workplace issues, it is evident that the EU's orientation is supportive of collective action.

6

Member States, the European Union, and the Workplace

The EU has always had a social dimension. However, when the organization was born, there was a hesitancy to assign it a role in this sector. Thus, social policy features a limited and distinctive pattern of development (Geyer 2000). Subsidiarity as related to it dictated that Member States were to be masters of activities in the social realm, but in matters related to economic integration, Community accords were to prevail. De Gooijer (2007) questions whether the choices made in reference to social and economic policy decision-making were congruent in that the two sectors are so closely interrelated. It was assumed that the social dimension of European integration would flow indirectly from the establishment of the common market. Such did not occur. Free movement created social problems that did not evaporate. Spillover from economic pursuits dictated that the EU assumes some responsibility for social policy from the Member States.

Social policy traditionally "refers to the set of public policies that influence the well-being and life chances of individuals" (Anderson 2015, p. 2). Moreover, conventional definitions stress the collective organization and financing of such policies. In the EU framework, social policy has had a narrower meaning, referring to "actions to improve working conditions and living standards for workers" (Scappucci 1998, p. 249). EU social policy has focused, for the most part, on the employed, their rights, and needs within the common market. Having limited financial and administrative resources, the EU's role in the social sector has been principally regulatory and other actors have dealt with the monetary aspects of social policy.

In general, health-at-work issues have been of central importance to the individual Member States and the EU. It is generally acknowledged that a congenial work environment has a positive influence on the health and well-being of employees as well as on performance and productivity. Given the nature of the nursing profession, good physical and mental health is important to the individual practitioner. Controls in the workplace are crucial to health status. Many of the injuries and accidents that occur in the provision of health-care services are preventable. However, efforts related to prevention are less than complete due to the interests of efficiency and time pressures. These present obstacles to learning procedures and methods of carrying out duties that could diminish nurses' maladies (De Troyer 2000). Moreover, the perception of workplace hazards is a serious concern. However, if employees are properly informed, these perils may be dealt with in appropriate fashion and tempered. Such depends on the communication capacities of management. It is noteworthy that a recent report notes that in the EU health-care arena, workers are very well informed of workplace health and safety risks. In fact, the percentage of workers in this sector who claim to be not well informed of workplace hazards is much less than in all the twenty-eight Member States (European Working Conditions Observatory 2014).

Risks at the workplace have always been greater among the Central and East European Member States. Major reasons for this have been the inadequacies of the infrastructure and general economic challenges. In addition, regulation has not functioned as hoped. Responsibilities were devolved to local governments and institutions before the appropriate administrative structures were in place and authorities were trained to maintain proper oversight. Furthermore, the power of the trade unions, as noted, was compromised. Thus, positive and safe work environments, in general, and, in particular, improvement of the basic infrastructure and government supervision of workplace conditions were not assigned priority on the political agenda (Rosskam and Leather 2006).

Since transition these Member States have reported fewer injuries at work, fewer work-related illnesses, and fewer days of work lost due to these conditions. However, there is a difference between the conditions enjoyed by employees on paper and the reality they live. These announced tendencies have been attributed to underreporting of the workplace situation. This has occurred because of management's reluctance to acknowledge liability. Also, the practice results from weak trade union structures that frequently do not have the necessary resources to maintain reporting channels. On the other hand, it has been suggested that before the transition in many of these Member States, there was an overreporting of this information and that health-care staff would take advantage of sick leave up to an informal norm.

Such practices were evidently set aside when job insecurity raised its head after transition.

The result is that in the pre and posttransition periods very few reliable data concerning the physical and psychosocial work environments, work-related diseases, and injuries and working days lost are available. Data problems on this subject matter are not limited to the Central and East European Member States. ICN (2008b) has noted that a majority of governments fail to gather precise and up-to-date information on workplace matters as they relate to nurses, so it can serve as a point of departure for the development of effective occupational health and safety policies. It labeled this failure "a cause of great concern." Safe and secure work places are a prerequisite for a positive practice environment and they reap benefits for management, nurses, and patients.

Member States feature a galaxy of regulations and laws concerned with working life and work security protection against accidents and illness. Most of these have resulted from policies and guidelines issued by the EU and other international associations, such as the ILO. Others were nurtured by internal efforts. Regardless of their origin, programs concerning safety and health at work are of utmost significance. For the most part, as noted in this discussion, they focus on various facets of working life, including working time, the content and demands of work, the physical and psychosocial environment, management and leadership matters, organizational features, and staff relationships, among other elements. Most of these projects are part of a general occupational health policy that applies to the workforce. Frequently, in the health-care sector, there are particular systems, such as those concerned with monitoring risk factors, prevention of needle-stick injuries, etc. Some Member States have long-standing programs in this area and for others, they are a recent innovation.

The scope of such schemes is vast and promotional, preventive, and curative approaches are adopted. Activities are focused on the individual worker, workplaces, and society as a whole. Moreover, efforts cover the entire span of working life, from entry into the world of work until retirement. Unfortunately, in some Member States, exemplified by Denmark, Greece, and Portugal, regulations have not been fully implemented (Büscher, Sivertsen, and White 2010; Büscher and Wagner 2005; Hämäläinen and Lindström 2006). Safety and health protection at the workplace is closely related to the health of the individual workers, patient safety and outcomes, the health of society, institutional and general productivity, work ability, the nature and length of participation in the workforce, and recruitment and retention, to cite a few elements. Thus, it is understandable why occupational health and safety are an important part of the nursing agenda in most Member States.

EU interest in the workplace and specifically, in occupational health and safety policy has roots in the historical foundations of the organization. Its activities in this area surfaced in the early 1960s, but its role was somewhat constrained, in part, due to the fragile legal basis for the development of measures, limited political and social interest, and the requisite of unanimous voting in the Council. For more than two decades, action was greater and more significant at the national level of government. However, within the EU, it was during this period that the structures and debates that were to facilitate the future development of policies to regulate occupational health and safety took place.

It was the Single European Act of 1986 and the three EU treaty reforms negotiated during the 1990s that changed the political landscape and paved the way for an active supranational role. The former transformed processes with the introduction of qualified majority voting, now the most widely adopted voting process in the EU, and the provision of a new cooperation procedure with the EP on health and safety directives. Treaty revisions, enlarging the powers of the organization, modified the level of competences. Removal of the requirement for unanimous agreement on health and safety instruments meant Member States could no longer exercise a veto to block them. Thus, the way was paved for the EU to assume a new role in social policy. In fact, its contributions to and impact on occupational health and safety became substantial. At the base of the Commission's proposals has been the belief that national and EU policies should stimulate an environment at the workplace that allows employees to fully participate in working life and enhances personal health and well-being as well as that of the total society.

There is a galaxy of EU legal and nonlegal documents that relate to health, hygiene, and safety at work, in general, and, in particular, to workers exposed to specific risks, several of which have been cited in this discussion. Since 2000, an integrative part of the European Social Agenda and the European Employment Guidelines has been an improvement in the quality of work. The Charter of Fundamental Social Rights of Workers of the European Union specifically refers to the workers' rights as they relate to freedom of movement, employment and remuneration, social protection, freedom of association and collective bargaining, improvement of living and working conditions, vocational training, health protection and safety at the workplace, equal treatment for men and women, protection of children and adolescents, information, consultation and participation for workers, elderly persons and disabled persons. Such emphasis on workers disregarded the needs of many population groups. Because of the nature of this document and others, the EU's approach to social policy has been labeled rights-based (Barnard and Deakin 2012).

Various EU measures have been concerned with minimum safety requirements for the use of equipment at the workplace, workers' use of personal protective equipment, back injury risks, protection of workers from risks related to exposure to chemical, physical, and biological agents; use of safety and health signs at the workplace, information and consultation processes, safety and health of pregnant employees and those who have recently given birth or are nursing their offspring, control of major accident hazards, social security, nondiscrimination and equality at the workplace, annual leaves, working times, etc. The list is long which is surprising because at first the Member States were unwilling to give the EU a meaningful role in this sector. However, their view changed. They came to believe that certain aspects of health policy, such as the health and safety of workers understood in the broadest sense, given their relationship to the internal market, were better regulated on their behalf at the supranational level (Falkner et al. 2005; Mossialos and McKee 2002). Eventually, competences were extended to a wider range of work issues.

The main areas of supranational concern are health and safety, other working conditions, and equality between males and females at the workplace. Von Wahl (2005) observes:

> equal employment policy has taken a permanent hold within the EU and within its treaties, institutions, networks, and programs. A European equal employment regime has emerged amid nations, market, and supranational forces, pushing each of the national regime clusters to make specific legal and institutional adjustments through nonredistributive policies to increase employment access, openness and a nominally equal playing field (p. 90).

EU measures only occasionally refer specifically to health-care professionals. However, in the framework of the organization's employment law, it is understood that these providers are workers in the same sense as any other employee in any sector. Thus, EU mandates, concerning, for example, health and safety at work, nondiscrimination, and employment rights in the event of restructuring of the workplace, apply to all employees in the health sector and elsewhere (Hervey and McHale 2004; Hervey and Vanhercke 2010).

Of the extensive quantity of health and safety legislation adopted by the EU, the stellar instrument is the Council's Framework Directive 89/391/EEC, passed on 12 June 1989. A "command and control" model had been used for the regulation of health and safety prior to the approval of this directive. Failure on the part of institutions to meet detailed prescriptive requirements resulted in criminal prosecution. The result was a program characterized by rigidity and an inability to confront structural, technological, and social change (Walters 2002). The Framework manifested a significant shift in regulatory policy. It stressed the regulation of process as opposed to the previous regulation of substance. Focusing on processes, certain requirements for the management of health and safety became obligatory for employers. Thus, a series of general obligations were to be assumed by employers and employees to encourage improvements in workers' health and safety interpreted broadly. The new orientation required the Member States to cast aside prescriptive detailed legislation in favor of objective-oriented norms (Hämäläinen and Lindström 2006; Shaw, Hunt, and Wallace 2007).

In terms of its substantive provisions, the directive assigns employers responsibility for guaranteeing the complete health and safety of workers and developing a prevention program containing provisions for information and training, appropriate organization and the necessary means for operation. It also refers to protective and preventive services and their organization as well as worker information concerning safety and health risks. Moreover, workers are to be consulted and participate in the resolution of all matters related to the health and safety of the workplace. They are also to receive adequate health and safety training appropriate to their position. At the same time, they have an obligation to assume responsibility for their own and their colleagues' health and safety. All in all, as is evident, the new approach of the EU to regulation featured measures focusing on processes that beforehand were thought to be in the realm of management. Specification and performance standards were relegated to a lesser position. The Framework Directive sparked and set the stage for other directives concerned with health and safety at the workplace. Regulatory principles focus on "workplace risk assessment, participation, and use of competence to support and deliver health and safety management at the enterprise level" (Walters

2002, p. 40). Reactions throughout the Member States to this change in orientation were mixed.

More recently, the European Commission in a Communication (Commission of the European Communities 2007) issued its strategy for promoting health and safety at the workplace. It envisions that EU policies as well as those of the Member States will establish working environments that enable employees to participate fully in working life until they become senior citizens. The objective is to realize circumstances in which work enriches individuals' health and well-being, rather than impacting them in negative fashion, as is so often the case. Principal items in the Commission's strategy refer to the integration of health and safety into education and training programs, proper implementation of EU legislation, the adaptation of the legal framework to changes in the workplace, development and implementation of national strategies, programs to modify worker behavior, the adoption of health-focused approaches by employers, improvement in the methods of tracking progress, and promotion of health and safety at the international level. The program is ambitious and it is shared by the European Agency for Safety and Health at Work, the European Pact for Mental Health, and the European Network for Workplace Health Promotion.

Reference to proper implementation of EU legislation results from the fact that the degree to which it has been implemented varies a great deal from one Member State to another. Thus, due to this situation, in order to secure the cited objectives, mention is made in the Communication of national strategies and the particular areas they should cover. Prevention is underscored as is promotion of the rehabilitation and reintegration of workers. Dealing with social and economic change is singled out for attention along with the reinforcement of policy coherence via coordination at the national and supranational levels of health and safety policy with other closely related ones.

The Commission's 2014–20 program on health and safety at work is also concerned with the implementation of rules in this sector. It hopes to witness an improvement. In addition, it calls for improvement in the prevention of old and new work-related diseases and full consideration of ageing in the EU's workforce.

The EU, in addition to its activities in the area of general health and safety at the workplace, has also focused on specific workplace issues. The Framework Agreement on Work-related Stress (European Trade Union Confederation 2004) concluded by the European cross-industry social partners serves as an example. Its aim is to increase awareness and understanding of the problem and to provide an action-oriented framework to ideally prevent, but, at least, to control it. The EU makes use of many different mechanisms in constructing its programs. This Framework Agreement is an autonomous one, meaning it is not a legal instrument. Thus, implementation must follow the rules and procedures of each country's national industrial relations system. As discussed elsewhere, in each, the roles of the trade unions, employers' organizations and public authorities vary. The implementation process is diverse from that utilized to transpose EU directives and as a result, comparable outcomes cannot be expected (European Commission 2011)

The Agreement was significant because it generated awareness and consensus among the Member States as to the nature of work-related stress which is a structural problem related to work organization that affects individuals in diverse ways. Moreover, in these nations, dialogue and policy development on the issue blossomed. As a result, a majority of them now feature a legal framework focused on psychosocial risks and/or stress. Unfortunately, the Agreement has not been implemented throughout the entire EU and in some Member States, as in other cases, there has been only partial implementation. Consequently, levels of protection vary (European Commission 2011; *Social Partners* 2008).

The European Agency for Health and Safety at Work, using the motto "Healthy Workplaces: Good for You. Good for Business," launched a multiyear Healthy Workplace Campaign on Risk Assessment. Its purpose is the promotion throughout the EU of an integrated management approach that considers the various phases of risk assessment. Objectives include achieving a reduction in the number of deaths resulting from work-related accidents or occupational illnesses. Also, the campaign is aimed at decreasing the number of accidents at the workplace that cause three or more days of leave. In April 2012, the agency initiated a "Working Together for Risk Prevention" campaign whose purpose is to encourage organizations and management to collaborate with employees and their representatives to improve health and safety for all.

In the context of the EU an alternative to the standard legislative procedure is social dialogue. It is principally related to the sphere of social policy. This process requires that the Commission consult management and labor in the formulation of social policy law. Such an obligation reserves a role for these two forces in the EU's policy-making process. This is most important. Moreover, European level agreements reached by the social partners can set standards for all Member States which may be assigned legal force.

Reference has been made to nurses' potential to undergo sharps injuries. After extensive negotiations between the European social partners, in 2009, agreement was reached on their prevention. Signed by the European Hospital and Healthcare Employers' Association and the European Federation of Public Services Unions, the accord aims at setting minimum standards for the prevention of needle stick and other sharp instrument injuries at work. It applies to all health-care providers employed in the public and private sectors as well as in any other site providing health services. The objective is to be accomplished through the use of risk assessment, risk prevention, training, information, and awareness raising and monitoring programs. As in other supranational initiatives, employee participation is mandated. Furthermore, the agreement is closely related to a primary aim of the Commission's aforementioned program to reduce workplace accidents throughout the EU by 25 percent. Implementation of the agreement was detailed in Council Directive 2010/32/EU. It was provided that Member States are responsible for developing the laws, regulations, and administrative provisions necessary for enforcement. In addition, each nation is to determine the nature of the sanctions to be applied when national norms pertaining to the agreement are violated. All necessary measures were to be in place by May 2013.

In this context, reference must again be made to Convention 149 and Recommendation 157 of the ILO (1977a, 1977b), both of which are concerned with the employment and working conditions of nurses. ILO conventions are legally binding instruments in ratifying countries and recommendations are nonbinding. The latter supplement conventions by providing additional orientation and guidance for national policy and action. In short, they serve as guides for implementation. These instruments are among the few that specifically refer to nurses. Although they were approved in 1977, the ILO classifies both documents as still of significance because, in many places, the conditions that nurtured them continue to exist. Their purpose was to supplement general international standards with those specific to nursing. Based on the notion that occupational health and safety laws and regulations should be congruent with nursing practice and the environment in which it is carried out, the Convention affirmed the need to adapt workplace practices to the special conditions of nurses' work world.

The Recommendation further developed measures to prevent, reduce, or eliminate hazards to nurses' health. It referred to establishment of a comprehensive national policy on occupational health, the creation of occupational health services, access to health surveillance, financial compensation for those exposed to special risks, and broad participation in all facets of protection provisions. The purpose of such initiatives was to reinforce nurses' rights and to offer guidelines to policy makers, employers, and employees in the development of nursing policies. Many aspects of nurses' realm outside of occupational health and safety were supported as well in these instruments. In terms of their content, both documents could have been written today.

A major requisite for the realization of EU goals concerning economic growth and integration, employment, and social cohesion is the elimination of all forms of workplace abuse. Various institutions of the EU have been involved in this effort as well. In fact, gender equality has always been central to EU social policy development. Also, problems of discrimination based on race and ethnic origin have been spoken to with force via Council Directive 2000/43/EC of 29 June 2000. This document stressed the need to foster a socially inclusive labor force based on the principle of equal treatment and it set forth minimum requirements for its achievement. Given the previous discussion concerning reasons for failure to report abuse, its mandate to Member States to protect victims from adverse treatment resulting from a complaint is noteworthy. Victimization was recognized. In addition, a general framework for equal treatment in employment has been established with Council Directive 2000/78/EC of 27 November 2000. This document specifically addresses access to employment, training opportunities, work conditions, equality before the law, and adequate means of protection against direct and indirect discrimination and it refers specifically to discrimination based on religion or belief, disability, age, or sexual orientation.

Of major importance is Directive 2006/54/EC, a work that serves as an umbrella in that it groups into one, several directives issued over time on many issues related to workplace abuse. It focuses on implementation of the principles of equal opportunity and equal treatment of both sexes in matters of employment and education. A galaxy of other documents, such as Directive 2002/73/EC of the European Parliament and of the Council of 23 September 2002, relate to many of the above-mentioned subjects, including promotion, training, access to employment, working conditions, and the protection of dignity. The list is extremely long.

As part of wider efforts to ensure equal opportunities and a healthy work environment, EU institutions have taken actions to promote greater awareness at all levels of the various facets of sexual harassment. More specifically, the Commission's Recommendation on the Protection of the Dignity of Women and Men at Work (92/131/EEC of 27 November 1991) examined issues that necessitate a change in male behavior. This particular document went beyond the equal opportunity objectives of EU law and it contained a code of practice to combat sexual harassment. Furthermore, it issued a call for Member States to implement this code in the public sector so as to serve as a model for the private sector. The problem is that, throughout the Member States, there are a variety of definitions as to what constitutes harassment and the situation becomes more complex, due to low levels of enforcement or penalty (von Wahl 2005). In addition to other policy statements, a Communication from the Commission (European Commission 2006) provides a roadmap for equality between men and women. Among the priority areas identified for action on the part of the EU were eradication of all forms of gender-based violence and elimination of gender stereotypes.

It was really the Amsterdam Treaty of 1997 that significantly increased the power of the EU to confront many of the facets of workplace violence as discussed here. This document amended the Treaty on European Union, the Treaties establishing the European Communities, as well as certain related acts. The Treaty of Rome prohibited discrimination on the basis of nationality (Article 6) and discrimination based on sex, but only in reference to equal pay (Article 119). The EU could only legislate on matters of equality according to these provisions. The principle on which they were based was reinforced in the Amsterdam agreement. It acknowledged that the responsibilities of the Commission now included the promotion of equality between the sexes. The word promotion should be stressed. Moreover, the EU was obligated to eliminate existing inequalities between men and women (Article 3). Not only was responsibility pinpointed, but the scope of action was enlarged in the more recent document. A stellar feature of this treaty was Article 13 which formally recognized human rights. There had been no direct reference to general antidiscrimination in previous documents. The Council was now empowered to take appropriate action to combat discrimination based on sex, race, or ethnic origin, religion or belief, disability, age, and sexual orientation. These new provisions widened the EU's field of action to include what had been strictly within the limits of national preserves.

EU institutions have taken seriously their efforts to erase the various types of workplace abuse and violence. In addition to developing policies on the subject, they conscientiously monitor the Member States' implementation of these efforts. The Commission has been especially proactive. Prominent concerns have been the Council Directive 2000/43/EC, the Race Equality Directive, and Council Directive 2000/78/EC, the Employment Equality Directive. This unit started proceedings against the Czech Republic, in 2007, because it believed that this Member State failed to transpose these directives in an appropriate manner. Moreover, in 2010, it referred Poland to the CJEU for failure to fully implement EU rules prohibiting discrimination on the basis of race or ethnic origin. The Commission has also issued warnings to the governments of Austria, Belgium, and Poland in specific reference to Directive 2006/54/EC. These advisories referred to these governments' failure to communicate appropriate national legislation implementing established EU norms against gender discrimination in employment.

In addition, the Commission has established an organ for the purpose of coordinating its efforts and those of the Member States. It founded the European Network of Equality Bodies which brings together under its aegis independent national gender equality units for the promotion of equality and the erasure of discrimination in sectors covered by the European Union Equal Treatment Directives. Also, of note, is the agreement signed by the social partners in April 2007, as part of the European social dialogue process. This was a framework accord to combat harassment and violence at the workplace. It was to be implemented within three years in accordance with procedures and practices specific to management and labor in the Member States.

All of these efforts and many others are valiant and of pertinence to nurses. However, in seeking to control violence at the workplace, special consideration should be given to a research finding which indicated that patients and nurses, having been involved in abusive behavior, had diverse views concerning the causes and management of this violence (Duxbury and Whittington 2005). Most studies of abusive behavior in the health sector have focused on the perspective of nurses, not patients. The views of the latter merit further intensive exploration and consideration in the design of policies to manage violence in healthcare institutions. Much has been done to combat the various types of workplace violence experienced by nurses, but unfortunately, much remains to be done.

Citation of these legal and nonlegal mechanisms, although few in terms of those that could be cited, indicates the seriousness of purpose and wide scope of interest, particularly on the part of the EU and other international organizations as well, in the state of conditions in nurses' world of work and their impact. These efforts must be recognized in conjunction with those at the national level. These endeavors and their orientation are significant in that they address many issues discussed in this volume.

The major dimensions of working conditions concerned with job quality are a determinant of the well-being of workers. These themes are a major thrust of the EU's social policy. The organization has shown ambition in this area. There are numerous directives, regulations, and recommendations that regulate employment and the workplace across the Member States. Equality, health and safety, and working conditions provide the rubrics for these efforts. In addition to the legal documents cited in this discussion, there are also those concerned with other working conditions, such as workplace ventilation, fire prevention, quality of lighting, conditions of work with visual display units, handling of heavy loads, etc. Excluded from EU harmonization are workers' remuneration, the right of association, the right to strike and the right to impose lockouts. EU social policy has focused on health and safety, other working conditions, and equality between males and females in the workplace. Of these three sectors, the first has received the most attention (Falkner et al. 2009). Given these efforts, nurses are guaranteed protection by European and Member States' employment law.

Directives establish the minimum standards for employment of individuals and they are supposed to be integrated into the domestic legislation of each Member State. Such does not take place uniformly. As a result, the latter can and does vary from minimum to maximum standards throughout the confines of the EU. This discussion has identified diversities in transposition. Research (Börzel et al. 2010) has found that some Member States fail to comply with EU laws more often than others. Most likely to do so are the powerful ones, especially those with less administrative capacity. On the other hand, the small Member States with efficient bureaucracies tend to be the best compliers. As noted, throughout the Member States, there are many divergent rules and standards related to the workplace. However, it must be recognized that they are less in number than what might have been without EU efforts.

Historically, social policy, especially that which concerned health and safety and work conditions, has been affiliated with the so-called hard regulations or directives. In fact, after 1990, use of this instrument increased significantly. Binding minimum norms have dominated the social policy arena and especially, the facet related to work conditions (Falkner et al. 2009). More recently, soft regulations and the Open Method of Coordination have been adopted in this field. In addition, the EU has also nurtured European-level social dialogue and the same process in the national and sectoral levels as it relates to work conditions (Adams and Kennedy 2006; Keune 2008).

Efforts have been undertaken at the supranational and national levels that relate to the creation of healthy workplaces. Promotion of positive practice environments is vital. It benefits job satisfaction and well being, health-care providers' and organizational performance, patient outcomes, innovations, professional recruitment and retention, the prevention of the adverse effects of psychosocial and other negative factors at work, and health-care delivery, in general. These advantages have been substantiated and they have been linked to the multifaceted efforts of a broad spectrum of actors, including nurses associations (Baumann 2007; International Council of Nurses et al. 2008b). Efforts should be multiple and coordinated, involving several sectors. Achievement of a healthy workplace broadly interpreted represents a "win–win" situation for all.

References[*]

Adams, E. (2011, June). "Public Health Systems Under Pressure." *ICHRN Newsletter* 5(1):1–2.

Adams, E., & Kennedy, A. (2006). *Positive Practice Environments: Key Considerations for the Development of a Framework to Support the Integration of International Nurses.* Geneva, Switzerland: International Centre on Nurse Migration.

Adnett, N., & Hardy, S. (2001). "Reviewing the Working Time Directive: Rationale, Implementation and Case Law." *Industrial Relations Journal* 32(2):114–125.

Afford, C., & Lessof, S. (2006). "The Challenge of Transition in CEE and the NIS of the Former USSR." In C.–A. Dubois, M. McKee, & E. Nolte (Eds.), *Human Resources for Health in Europe* (pp. 193–213). Maidenhead, Berkshire, England: Open University Press.

"Agency Nurse Plans Cause Disruption in Ireland." (2011, June). *ICHRN Newsletter* 5(1):4–5.

Agenda for Change Project Team. (2004). *Agenda for Change: Final Agreement.* London: Department of Health.

Ahlberg, K., & Bruun, N. (2005). "Sweden: Transition Through Collective Bargaining." *Bulletin of Comparative Labour Relations* (56):117–143.

Aiken, L. H. (2007). "Nurse Staffing Impact on Organizational Outcomes." In D. J. Mason, S. K. Leavitt, & M. W. Chaffee (Eds.), *Policy and Politics in Nursing and Health Care* (pp. 550–559). St Louis, MO: Saunders Elsevier.

Aiken, L. H. (2011). *RN4CAST: Evidence from Europe and the U.S. for Improving Nurse Retention and Patient Outcomes.* Paper prepared for delivery at the International Society for Quality in Health Care 28th International Conference, Hong Kong, 14–17 September, 2011.

Aiken, L. H., Clarke, S. P., & Sloane, D. M. (2002). "Hospital Staffing, Organization, and Quality of Care: Cross-National Findings." *International Journal for Quality in Health Care* 14(1):5–13.

Aiken, L., Clarke, S. P., Sloane, D. M., Sochalski, J., & Silber, J. H. (2002). "Hospital Nurse Staffing and Patient Mortality, Nurse Burnout, and Job Dissatisfaction." *JAMA: The Journal of the American Medical Association* 288(16):1987–1993.

Aiken, L., & Sloane, D. (2002). "Hospital Organization and Culture." In M. McKee, & J. Healy (Eds.), *Hospitals in a Changing Europe* (pp. 265–278). Buckingham, England and Philadelphia, PA: Open University Press.

---

[*]Documents issued by European Union institutions may be found on the official web site of the European Union (www.europa.eu). Those issued by Member States may be located on the web sites of the individual national government concerned. Dates are cited for materials retrieved from the internet when a site has been archived or the particular work is no longer available.

Albreht, T. (2011). "Addressing Shortages: Slovenia's Reliance on Foreign Health Professionals, Current Developments and Policy Responses." In M. Wismar, C. B. Maier, I. A. Glinos, G. Dussault, & J. Figueras (Eds.), *Health Professional Mobility and Health Systems: Evidence From 17 European Countries* (pp. 511–538). Copenhagen, Denmark: World Health Organization on behalf of the European Observatory on Health Systems and Policies.

Albreht, T., Turk, E., Toth, M., Ceglar, J., Marn, S., Pribaković, R., et al. (2009). "Slovenia: Health System Review." *Health Systems in Transition* 11(3):1–168.

Alda, K. (2006, September 6). "Czech Nurses Flocking to Austria." *The Prague Post*. Retrieved from www.praguepost.com

Alexis, O., Vydelingum, V., & Robbins, I. (2007). "Engaging with a New Reality: Experiences of Overseas Minority Ethnic Nurses in the NHS." *Journal of Clinical Nursing* 16(12):2221–2228.

Alford, C. W. (2003). *Corrosive Reform: Failing Health Systems in Eastern Europe.* Geneva, Switzerland: International Labour Office.

Allinger, B. (2014, January 28). *Austria: Tackling Low Pay for Part-Time Workers.* Retrieved from www.eurofound.europa.eu

Amoah, C. F. (2011). "The Central Importance of Spirituality in Palliative Care." *International Journal of Palliative Nursing* 17(7):353–358.

An Bord Altranais & National Council for the Professional Development of Nursing and Midwifery. (2005). *Final Report 2005: Review of Nurses and Midwives in the Prescribing and Administration of Medicinal Products.* Dublin, Ireland: Authors.

Anderson, K. M. (2015). *Social Policy in the European Union.* London: Palgrave.

Arnold, J., Loan-Clarke, J., Coombs, C., Park, J., Wilkinson, A., & Preston, D. (2003). *Looking Good?: The Attractiveness of the NHS as an Employer to Potential Nurses and Allied Health Professional Staff: Final Report: A Report Prepared for the Department of Health Based on Research Conducted as Part of the Human Resources Research Initiative.* Retrieved from www.lboro.ac.uk

Arrowsmith, J., & Mosse, P. (2000). "Health Care Reform and the Working Time of Hospital Nurses in England and France." *European Journal of Industrial Relations* 6(3):283–306.

Asenova, D., & McKinnon, R. (2007). "The Bulgarian Pension Reform: Post-Accession Issues and Challenges." *Journal of European Social Policy* 17(4):389–396.

Associated Press. (2010, December 8). "Romania Gov't Cuts Maternity Leave." *Boston Globe*. Retrieved from www.boston.com

Audric, S., Niel, X., Sicart, D., & Vilain, A. (2001). "Les professions de santé: éléments d'informations statistiques [Health care professions: Elements of statistical information]." *Dossiers solidarité et santé*, N°. 1:115–136.

B., P. D. (2007, 10-16 luglio). "Rinnovi contrattuali, si parte [Contract renewals are beginning]." *Il Sole 24 Ore: Sanità*, p. 10.

Babić-Banaszak, A., Kovacić, L., Mastilica, M., Babić, S., Ivanković, D., & Budak, A. (2001). "The Croatian Health Survey – Patient's Satisfaction with Medical Service in Primary Health Care in Croatia." *Collegium Antropologicum* 25(2):449–458.

Bach, S. (1999). "From National Pay Determination to Qualified Market Relations: NHS Pay Bargaining Reform." *Historical Studies in Industrial Relations* 8:99–115.

Bach, S. (2003). *International Migration of Health Workers: Labour and Social Issues* (International Labour Office Working Paper No. 209). Geneva, Switzerland: International Labour Office.

References

Bach, S. (2004). "Employee Participation and Union Voice in the National Health Service." *Human Resource Management Journal* 14(2):3–19.

Bach, S. (n.d. -a). *Labour and Social Dimensions of Privatization and Restructuring: Health Services (Prepared for the International Labour Office Action Programme on Privatization, Restructuring and Economic Democracy).* n.p.: International Labour Organization.

Bach, S. (n.d. -b). *Restructuring and Privatization of Health Care Services: Selected Cases in Western Europe (Prepared for the International Labour Office Action Programme on Privatization, Restructuring and Economic Democracy).* n.p.: International Labour Organization.

Bae, S.-H., Mark, B., & Fried, B. (2010). "Impact of Nursing Unit Turnover on Patient Outcomes in Hospitals." *Journal of Nursing Scholarship* 42(1):40–49.

Bakker, A. B., Killmer, C. H., Siegrist, J., & Schaufeli, W. B. (2000). "Effort-Reward Imbalance and Burnout Among Nurses." *Journal of Advanced Nursing* 31(4):884–891.

Balabanova, D., & McKee, M. (2002). "Understanding Informal Payments for Health Care: The Example of Bulgaria." *Health Policy* 62:243–273.

Ball, J., & Pike, G. (2003). *Nurses in the Independent Sector: Results from the RCN Membership Surveys 2001/02.* London: Royal College of Nursing.

Ball, J., & Pike, G. (2005). *Nurses in Northern Ireland 2005: Results for Northern Ireland from RCN Employment Survey 2005.* London: Royal College of Nursing.

Ball, J., & Pike, G. (2006a). *At Breaking Point? A Survey of the Well-Being and Working Lives of Nurses in 2005.* London: Royal College of Nursing.

Ball, J., & Pike, G. (2006b). *Results from an On-Line Survey of Bank and Agency Nurses.* London: Royal College of Nursing.

Ball, J., & Pike, G. (2007). *Independent Sector Nurses in 2007: Results by Sector from the RCN Annual Employment Survey 2007.* London: Royal College of Nursing.

Ball, J., & Pike, G. (2009). *Past Imperfect, Future Tense: Nurses' Employment and Morale in 2009.* London: Royal College of Nursing.

Ballebye, M., & Nielsen, H. O. (2009, November 17). *Working Time in the European Union: Denmark.* Retrieved from www.eurofound.europa.eu

Ban, C. (2002, 17–23 dicembre). "Il mobbing attacca in corsia [Mobbing assails hospital wards]." *Il Sole 24 Ore: Sanità*, p. 36.

Barnard, C., & Deakin, S. (2012). "Social Policy and Labor Market Regulation." In E. Jones, A. Menon, & S. Weatherhill (Eds.), *The Oxford Handbook of the European Union* (pp. 542–555). Oxford: Oxford University Press.

Barnes, S. H., Farah, B. G., & Heunks, F. (1979). "Personal Dissatisfaction." In S. H. Barnes, & M. Kaase (and Allerback, K. R., Farah, B., Heunks, F., Inglehart, R., Jennings, M. K., Klingemann, H. D., et al.) (Eds.), *Political Action: Mass Participation in Five Western Democracies* (pp. 381–407). Beverly Hills, CA and London: Sage Publications.

Barosová, M. (2005, September 6). *Nurses are Protesting.* Retrieved from www.eurofound.europa.eu

Barros, P., Machado, S. R., & Simões. J. (2011). "Portugal: Health System Review." *Health Systems in Transition* 13(4):1–156.

Barros, P., & Simões, J. de A. (2007). "Portugal: Health System Review." *Health Systems in Transition* 9(5):1–140.

Bartoloni, M. (2007, 27 febbraio -5 marzo). "I rischi di chi lavora in corsia [Risks for he who works in hospital wards]." *Il Sole 24 Ore: Sanità*, p. 31.

279

Basso, R., & Salmaso, D. (2004). "La soddisfazione lavorativa dell'infermiere di assistenza domiciliare: Un indagine conoscitiva [A study of home care nurses' work satisfaction]." *Professioni Infermieristiche* 57(3):181–186.

Baumann, A. (2007). *Positive Practice Environments: Quality Workplaces = Quality Patient Care*. Geneva, Switzerland: International Council of Nurses.

Baumann, A. (2010). *The Impact of Turnover and the Benefit of Stability in the Nursing Workforce*. Geneva, Switzerland: International Council of Nurses.

Beekman, R. (2007, December 14). "Bulgarian Nurses Protest Over Salary, Exodus Medical Workers." *The Sofia Echo*. Retrieved from www.sofiaecho.com

Beese, B. (2006, September 6). *New Collective Agreement for Public Sector*. Retrieved from www.eurofound.europa.eu/eiro/2006/06/articles/de0606029i. htm

Beishon, S., Satnam, V., & Hagell, A. (1995). *Nursing in a Multi-Ethnic NHS*. London: Policy Studies Institute.

Belcher, D. K., & Hart, B. G. (2005). "Perspectives on Nursing Education in Poland." *International Journal of Nursing Education Scholarship* 2(1):Article 32. Retrieved from www.bepress.com/ijnes

Bennett, J., Davey, B., & Harris, R. (2007). *Nurses Working in Mid-Life: Final Report*. London: Nursing Research Unit King's College.

Berg, A. (1999, May 28). *Nurses Resign to Seek Better Pay and Conditions*. Retrieved from www.eurofound.europa.eu

Berry, P. A., Gillespie, G. L., Gates, D., & Schofer, J. (2012). "Novice Nurse Productivity Following Workplace Bullying." *Journal of Nursing Scholarship* 44(1):80–87.

Bessière, S. (2005). "La féminisation des professions de santé en France: Données de cadrage [Feminization of the health-care professions in France: Structural data]." *Revue Française des Affaires Sociales* 59(1):19–33.

Bilefsky, D. (2009, June 14). "Wanted: Czech Nurses. Bonus: Free Breast Implants." *New York Times*. Retrieved from www.nytimes.com

Bjorn, T. L. (2012, September 28). *New Studies on the Long-Term Effects of Bullying*. Retrieved from www.eurofound.europa.eu

Björnsdóttir, K., & Thome, M. (2006). "Specialist in Nursing: Role, Regulation and Education." *Nursing Journal* 1(1):28–36.

Blais, K. K., Hayes, J. S., Kozier, B., & Erb, G. (2006). *Professional Nursing Practice: Concepts and Perspectives*. Upper Saddle River, NJ: Pearson Prentice Hall.

Blanke, T. (2005a). "Foreword: Collective Bargaining and Wages in Comparative Perspective: Germany, France, the Netherlands and Sweden and United Kingdom." *Bulletin of Comparative Labour Relations* (56): ix–x.

Blanke, T. (2005b). "Outlook – Chances of European Harmonization or Coordination of Collective Wage Formation." *Bulletin of Comparative Labour Relations* (56):159–168.

Blanke, T., & Rose, E. (2005). "Erosion or Renewal? The Crisis of Collective Wage Formation in Germany." *Bulletin of Comparative Labour Relations* (56):5–29.

Blum, K. (2006). *Nurse Practitioners in Eastern Germany*. Gütersloh, Germany: Health Policy Monitor.

Boerma, W., & Genet, N. (2012). "Introduction and Background." In N. Genet, W. Boerma, M. Kroneman, A. Hutchinson, & R. B. Saltman (Eds.), *Home Care Across Europe: Current Structure and Future Challenges* (pp. 1–23). Copenhagen, Denmark: World Health Organization.

Boerma, W. G. W. (2006). "Coordination and Integration in European Primary Care." In R. B. Saltman, A. Rico, & W. G. W. Boerma (Eds.), *Primary Care in the Driver's Seat? Organizational Reform in European Primary Care* (pp. 3–21). Maidenhead, Berkshire, England: Open University Press.

Bonanni, A. (2010, 4 giugno). "Pensioni, ultimatum Ue all'Italia [Pensions, EU ultimatum to Italy]." *La Repubblica*, p. 20.

Bonitz, D. (2000). *Sick Leave Data for Jobs in German Hospitals as an Indicator of Health Impairing Working Conditions.* Presentation at the TUTB-SALTSA Conference, 25–27 September 2000, Brussels, Belgium.

van der Boom, H. (2008). *Home Nursing in Europe.* Amsterdam: Aksant

Borg, A. (2012, January 6). *Unions' Role in Combating Workplace Discrimination.* Retrieved from www.eurofound.europa.eu

Börzel, T. A., Hofmann, T., Panke, D., & Sprungk, C. (2010). "Obstinate and Inefficient: Why Member States Do Not Comply with European Law." *Comparative Political Studies* 43(11):1363–1390.

van den Bossche, S. (2005, October 24). *Workplace Violence Stabilising in the Netherlands.* Retrieved from www.eurofound.europa.eu

Bourbonniere, M., Feng, Z., Intrator, O., & Others. (2006). "The Use of Contract Licensed Nursing Staff in U.S. Nursing Homes." *Medical Care Research and Review* 63(1):88–109.

Bourgeault, I. L., Kuhlmann, E., Neiterman, E., & Wrede, S. (2008). *How Can Optimal Skill Mix Be Effectively Implemented and Why?* Copenhagen, Denmark: WHO Regional Office for Europe.

Bourgueil, Y., Marek, A., & Mousques, J. (2005*). La participation des infirmières aux soins primaires dans six pays européens et au Canada [Nurses' participation in primary care in six European countries and Canada]* (No. 406). Paris: Observatoire National de la Démographie des Professions de Santé (ONDPS).

Bouten, R., & Versieck, K. (1995). *Manpower Problems in the Nursing/Midwifery Profession in the EC*: Vol. 2. *Country Reports: Italy, Ireland, Luxembourg, Netherlands, Portugal, United Kingdom.* Leuven, Belgium: Katholieke Universiteit Leuven & Hoger Instituut voor de Arbeid.

Breuil-Genier, P. (2003). *Honoraires et revenus des professions de santé en milieu rural ou urbain [Health-care professionals' honoraria and income in rural or urban areas]* (No. 254). Paris: Observatoire National de la Démographie des Professions de Santé (ONDPS).

Brewer, C. S., Kovner, C. T., Wu, Y. W., & Others. (2006). "Factors Influencing Female Registered Nurses' Work Behaviour." *Health Services Research* 41(3):860–886.

Bridges, J., & Hyde, P. (2007). "Outcomes of Variation in Hospital Nurse Staffing in English Hospitals: More Nurses, Working Differently?" *International Journal of Nursing Studies* 44(2):171–174.

"British Nurses Stressed Out, Underpaid, Undervalued and Their Sex Lives Suffer." (2007, May 29). *The Medical News.* Retrieved from www.news-medical.net/news/2007/05/29/25699.aspx

Bromo, C., & Bartolucci, G. (2005). "Il mobbing nell'ambiente infermieristico: Indagine esplorativa in una ASL Toscana [Mobbing in the nursing sector: An exploratory study of a Tuscan ASL]." *Professioni Infermieristiche* 58(4):208–214.

Brown, A., & Kirpal, S. (2004). "'Old Nurses with New Qualifications are Best': Competing Ideas About the Skills That Matter in Nursing in Estonia, France,

Germany and the United States." In C. Warhurst, I. Grugulis, & E. Keep (Eds.), *The Skills That Matter* (pp. 225–241). Basingstoke, England: Palgrave MacMillan.

Bruyneel, L. (2011). *Patients' Perception of Hospital Care and Its Relation to Nursing Workforce Factors.* Presentation at the ICN Conference on Nurses Driving Access, Quality and Health, Valletta, Malta, 2–8 May, 2011.

Buchan, J. (2004, June 7). "What Difference Does ("Good") HRM Make?" *Human Resources for Health*, pp. 1–7. Retrieved from www.ncbi.nlm.nih.gov/pmc/articles/PMC425601

Buchan, J. (2007). *Nurse Workforce Planning in the UK: A Report for the Royal College of Nursing.* London: Royal College of Nursing.

Buchan, J., & Calman, L. (2005). *Skill-Mix and Policy Change in the Health Workforce: Nurses in Advanced Roles* (OECD Health Working Papers No. 17). Paris: Organisation for Economic Co-operation and Development.

Buchan, J., & Dal Poz, M. R. (2002). "Skill Mix in the Health Care Workforce: Reviewing the Evidence." *Bulletin of the World Health Organization* 80(7): 575–580.

Buchan, J., & Evans, D. (2008). "Assessing the Impact of a New Health Sector Pay System Upon NHS Staff in England." *Human Resources for Health* 6:12. Retrieved from www.human-resources-health.com/content/6/1/12

Buchan, J., & Maynard, A. (2006). "United Kingdom." In B. Rechel, C.-A. Dubois, & M. McKee (Eds.), *The Health Care Workforce in Europe: Learning from Experience* (pp. 129–142). Copenhagen, Denmark: WHO Regional Office for Europe on behalf of the European Observatory on Health Systems and Policies.

Buchan, J., O'May, F., & Dussault, G. (2013). "Nursing Workforce Policy and the Economic Crisis: A Global Overview." *Journal of Nursing Scholarship* 45(3):298–307.

Buchan, J., & Seccombe, I. (2006). *From Boom to Bust? The UK Nursing Labour Market Review 2005/6.* London: Royal College of Nursing.

"Bulgaria has the Longest Maternity Leave in the EU." (2008, October 5). *Bulgaria Gazette.* Retrieved from www.bulgariagazette.com/bulgaria-has-the-longest-maternity-leave-in-the-eu

Burau, V. (1999). "The Politics of Internal Boundaries – A Comparative Analysis of Community Nursing in Britain and Germany: Some Preliminary Observations." In I. Hellberg, M. Saks, & C. Benoit (Eds.), *Professional Identities in Transition: Cross-Cultural Dimensions* (pp. 239–253). Göteborg, Sweden: Göteborg University.

Büscher, A., Sivertsen, B., & White, J. (2010). *Nurses and Midwives: A Force for Health.* Copenhagen, Denmark: WHO Regional Office for Europe.

Büscher, A., & Wagner, L. (2005). *Munich Declaration: Nurses and Midwives: A Force for Health – Analysis of Implementation of the Munich Declaration 2004.* Copenhagen, Denmark: WHO Regional Office for Europe.

Busse, R., & Blümel, M. (2014). "Germany: Health Systems Review." *Health Systems in Transition* 16(2):1–296.

Busse, R., & Schlette, S. (Eds.). (2004). *Health Policy Developments: Focus on Health and Aging, Pharmaceutical Policy and Human Resources.* Gütersloh, Germany: Verlag Bertelsmann Stiftung.

Cabrita, J., & Galli da Bino, C. (2013, June 26). *EU Countries: Developments in Collectively Agreed Working Time: 2012.* Retrieved from www.eurofound.europa.eu

References

Camerino, D., Conway, P. M., van der Heijden, B. I. J. M., Estryn-Behar, M., Consonni, D., Gould, D., et al. (2006). "Low-Perceived Work Ability, Ageing and Intention to Leave Nursing: A Comparison Among 10 European Countries." *Journal of Advanced Nursing* 56(5):542–552.

Camerino, D., Conway, P. M., van der Heijden, B. I. J. M., Estryn-Behar, M., Costa, G., & Hasselhorn, H.-M. (2008a). "Age-Dependent Relationships Between Work Ability, Thinking of Quitting the Job, and Actual Leaving Among Italian Nurses: A Longitudinal Study." *International Journal of Nursing Studies* 45(11):1645–1659.

Camerino, D., Conway, P. M., Sartori, S., Campanini, P., Estryn-Behar, M., van der Heijden, B. I., et al. (2008b). "Factors Affecting Work Ability in Day and Shift-Working Nurses." *Chronobiology International* 25(2):425–442.

Camerino, D., Estryn-Behar, M., Conway, P. M., van der Heijden, B. I. J. M., & Hasselhorn, H.-M. (2008c). "Work-Related Factors and Violence Among Nursing Staff in the European NEXT Study: A Longitudinal Cohort Study." *International Journal of Nursing Studies* 45(1):35–50.

Carley, M. (2007, July 19). *Working Time Developments – 2006*. Retrieved from www.eurofound.europa.eu

Carley, M. (2008, July 1). *Developments in Industrial Action: 2003–2007*. Retrieved from www.eurofound.europa.eu

Carley, M. (2009, July 24). *Working Time Developments – 2008*. Retrieved from www.eurofound.europa.eu

Carley, M., McKay, S., Miller, J.-M., & Biletta, I. (2010). *Industrial Relations Developments in Europe: 2009*. Retrieved from www.eurofound.europa.eu/eiro/studies/tn1004019s/tn1004019s.htm

Carvel, J. (2007, April 18). "Nurses Back Industrial Action Over Pay." *The Guardian*, p. 12.

de Castro, A. B., Fujishiro, K., Rue, T., Tagalog, E. A., Samaco-Paquiz, L. P. G., & Gée, G. C. (2010). "Associations Between Work Schedule Characteristics and Occupational Injury and Illness." *International Nursing Review* 57(2):188–194.

Centeno, C., Clark, D., Lynch, T., Rocafort, J., Greenwood, A., Flores, L. A., et al. (2007). *EAPC Atlas of Palliative Care in Europe*. n.p.: IAHPC Press.

Chadwick, R., & Thompson, A. (2000). "Professional Ethics and Labor Disputes: Medicine and Nursing in the United Kingdom." *Cambridge Quarterly of Healthcare Ethics* 9(4):483–497.

Chan, Z. C. Y., & Lai, W.-F. (2010). "A Hong Kong Perspective on Ways to Improve Nurse Retention." *Nursing Standard* 24(35):24, 35–40.

Chappell, D., & Di Martino, V. (2006). *Violence At Work* (3rd ed.). Geneva, Switzerland: International Labour Office.

Chard, R. E. (2004). *The Mediating Effect of Public Opinion on Public Policy: Exploring the Realm of Health Care*. Albany, NY: State University of New York Press.

Cherry, B., & Jacob, S. R. (2005). *Contemporary Nursing: Issues, Trends, & Management* (3rd ed.). St. Louis, MO: Elsevier Mosby.

Chevreul, K., Durand-Zaleski, I., Bahrami, S., Hernandez-Quevedo, C., & Mladovsky, P. (2010). "France: Health System Review." *Health Systems in Transition* 12(6):1–291.

Christensen, G. (2009). *EU Workforce for Health: Challenges and Perspectives*. Presentation by the President of the European Federation of Nurses Associations, Nicosia, Cyprus, 23 March 2009.

Christiansen, R. H., & Nielsen, H. O. (2010, February 5). *Negative Health Outcomes Resulting from Bullying in the Workplace.* Retrieved from www.eurofound. europa.eu

Clews, G. (2009, April 14). "NHS Stress Driving Up Nurse Sick Leave Levels." *Nursing Times.* Retrieved from www.nursingtimes.net

Code of Practice on Industrial Action: Procedure for Authorising RCN Industrial Action – Guidance for Members and Staff. (n.d.). London: Royal College of Nursing.

Commission of the European Communities. (2000). *Report: Industrial Relations in Europe –2000.* COM(2000)113 final, Brussels, 6 March 2000.

Commission of the European Communities. (2001). *Communication from the Commission to the Council, the European Parliament, the Economic and Social Committee of the Regions. Employment and Social Policies: A Framework for Investing in Quality.* COM(2001)313 final, Brussels, 20 June 2001.

Commission of the European Communities. (2007, February 21). *Communication from the Commission to the European Parliament, the Council, the European Economic and Social Committee and the Committee of the Regions. Improving Quality and Productivity at Work: Community Strategy 2007-2012 on Health and Safety at Work.* COM(2007)62 final, Brussels, 21 February 2007.

Commission of the European Communities. (2008, October 3). *Report from the Commission to the European Parliament, the Council, the European Economic and Social Committee and the Committee of the Regions: Implementation of the Barcelona Objectives Concerning Childcare Facilities for Pre-School-Age Children.* SEC(2008)2597; COM(2008)638 final, Brussels, 3 October 2008.

Commission Recommendation 92/131/EEC of 27 November 1991 on the Protection of the Dignity of Women and Men at Work.

Com-Ruelle, L., Midy, F., & Ulmann, P. (2000). *La profession infirmière en mutation: Eléments de réflexion à partir d'exemples europeéns [The changing nursing profession: Elements for thought beginning with European examples].* Paris: Centre de Recherche d'Étude et de Documentation en Economie de la Santé (CREDES).

Coomber, B., & Barriball, K. L. (2007). "Impact of Job Satisfaction Components on Intent to Leave and Turnover for Hospital-Based Nurses: A Review of the Research Literature." *International Journal of Nursing Studies* 44(2):297–314.

Corens, D. (2007). "Health Systems Review: Belgium." *Health Systems in Transition* 9(2):1–172.

Corral, A., & de Munain, J. R. (2006). *Sexual Harassment of Women in the Workplace.* Retrieved from www.eurofound.europa.eu

Council Decision 2008/618/EC of 15 July 2008 on Guidelines for the Employment Policies of the Member States.

Council Directive 89/391/EEC of 12 June 1989 on the Introduction of Measures to Encourage Improvements in the Safety and Health of Workers at Work.

Council Directive 92/85/EEC of 19 October 1992 on the Introduction of Measures to Encourage Improvements in the Safety and Health at Work of Pregnant Workers and Workers Who have Recently Given Birth or are Breastfeeding (Tenth Individual Directive Within the Meaning of Article 16(1) of Directive 89/391/EEC).

Council Directive 93/104/EC of 23 November 1993 Concerning Certain Aspects of the Organisation of Working Time.

Council Directive 96/34/EC of 3 June 1996 on the Framework Agreement on Parental Leave Concluded by UNICE, CEEP, and the ETUC.

Council Directive 97/81/EC of 15 December 1997 Concerning the Framework Agreement on Part-time Work Concluded by UNICE, CEEP and the ETUC.

Council Directive 98/49/EC of 29 June 1998 on Safeguarding the Supplementary Pension Rights of Employed and Self-Employed Persons Moving within the Community.

Council Directive 2000/43/EC of 29 June 2000 Implementing the Principle of Equal Treatment Between Persons Irrespective of Racial or Ethnic Origin.

Council Directive 2000/78/EC of 27 November 2000 Establishing A General Framework for Equal Treatment in Employment and Occupation.

Council Directive 2010/18/EU of 8 March 2010 Implementing the Revised Framework Agreement on Parental Leave Concluded by BUSINESSEUROPE, UEAPME, CEEP and ETUC and Repealing Directive 96/34/EC.

Council Directive 2010/32/EU of 10 May 2010 Implementing the Framework Agreement on Prevention from Sharp Injuries in the Hospital and Healthcare Sector Concluded by HOSPEEM and EPSU.

Council Recommendation 92/241/EEC of 31 March 1992 on Child Care.

Council Regulation (EEC) No. 1408/71 of the Council of 14 June 1971 on the Application of Social Security Schemes To Employed Persons and Their Families Moving Within the Community.

Council Regulation (EC) 118/97 of 2 December 1996 Amending and Updating Regulation (EEC) No. 1408/71 on the Application of Social Security Schemes to Employed Persons, To Self-Employed Persons and To Members of Their Families Moving Within the Community and Regulation (EEC) No. 154/72 Laying Down the Procedure for Implementing Regulation (EEC) No. 1408/71.

Cowart, M. E., & Speake, D. L. (1992). "Community Employment Settings." In M. E. Cowart, & W. E. Serow (Eds.), *Nurses in the Workplace* (pp. 134–151). Newbury Park, CA: SAGE Publications.

Cox, K. B. (2001). "The Effects of Unit Morale and Interpersonal Relations on Conflict in the Nursing Unit." *Journal of Advanced Nursing* 35(1):17–25.

Création d'une instance professionnelle infirmière: Réflexions et propositions de la fédération CFDT santé-sociaux [Setting up a professional nursing process: The social-medical CFDT Federation's reflections and propositions]. (2007). Paris: Fédération nationale des syndicates CFDT santé-sociaux.

Cristovam, M. L. (2001). *Unions Protest Against New Management Models for Public Services.* Retrieved August 20, 2009 from www.eurofound.europa.eu/eiro/2001/03/features/pt0103139f.htm

Croatia. Ministry of Economy, Labour and Entrepreneurship. (2009). *Labour Act of 4 December 2009 (Text No. 3635).*

Croatia. Ministry of Economy, Labour and Entrepreneurship. (2011). *Act on Amendments to the Labour Act Official Gazette 61/11 or Labour Act of 20 May 2011 to Amend and Supplement the Labour Act (Text No. 1353).*

Croatian Nursing Council. (n.d.). *Code of Ethics.* Retrieved from www.hkms.hr/documents/CNC_code_of_ethics.pdf

Currie, J., Chiarella, M., & Buckley, T. (2013). "An Investigation of the International Literature on Nurse Practitioner Private Practice Models." *International Nursing Review* 60(4):435–447.

Curtarelli, M., Fric, K., Galli da Bino, C., Aumayr-Pintar, C., Cabrita, J., Kerkhofs, P., et al. (2013, December 12). *Industrial Relations and Working Conditions Developments in Europe: 2012.* Retrieved from www.eurofound.europa.eu

Curtis, E. A. (2007). "Job Satisfaction: A Survey of Nurses in the Republic of Ireland." *International Nursing Review* 54(1):92–99.

"Czech Hospital Nurses to See 15% Pay Raise." (2009, April 27). *Prague Daily Monitor.* Retrieved from www.praguemonitor.com

Cziria, L. (2006, July 3). *Hospital Workers Strike Over Pay and Overtime.* Retrieved from www.eurofound.europa.eu/eiro/2006/05/articles/sk0605029i.htm

Cziria, L. (2012, November 29). *Slovakia: Annual Review: 2011. Retrieved from* www.eurofound.europa.eu/comparative/tn1203020s/sk1203029q.htm

Cziria, L. (2013, June 18). *Slovakia: Impact of the Crisis on Industrial Relations.* Retrieved from www.eurofound.europa.eu/eiro/studies/tn1301019s/sk1301019q.htm

Dallender, J., Nolan, P., Soares, J., Thomsen, S., & Arnetz, B. (1999). "A Comparative Study of the Perceptions of British Mental Health Nurses and Psychiatrists of Their Work Environment." *Journal of Advanced Nursing* 29(1):36–43.

D'Árgenio, A. (2007, 14 marzo). "Parità di stipendio tra uomo e donna [Equal pay for men and women]." *La Repubblica*, p. 33.

D'Árgenio, A. (2008, 14 novembre). "In pensione a 60 anni donne discriminate: La UE condanna l'Italia [In pension at age 60, women discriminate: The EU condemns Italy]." *La Repubblica*, p. 22.

Daskalova, N. (2006). *Social Dialogue Develops in Healthcare Sector.* Retrieved from www.eurofound.europa.eu/eiro/2006/01/feature/bg0601201f.htm

Daskalova, N., Tornev, L., Ivanova, Y., Nikolova, A., Naydenova, Z., & Trakieva, D. (2005). *Health Care Reforms and Privatization – Social and Economic Consequences: Case of Bulgaria.* n.p.: Global Policy Network.

Davaki, K., & Mossialos, E. (2005). "Plus ça change [More change:]: Health Sector Reforms in Greece." *Journal of Health Politics, Policy and Law* 30(12):143–167.

Dawoud, D., & Maban, J. (2008). *Nurses in Society: Starting the Debate – Written Evidence.* London: King's College London, National Nursing Research Unit.

De Gieter, S., De Cooman, R., Pepermans, R., Caers, R., Du Bois, C., & Jegers, M. (2006). "Identifying Nurses' Rewards: A Qualitative Categorization Study in Belgium." *Human Resources for Health* 4:15. Retrieved from www.human-resources-health.com/content/4/1/15

Delamaire, M.-L., & Lafortune, G. (2010). *Nursing in Advanced Roles: A Description of Experiences in 12 Developed Countries* (OECD Health Working Papers. No. 54). n.p.: OECD Publishing.

"Demi-victoire pour les syndicats danois de la fonction publique [Half-victory for Danish trade unions related to public offices]." (2007, 28 décembre). *Le Monde.* Retrieved from www.lemonde.fr

Dent, M. (2003a). "Nurse Professionalisation and Traditional Values in Poland and Greece." *The International Journal of Public Sector Management* 16(2):153–162.

Dent, M. (2003b). *Remodelling Hospitals and Health Professions in Europe: Medicine, Nursing and the State.* Basingstoke, Hampshire, England: Palgrave Macmillan.

De Raeve, P. (2009). *Nurses' Views on the EU Challenges for Long-Term Care.* Presentation prepared for II International Congress on Long Term Care and Quality of Life, 11–13 May 2009, Pamplona, Spain.

De Troyer, M. (2000). *The Hospital Sector in Europe: Introductory Report.* Presentation at TUTB-SALTSA Conference, 25–27 September 2000, Brussels, Belgium.

De Troyer, M. (Ed.). (2001). "The Hospital Sector in Europe – Introductory Report." *TUTB: Newsletter of the European Trade Union Technical Bureau for Health and Safety,* No. 15–16, 50–51.

Dhaliwal, S., & McKay, S. (2008*). The Work-Life Experience of Black Nurses in the UK: A Report for the Royal College of Nursing.* London: Royal College of Nursing.

Dierick-van Daele, A. T. M., Metsemakers, J. F. M., Derckx, E. W. C. C., Spreeuwenberg, C., & Vrijhoef, H. J. M. (2009). "Nurse Practitioners Substituting for General Practitioners: Randomized Controlled Trial." *Journal of Advanced Nursing* 65(2):391–401.

Dierick-van Daele, A. T. M., Spreeuwenberg, C., Derckx, E. W. C. C., van Leeuwen, Y., Toemen, T., Legius, M., et al. (2010). "The Value of Nurse Practitioners in Dutch General Practices." *Quality in Primary Care* 18(4):231–241.

van Dijk, J. K. (2003, December). "NP Update." *Health Policy Monitor.* Retrieved January 4, 2007 from www.hpm.org

Di Martino, V. (2002). *Workplace Violence in the Health Sector: Country Case Studies – Brazil, Bulgaria, Lebanon, Portugal, South Africa, Thailand and an Additional Australian Study* (Working Paper of the Joint ILO/ICN/WHO/PSI Programme on Workplace Violence in the Health Sector).

Di Martino, V. (2003). *Relationship Between Work Stress and Workplace Violence in the Health Sector.* Geneva, Switzerland: ILO/ICN/WHO/PSI Joint Programme on Workplace Violence in the Health Sector.

Dimitriv, R. (2007). *Romanian Industrial Relations Law.* Antwerp, Belgium: Intersentia.

Dimond, B. (1997). "Strikes, Nurses and the Law in the UK." *Nursing Ethics* 4(4):269–276.

Directive 2002/14/EC of the European Parliament and of the Council of 11 March 2002 Establishing A General Framework for Informing and Consulting Employees in the European Community- Joint Declaration of the European Parliament, the Council and the Commission on Employee Representation.

Directive 2002/73/EC of the European Parliament and of the Council of 23 September 2002 Amending Council Directive 76/207/EEC on the Implementation of the Principle of Equal Treatment for Men And Women as Regards Access to Employment, Vocational Training and Promotion, and Working Conditions.

Directive 2003/41/EC of the European Parliament and of the Council of 3 June 2003 on the Activities and Supervision of Institutions for Occupational Retirement Provision.

Directive 2003/88/EC of the European Parliament and of the Council of 4 November 2003 Concerning Certain Aspects of the Organization of Working Time.

Directive 2006/54/EC of the European Parliament and of the Council of 5 July 2006 on the Implementation of the Principle of Equal Opportunities and Equal Treatment of Men and Women in Matters of Employment and Occupation (Recast).

Directive 2008/104/EC of the European Parliament and of the Council of 19 November 2008 on Temporary Agency Work.

Dison, C. C. (1992). "An Action Plan for Nurse Executives." In M. E. Cowart, & W. J. Serow (Eds.), *Nurses in the Workplace* (pp. 219–234). Newbury Park, CA: SAGE Publications.

Dollard, M. F., & Neser, D. Y. (2013). "Worker Health is Good for the Economy: Union Density and Psychosocial Safety Climate As Determinants of Country Differences in Worker Health and Productivity in 31 European Countries." *Social Science and Medicine* 92:114–123.

Domagala, A., Pomykalska, E., Rys, A., & Zajic, M. (1999). *Public Service Reforms and Their Impact on Health Sector Personnel in Poland.* Kraków, Poland: University Public Health Foundation.

Donnelly, L. (2012, March 11). "Nurses Could be Given Limits on Number of Patients They Care for." *The Telegraph.* Retrieved from www.telegraph.co.uk/health/healthnews/9135722/Nurses-could-be-given-limits-on-number-of-patients-they-care-for.html

Downing, J., & Ling, J. (2012). "Education in Children's Palliative Care Across Europe and Internationally." *International Journal of Palliative Nursing* 18(3):115–120.

Dragu, A. (2006, April 28). "Six of Slovakia's Largest Hospitals Struggling with Protesting Staff." *Insight Central Europe.* Retrieved April 30, 2008, from www.incentraleurope.radio.cz

dsegretain. (2009, February 26). "The Greek Health System Collapses." *France 24 International News.* Retrieved February 26, 2009, from www.france24.com/en

Dubois, C.-A., McKee, M., & Nolte, E. (2006). "Analysing Trends, Opportunities and Challenges." In C.-A. Dubois, M. McKee, & E. Nolte (Eds.), *Human Resources for Health in Europe* (pp. 15–40). Maidenhead, Berkshire, England: Open University Press.

Dubois, C.-A., Nolte, E., & McKee, M. (2006). "Human Resources for Health in Europe." In C.-A. Dubois, M. McKee, & E. Nolte (Eds.), *Human Resources for Health in Europe* (pp. 1–14). Maidenhead, Berkshire, England: Open University Press.

Dubois, C.-A., Singh, D., & Jinani, I. (2008). "The Human Resource Challenge in Chronic Care." In E. Nolte, & M. McKee (Eds.), *Caring for People with Chronic Conditions: A Health System Perspective* (pp. 143–171). Maidenhead, Berkshire, England: Open University Press.

Duddle, M., & Boughton, M. (2007). "Intraprofessional Relations in Nursing." *Journal of Advanced Nursing* 59(1):29–37.

Dumont, J.-C., & Zurn, P. (2007). "Immigrant Health Workers in OECD Countries in the Broader Context of Highly Skilled Migration." *International Migration Outlook*, Part III, 161–228.

Dunin, A. (2007, July 6). *Intel Brief: Polish Health Care Crisis.* Retrieved May 22, 2008, from www.isn.ethz.ch

Durán, A., Lara, J. L., & van Waveren, M. (2006). "Spain: Health System Review." *Health Systems in Transition* 8(4):1–208.

Dussault, G., Buchan, J., Sermeus, W., & Padaiga, Z. (2010). *Assessing Future Health Workforce Needs.* Copenhagen, Denmark: The Regional Office for Europe of the World Health Organization.

Dussault, G., Buchan, J., & Wismar, M. (2013). *The Economic Crisis in the EU: Impact on Health Workforce Mobility: Meeting of the Working Group on Health Workforce, 12 April 2013.* Brussels, Belgium: European Commission.

Düvel, W., Schömano, I., Gradev, G., & Clauwaert, S. (2004). *Labour Dispute Settlement: A Comparative Legal Overview of Extra-Judicial and Judicial Procedures in the European Union, Switzerland and the Countries of South Eastern Europe.* Brussels, Belgium: European Trade Union Institute.

Duxbury, J., & Whittington, R. (2005). "Causes and Management of Patient Aggression and Violence: Staff and Patient Perspective." *Journal of Advanced Nursing* 50(5):469–478.

Džakula, A., Sagan, A., Pavić, N., Lončarek, K., & Sekelj-Kauzlarić, K. (2014). "Croatia: Health System Review." *Health Systems in Transition* 16(3):1–162.

EAPC (European Association for Palliative Care) "Task Force on the Development of Palliative Care in Europe." (n.d.). *Country Information.* Retrieved January 21, 2013 from www.eapc-taskforce-development.eu/country.php

ECORYS Research and Consulting. (2010). *Sector Councils on Employment and Skills at EU Level: Country Reports – Prepared for European Commission, DG Employment, Social Affairs and Equal Opportunities.* Rotterdam, The Netherlands: Author.

"Editorial." (2008, 18 marzo). *Diario Enfermero*, No. 200. Retrieved May 15, 2008, from www.enfermundi.com/boletino.ge

Edwards, C., & Robinson, O. (2004). "Evaluating the Business Case for Part-Time Working Amongst Qualified Nurses." *British Journal of Industrial Relations* 42(1):167–183.

Ehrenfeld, M. (1998). "Nursing and Home Care in Europe." *International Nursing Review* 45(2): 61–64.

Eke, E., Girasek, E., & Szócska, M. (2011). "From Melting Pot to Laboratory of Change in Central Europe: Hungary and Health Workforce Migration." In M. Wismar, C. B. Maier, I. A. Glinos, G. Dussault, & J. Figueras (Eds.), *Health Professional Mobility and Health Systems: Evidence from 17 European Countries* (pp. 365–394). Copenhagen, Denmark: World Health Organization on behalf of European Observatory on Health Systems and Policies.

Ellefsen, B. (2002). "The Experience of Collaboration: A Comparison of Health Visiting in Scotland and Norway." *International Nursing Review* 49(3):144–153.

Ellins, J., & Ham, C. (2009). *NHS Mutual: Engaging Staff and Aligning Incentives to Achieve Higher Levels of Performance.* London: The Nuffield Trust.

England: Department of Health, Professional Leadership-CNO's Directorate. (2011). *The Government's Response to the Recommendations in Frontline Care: The Report of the Prime Minister's Commission on the Future of Nursing and Midwifery in England.* Retrieved from www.gov.uk/government/publications/the-governments-response-to-the-recommendations-in-front-line-care

Ensor, T. (2000). "The Unofficial Business of Health Care in Transitional Europe." *Eurohealth* 6(2):35–37.

Ensor, T., & Witter, S. (2001). "Health Economics in Low Income Countries: Adapting to the Reality of the Unofficial Economy." *Health Policy* 57:1–13.

Estryn-Behar, M., van der Heijden, B., Camerino, D., Fry, C., Le Nézet, O., Conway, P. M., et al. (2008). "Violence Risks in Nursing – Results from the European 'NEXT' Study." *Occupational Medicine* 58:107–114.

Estryn-Behar, M., Le Nézet, O., Affre, A., Arbieu, P., Bedel, M., Bonnet, N., et al. (2003a). "Intent to Leave Nursing in France." In H.-M. Hasselhorn, P. Tackenberg, & B. H. Müller (Eds.), *Working Conditions and Intent to Leave the Profession Among Nursing Staff in Europe* (pp. 159–170). (SALTA-JOINT PROGRAMME FOR WORKING LIFE RESEARCH IN EUROPE, Report No. 7). Retrieved January 5, 2007, from www.arbetslivsinstitutet.se

Estryn-Behar, M., Le Nézet, O., Bonnet, N., Bedel, M., Gadier, G., Fayet, C., et al. (2002). *Le personnel soignant en France [Nursing staff in France].* Retrieved from www.next.uni-wuppertal.de

Estryn-Behar, M., Le Nézet, O., & Jasseron, C. (2005). *Health and Satisfaction of Healthcare Workers in France and Europe: Results of the PRESST-NEXT Study,* Retrieved from www.next.uni-wuppertal.de

Estryn-Behar, M., Le Nézet, O., Laine, M., Pokorski, J., Caillard, J.-F., & the NEXT-Study Group. (2003b). "Physical Load Among Nursing Personnel." In H.-M. Hasselhorn, P. Tackenberg, & B. H. Müller (Eds.), *Working Conditions and Intent to Leave the Profession Among Nursing Staff in Europe* (pp. 94–100). (SALTA-JOINT PROGRAMME FOR WORKING LIFE RESEARCH IN EUROPE, Report No. 7). Retrieved January 5, 2007, from www.arbetslivsinstitutet.se

ETUI-REHS Research Department. (2005). *Acquis Communautaire Related to Pensions.* n.p.: Pragma Consulting.

Eurofound. (2012). *Croatia: Industrial Relations Profile.* Dublin, Ireland: Author.

European Commission. (1991). *Commission Recommendation 92/131/EEC of 27 November 1991 on the Protection of the Dignity of Women and Men at Work*

European Commission. (2006). *Communication from the Commission to the Council, the European Parliament, the European Economic and Social Committee and the Committee of the Regions: A Roadmap for Equality Between Women and Men: 2006–2010.* COM(2006)92 final. Brussels, 1 March 2006.

European Commission. (2008). *Childcare Services in the EU* (Memo/08/592). Brussels, 3 October 2008.

European Commission. (2011). *Commission Staff Working Paper: Report on the Implementation of the European Social Partners' Framework Agreement on Work-Related Stress.* SEC(2011)241 final. Brussels, 24 February 2011.

European Commission. (2012a). *Commission Decision of 5 July 2012 on Setting Up a Multisectoral and Independent Expert Panel to Provide Advice on Effective Ways of Investing in Health* (2012/c 198/06).

European Commission. (2012b). *Commission Staff Working Document on An Action Plan for the EU Health Workforce Accompanying the Document Communication from the Commission to the European Parliament, the Council, the European Economic and Social Committee and the Committee of the Regions: Towards a Job Rich Recovery.* SWD(2012)93 final. Strasbourg, 18 April 2012.

European Commission. (2013). *Tackling the Gender Pay Gap in the European Union.* Luxembourg: Publications Office of the European Union.

European Commission: Directorate- General for Employment and Social Affairs. (2004). *Industrial Relations in Europe: 2004.* Luxembourg: Office for Official Publications of the European Communities.

European Commission: Directorate-General for Employment, Social Affairs and Equal Opportunities. (2006). *Adequate and Sustainable Pensions: Synthesis Report 2006.* Luxembourg: Office for Official Publications of the European Communities.

European Commission: Directorate-General for Employment, Social Affairs and Equal Opportunities. (2007). *Joint Report on Social Protection and Social Inclusion.* Luxembourg: Office for Official Publications of the European Communities.

European Commission: Directorate-General for Employment, Social Affairs, and Equal Opportunities-Unit F-1. (2006). *Industrial Relations in Europe: 2006.*

European Commission: Directorate-General for Employment, Social Affairs and Equal Opportunities-Unit G-4. (2010). *Trade Union Practices on Anti-Discrimination and Diversity Study: Innovative and Significant Practices in Fighting Discrimination and Promoting Diversity*. Luxembourg: Publications Office of the European Union.

European Commission: Directorate-General Employment, Social Affairs and Inclusion. (2010). *Sector Councils on Employment and Skills at EU Level*.

European Commission: Vinay-Prospecta, P. (1997). *Women in Decision-Making in the Health Institutions of the European Union* (V/5806/97). Brussels: Directorate-General for Employment, Industrial Relations and Social Affairs.

European Council of Nursing Regulators. (n.d.). *FEPI Response to European Commission's Green Paper on the European Workforce for Health*. Brussels, Belgium: Author.

European Federation of Nurses Associations. (2007). *EFN Position Paper on the Prevention of Sharp Injuries*. Retrieved from www.efnweb.be/wp-content/uploads/2011/09/EFN-Policy-Statement-on-Sharps-injuries-EN-final-rev062007.pdf

European Federation of Nurses Associations. (2008). *Activity Report: Working Year 2008*. Retrieved from www.efnweb.be/wp-content/uploads/2011/09/EFN-Activity-Report-2008-EN.pdf

European Federation of Nurses Associations. (2012). *Caring in Crisis: The Impact of the Financial Crisis on Nurses and Nursing: A Comparative Overview of 34 European Countries*. Retrieved from www.efnweb.be

European Federation of Public Service Unions. (n.d.). *Estonia: Health Care Reforms*. Retrieved from www.epsu.org/a/2242

European Foundation for the Improvement of Living and Working Conditions. (2007a). *Gender and Working Conditions in the European Union*. Luxembourg: Office for Official Publications of the European Communities.

European Foundation for the Improvement of Living and Working Conditions. (2007b). *Working Conditions in the European Union*. Luxembourg: Office for Official Publications of the European Communities.

European Foundation for the Improvement of Living and Working Conditions. (2009a). *Industrial Relations Developments in Europe: 2008*. Luxembourg: Office for Official Publications of the European Communities.

European Foundation for the Improvement of Living and Working Conditions. (2009b). *Sweden: A Country Profile*. Dublin, Ireland: Author.

European Foundation for the Improvement of Living and Working Conditions. (2009c). *Working Conditions in the European Union: Working Time and Work Intensity*. Luxembourg: Office for Official Publications of the European Communities.

"European Nurses Fighting for Pay Increases." (2008, May 1). *EFN News*. Retrieved March 23, 2010, from www.efnweb.be

European Observatory on Health Care Systems. (1999). *Health Care Systems in Transition: Hungary*. Copenhagen, Denmark: WHO Regional Office for Europe.

European Observatory on Health Care Systems. (n.d.) *Policy Brief: The Significance of Hospitals*. n.p.: Author.

European Parliament- Directorate General for Internal Policies. (2010). *Costs and Benefits of Maternity and Paternity Leave. Workshop* FEMM/EMPL. Brussels, European Parliament, 5 October 2010.

European Parliament: Policy Department-Economic and Scientific Policy. (2008). *Palliative Care in the European Union* (IP/A/ENVI/ST/2007-22).

European Parliament: Press Service. (2010, October 21). EP: EU Maternity Leave Like the Polish One.

European Trade Union Confederation. (2004). *Accord-cadre sur le stress au travail (Proposition finale conjointe du 27 mai 2004) [Framework agreement on stress at work (Final proposal of May 27, 2004)]*. Retrieved from www.dgdr.cnrs.fr/drh/protect-soc/documents/fiches_rps/ue_accord_cadre_8_octobre_2004.pdf

European Trade Union Confederation. (2008). *Working Time Directive*. Retrieved from www.etuc.org/working-time-directive

European Working Conditions Observatory. (2014). *Human Health Sector: Working Conditions and Job Quality*. Luxembourg: Publications Office of the European Union.

Evans, J. M., Lippoldt, D. C., & Marianna, P. (2001). *Trends in Working Hours in OECD Countries* (Occasional paper No. 45, Directorate for Education, Employment, Labour and Social Affairs, Employment, Labour and Social Affairs Committee). Paris: Organisation for Economic Co-operation and Development.

Falkner, G., Treib, O., Hartlapp, M., & Leiber, S. (2005). *Complying with Europe: EU Harmonization and Soft Law in the Member States*. Cambridge, England: Cambridge University Press.

Falkner, G., Treib, O., Hartlapp, M., & Leiber, S. (2009). *EU Social Policy Over Time: The Role of Directives*. Cambridge, England: Cambridge University Press.

Farrell, G. A. (2001). "From Tall Poppies to Squashed Weeds: Why Don't Nurses Pull Together More?" *Journal of Advanced Nursing* 35(1):26–33.

Fawcett-Henesy, A. (2000/01). "Nursing in the WHO European Region in the 21st Century." *Eurohealth* 6(5):29–31.

Federation of European Employers. (2004). *Industrial Relations Across Europe 2004*. Retrieved from www.fedee.com

Federation of European Employers. (2011). *Industrial Relations Across Europe*. Retrieved from www.fedee.com

Ferrinho, P., Biscaia, A., Fronteira, I., Craveiro, I., Antunes, A. R., Conceição, C., et al. (2003). "Patterns of Perceptions of Workplace Violence in the Portuguese Health Care Sector." *Human Resources for Health* 1(11). Retrieved from www.human-resources-health.com/content/1/1/11

Filej, B., Skela-Savič, B., Vicic, V. H., & Hudorovic, N. (2009). "Necessary Organizational Changes According to [the] Burke-Litwin Model in the Head Nurses System of Management in Health Care and Social Welfare Institutions – The Slovenia Experience." *Health Policy* 90:166–174.

Finland. Ministry of Labour. (2003). *Industrial Relations and Labour Legislation in Finland*. n.p.: Author.

Flexible Career Options Introduced in the Flemish Not-for-Profit Sector. (2000). Retrieved from www.eurofound.europa.eu

Flinkman, M., Laine, M., Leino-Kilpi, H., Hasselhorn, H.-M., & Salantera, S. (2008). "Explaining Young Registered Finnish Nurses' Intention to Leave the Profession: A Questionnaire Survey." *International Journal of Nursing Studies* 45(5):727–739.

Flottorp, S. A., Jamtvedt, G., Gibis, B., & McKee, M. (2010). *Using Audit and Feedback to Health Professionals to Improve the Quality and Safety of Health Care*. Copenhagen, Denmark: WHO Regional Office for Europe.

Ford, S. (2009, June 2). "Working Time Directive Tsar Says the 48-Hour Week is Good for Nursing." *Nursing Times*. Retrieved from www.nursingtimes.net

Forde, C., & Slater, G. (2005). "Agency Working in Britain: Character, Consequences and Regulation." *British Journal of Industrial Relations* 43(2):249–271.

Formation et trajectoires professionnelles des infirmiers [Nurses' training and professional pathways]. (2011, 11 janvier). Retrieved from www.infirmiers.com

Frijters, P., Shields, M. A., & Price, S. W. (2007). "Investigating the Quitting Decision of Nurses: Panel Data Evidence from the British National Health Service." *Health Economics* 16(1):57–74.

Friss, L. (1989). *Strategic Management of Nurses: A Policy-Oriented Approach.* Owings Mills, MD: The AUPHA Press.

Front Line Care: Report by the Prime Minister's Commission on the Future of Nursing and Midwifery in England. (2010). London: Prime Minister's Commission on the Future of Nursing and Midwifery in England.

Furlan, M. (2006, 21–27 novembre). "Nuovi infermieri, vecchi ruoli [New nurses, old roles]." *Il Sole 24 Ore: Sanità*, p. 2.

Fusani, C. (2005, 16 ottobre). "In piazza contro le liberalizzazioni [In the square against liberalization]." *La Repubblica*, p. 11.

Gaal, P. (2004). *Health Care Systems in Transition: Hungary.* Copenhagen, Denmark: WHO Regional Office for Europe on behalf of the European Observatory on Health Systems and Policies.

Gaal, P., Belli, P. C., McKee, M., & Szócska, M. (2006). "Informal Payments for Health Care: Definitions, Distinctions and Dilemmas." *Journal of Health Politics, Policy and Law* 31(2):251–293.

Gaal, P., Evetovits, T., & McKee, M. (2006). "Informal Payment for Health Care: Evidence from Hungary." *Health Policy* 77:86–102.

Gaal, P., & McKee, M. (2004). "Informal Payment for Health Care and the Theory of 'INXIT'." *International Journal of Health Planning and Management* 19(2):163–178.

Gajdzica, M. (2007, May). "Wages in the Slovak Healthcare Sector." *Into Balance*, p. 4. Retrieved from www.hpi.sk/cdata/IntoBalance/english/IntoBalance_05-2007_en.pdf

Galan, A., Olsavszky, V., & Vladescu, C. (2011). "Emergent Challenge of Health Professional Emigration: Romania's Accession to the EU." In M. Wismar, C. B. Maier, I. A. Glinos, G. Dussault, & J. Figueras (Eds.), *Health Professional Mobility and Health Systems: Evidence from 17 European Countries* (pp. 449–477). Copenhagen, Denmark: World Health Organization on behalf of European Observatory on Health Systems and Policies.

Gallie, D. & Russell, H. (2009). "Work-Family Conflict and Working Conditions in Western Europe." *Social Indicators Research* 93(3):445–467.

Gancedo, P.M. (2006, January 11). *Strike in the Private Health Sector in Madrid Due to Collective Bargaining Disagreement.* Retrieved from www.eurofound.europa.eu

Geiger-Brown, J., & Trinkoff, A. (2010). "Is It Time to Pull the Plug on 12-Hour Shifts? Part 1. The Evidence." *The Journal of Nursing Administration* 40(3): 100–102.

Genet, N., Hutchinson, A., Naiditch, M., Garms-Homolova, V., Fagerström, C., Melchiorre, M., et al. (2012). "Management of the Care Process." In N. Genet, W. Boerma, M. Kroneman, A. Hutchinson, & R. B. Saltman (Eds.), *Home Care*

Across Europe: Current Structure and Future Challenges (pp. 71–104). Copenhagen, Denmark: World Health Organization.

German Nurses Association. (n.d.). *Health Care in Germany.* Retrieved June 19, 2010, from www.dbfk.de

Geyer, R. R. (2000). *Exploring European Social Policy.* Cambridge, United Kingdom: Polity Press.

Gillies, D. A. (1994). *Nursing Management: A Systems Approach* (3rd ed.). Philadelphia: W. B. Saunders Company.

Girot, E. A., & Rickaby, C. E. (2008). "Education for New Role Development: The Community Matron in England." *Journal of Advanced Nursing* 64(1):38–48.

Glasberg, A. L., Eriksson, S., & Norberg, A. (2007). "Burnout and 'Stress of Conscience' Among Health-Care Personnel." *Journal of Advanced Nursing* 57(4):392–403.

Glenngård, A. H., Hjalte, F., Svensron, M., Anell, A., & Bankauskaite, V. (2005). *Health Systems in Transition: Sweden.* Copenhagen, Denmark: WHO Regional Office for Europe on behalf of the European Observatory on Health Systems and Policies.

Global Health Workforce Alliance. (2008). *Guidelines: Incentives for Health Professionals.* Geneva, Switzerland: Global Health Workforce Alliance –World Health Organization.

Golna, C., Pashardes, P., Allin, S., Theodorou, M., Merkur, S., & Mossialos, E. (2004). *Health Care Systems in Transition: Cyprus.* Copenhagen, Denmark: WHO Regional Office for Europe on behalf of the European Observatory on Health Systems and Policies.

Golubic, R., Milosevic, M., Knezevic, B., & Mustajbegovic, J. (2009). "Work-Related Stress, Education and Work Ability Among Hospital Nurses." *Journal of Advanced Nursing* 65(10):2056–2066.

Goodwin, N. (2006). *Leadership in Health Care: A European Perspective.* London and New York: Routledge.

de Gooijer, W. (2007). *Trends in EU Health Care Systems.* New York: Springer.

Górajek-Jóźwik, J. (2004). "Primary Nursing in Poland: Theory and Experience." *Journal of Nursing Management* 12(5):317–321.

Gordon, S. (2005). *Nursing Against the Odds: How Health Care Cost Cutting, Media Stereotypes, and Medical Hubris Undermine Nurses and Patient Care.* Ithaca, NY: Cornell University Press.

Gordon, S., Buchanan, J., & Bretherton, T. (2008). *Safety in Numbers: Nurse-to-Patient Ratios and the Future of Health Care.* Ithaca, NY and London: ILR Press.

Gould, D., Fontenla, M., Anderson, S., Conway, L., & Hinds, K. (2003). "Intention to Leave Nursing in the United Kingdom." In H.-M. Hasselhorn, P. Tackenberg, & B. H. Müller, (Eds.), *Working Conditions and Intent to Leave the Profession Among Nursing Staff in Europe* (pp. 171–181). (SALTA-JOINT PROGRAMME FOR WORKING LIFE RESEARCH IN EUROPE, Report No. 7). Retrieved January 5, 2007, from www.arbetslivsinstitutet.se

Greenwood, J. (1998). "The Professions." In J. Greenwood, & M. Aspinwall (Eds.), *Collective Action in the European Union: Interests and the New Politics of Associability* (pp. 126–148). London: Routledge.

Groenewegen, P. P. (2008, October). "Update on Nurse Practitioners." *Health Policy Monitor.* Retrieved May 14, 2009, from www.hpm.org

Gronroos, E., & Perala, M.-L. (2008). "Self-Reported Competence of Home Nursing Staff in Finland." *Journal of Advanced Nursing* 64(1):27–37.

Gunnarsdóttir, S., & Rafferty, A. M. (2006). "Enhancing Working Conditions." In C.-A. Dubois, M. McKee, & E. Nolte (Eds.), *Human Resources for Health in Europe* (pp. 155–172). Maidenhead, Berkshire, England: Open University Press.

Gurková, E., Čáp, J., Žiaková, K., & Ďurišková, M. (2012). "Job Satisfaction and Emotional Subjective Well-Being Among Slovak Nurses." *International Nursing Review* 59(1):94–100.

Gurková, E., Soósová, M. S., Harková, S., Žiaková, K., Serfelová, R., & Zamboriová, M. (2013). "Job Satisfaction and Leaving Intentions of Slovak and Czech Nurses." *International Nursing Review* 60(1):112–121.

Hale, D. (2007). "International Comparisons of Labour Disputes in 2005." *Economic & Labour Market Review* 1(4):23–31.

Hallin, K., & Danielson, E. (2007). "Registered Nurses' Experiences of Daily Work, a Balance Between Strain and Stimulation: A Qualitative Study." *International Journal of Nursing Studies* 44(7):1221–1230.

Hämäläinen, R. M., & Lindström, K. (2006). "Health in the World of Work." In T. Stahl, M. Wismar, E. Ollila, E. Lantinen, & K. Leppo (Eds.), *Health in All Policies: Prospects and Potentials* (pp. 64–92). n.p.: Finnish Ministry of Social Affairs and Health.

Hammett, R. S., Seidman, J., & London, J. (1957). "The Slowdown as a Union Tactic." *The Journal of Political Economy* 65(2):126–134.

Hardill, I., & MacDonald, S. (2000). "Skilled International Migration: The Experience of Nurses in the UK." *Regional Studies* 34(7):681–692.

Hartmann, L., Ulmann, P., & Rochai, L. (2006). "GPs and Access to Out-of-Hours Services in Six European Countries (Germany, Spain, France, Italy, the United Kingdom and Sweden)." *Revue Française des Affaires Sociales* 60(2–3):89–111.

Hasselhorn, H.-M., Conway, P. M., Widerszal-Bazyl, M., Simon, M., Tackenberg, P., Schmidt, S., et al. (2008). "Contribution of Job Strain to Nurses' Consideration of Leaving the Profession- Results from the Longitudinal European Nurses' Early Exit Study." *Scandinavian Journal of Work, Environment & Health Supplements* 6:75–82.

Hasselhorn, H.-M., Müller, B. H., & Tackenberg, P. (2005). *NEXT: Scientific Report July 2005: A Research Project Funded by the European Commission.* Wuppertal, Germany: University of Wuppertal.

Hasselhorn, H.-M., Tackenberg, P., Buscher, A., Simon, M., Kümmerling, A., & Müller, B. H. (2005). *Work and Health of Nurses in Europe: Results from the NEXT-Study.* Retrieved from www.next.uni-wuppertal.de

Hasselhorn, H.-M., Tackenberg, P., Buscher, A., Stelzig, S., Kümmerling, A., & Müller, B. H. (2003). "Intent to Leave Nursing in Germany." In H.-M. Hasselhorn, P. Tackenberg, & B. H. Müller (Eds.), *Working Conditions and Intent to Leave the Profession Among Nursing Staff in Europe* (pp. 136–145). (SALTA-JOINT PROGRAMME FOR WORKING LIFE RESEARCH IN EUROPE, Report No. 7). Retrieved January 5, 2007, from www.arbetslivsinstitutet.se

Hasselhorn, H.-M., Tackenberg, P., & Müller, B. H. (2003). "Intent to Leave Nursing in the European Nursing Profession." In H.-M. Hasselhorn, P. Tackenberg, & B. H. Müller (Eds.), *Working Conditions and Intent to Leave the Profession Among Nursing Staff in Europe* (pp. 115–124). (SALTA-JOINT PROGRAMME

FOR WORKING LIFE RESEARCH IN EUROPE, Report No. 7). Retrieved January 5, 2007, from www.arbetslivsinstitutet.se

Hasselhorn, H.-M., Tackenberg, P., & Peter, R. (2004). "Effort-Reward Imbalance Among Nurses in Stable Countries and in Countries in Transition." *International Journal of Occupational and Environmental Health* 10(4):401–408.

Hasselhorn, H.-M., Widerszal-Bazyl, M., & Radkiewicz, P. (2003). "Effort, Reward- and Effort-Reward-Imbalance in the Nursing Profession in Europe." In H.-M. Hasselhorn, P. Tackenberg, & B. H. Müller (Eds.), *Working Conditions and Intent to Leave the Profession Among Nursing Staff in Europe* (pp. 108–114). (SALTA-JOINT PROGRAMME FOR WORKING LIFE RESEARCH IN EUROPE, Report No. 7). Retrieved January 5, 2007, from www.arbetslivsinstitutet.se

Hayes, L. J., O'Brien-Pallas, L., Duffield, C., Shamian, J., Buchan, J., Hughes, F., et al. (2006). "Nurse Turnover: A Literature Review." *International Journal of Nursing Studies* 43(2):237–263.

Hays, M. M. (2002). "An Exploratory Study of Supportive Communication During Shift Report." *Southern Online Journal of Nursing Research* 3(3):1–14. Retrieved from www.resourcenter.net/images/SNRS/Files/SOJNR_articles/iss03vol03.pdf

Hays, M. M. (2005). "Dissonance and Powerlessness in Nursing: Its Affect on the Working Environment." In M. Tavakoli, & H. T. O. Davies (Eds.), *Reforming Health Systems: Analysis and Evidence [of] Strategic Issues on Health Care Management – Proceedings of the 2004 Strategic Issues on Health Care Management Conference at the University of St. Andrews, 2–4 September 2004* (pp. 221–229). St. Andrews, Scotland: University of St. Andrews.

Health Care in Central and Eastern Europe: Reform, Privatization and Employment in Four Countries. A Draft Report to the International Labour Office InFocus Programme on Socio-Economic Security and Public Service International. (2001). Geneva, Switzerland: International Labour Office.

Health Chapters of the Hungarian Human Resources Development Operational Programme 2004–2006. n.d. Retrieved from www.eum.hu/english/national-development/national-development

Hegedus, K. (2002). *Hospice Movement in Hungary and Experiences with Hospital Supportive Teams.* Paper presented at the V Symposium on Hospice and Palliative Care, March 21, 2002.

van der Heijden, B. I. J. M., Demerouti, E., Bakker, A. B., & the NEXT Study Group coordinated by H.-M. Hasselhorn. (2008). "Work-Home Interference Among Nurses: Reciprocal Relationships with Job Demands and Health." *Journal of Advanced Nursing* 62(5):572–584.

Heitlinger, A. (1998). "Czech Nursing During and After Communism." In V. Olgiati, L. Orzack, & M. Saks (Eds.), *Professions, Identity and Order in Comparative Perspective* (pp. 123–148). Oñati, Spain: The International Institute for the Sociology of Law.

Heitlinger, A., & Trnka, S. (1998). *Young Women of Prague.* Houndmills and London: Macmillan Press Ltd.

Help Wanted? Providing and Paying for Long-Term Care. (2011). Paris: Organisation for Economic Co-operation and Development.

Hervey, T., & Vanhercke, B. (2010). "Health Care and the EU: The Law and Policy Patchwork." In E. Mossialos, G. Permanand, R. Baeten, & T. K. Hervey (Eds.), *Health Systems Governance in Europe: The Role of European Union Law and Policy* (pp. 84–133). New York: Cambridge University Press.

Hervey, T. K., & McHale, J. V. (2004). *Health Law and the European Union.* New York: Cambridge University Press.

Hinno, S., Partanen, P., & Vehviläinen-Julkunsen, K. (2011). "Hospital Nurses' Work Environment and Quality of Care Provided and Career Plans." *International Nursing Review* 58(2):255–262.

Hlavačka, S., Wágner, R., & Riesberg, A. (2004). *Health Care Systems in Transition: Slovakia.* Copenhagen, Denmark: WHO Regional Office for Europe on behalf of the European Observatory on Health Systems and Policies.

Höckertin, C., & Härenstam, A. (2006). "The Impact of Ownership on Psychosocial Working Conditions: A Multilevel Analysis of 60 Workplaces." *Economic and Industrial Democracy* 27(2):245–284.

Hofmarcher, M. M., & Quentin, W. (2013). "Austria: Health System Review." *Health Systems in Transition* 15(7):1–291.

Hofmarcher, M. M., & Rack, H. M. (2006). "Austria: Health System Review." *Health Systems in Transition* 8(3):1–247.

Holt, E. (2010). "Poland's Nurses Warn of Crisis in Profession." *The Lancet* 375 (9719):972.

Hood, L. J., & Leddy, S. K. (2006). *Leddy & Pepper's Conceptual Bases of Professional Nursing* (6th ed.). Philadelphia, PA: Lippincott Williams & Wilkins.

Hristov, Z., Tomev, L., Kircheva, D., Daskalova, N., Mihailova, T., Ivanova, V., et al. (2003). *Work Stress in the Context of Transition: A Case Study of Education, Health and Public Administration in Bulgaria.* Budapest, Hungary: International Labour Office.

Hubačová, L., Križanová, D., Šulcová, M., & Wsólová, L. (2000). *Health Status of Employees in Selected Health Care Departments in the Slovak Republic.* Poster session presented at the TUTB-SALTA Conference, 25–27 September 2000, Brussels, Belgium.

Hudek-Knezević, J., Maglica, B. K., & Krapić, N. (2011). "Personality, Organizational Stress, and Attitudes Toward Work as Perspective Predictors of Professional Burnout in Hospital Nurses." *Croatian Medical Journal* 52(4):538–549.

Hughes, R. G., & Claney, C. M. (2009). "Complexity, Bullying, and Stress: Analyzing and Mitigating a Challenging Work Environment for Nurses." *Journal of Nursing Care Quality* 24(3):180–183.

Hultsjö, S., & Hjelm, K. (2005). "Immigrants in Emergency Care: Swedish Health Care Staff's Experience." *International Nursing Review* 52(4):276–285.

Human Resources in the Health Sector of Estonia. (2008). Presentation at the WHO European Ministerial Conference on Health Systems: "Health Systems: Health and Wealth," Tallinn, Estonia, 25–27 June, 2008.

Hungary-Austria: Nursing Emergency. (2006, September 28). Retrieved from www. wieninternational.at/en/node/1591/print

Hutt, R., & Buchan, J. (2005). *Trends in London's NHS Workforce: An Updated Analysis of Key Data.* London: King's Fund.

Ibison, D. (2007, November 13). "Finland's Nurses Braced for Forced Return to Work." *Financial Times.* Retrieved from www.ft.com

ILO (International Labour Organization). (1944). *Medical Care Recommendation, 1944. (No. 69).*

ILO (International Labour Organization). (1977a). *Nursing Personnel Convention, 1977 (No. 149). Convention Concerning Employment and Conditions of Work and Life of Nursing Personnel.*

ILO (International Labour Organization). (1977b). *Nursing Personnel Recommendation, 1977 (No. 157). Recommendation Concerning Employment and Conditions of Work and Life of Nursing Personnel.*

ILO (International Labour Organization). (n.d.). *Workplace Violence.* Retrieved from www.ilo.org/public/english/dialogue/sector/sectors/health/violence.htm

ILO/PSI *(International Labour Organization/Public Services International) Workshop on Employment and Labour Practices in Health Care in Central and Eastern Europe, Prague, Czech Republic, 15–17 May 1997.* (n.d.). Geneva, Switzerland: International Labour Office.

ILO (International Labour Organization) Sectoral Activities Program. (n.d.). *Joint Meeting on Terms of Employment and Working Conditions in Health Sector Reforms: Note on the Proceedings, Geneva, Switzerland, 21–25 September 1998.* Geneva, Switzerland: International Labour Office.

"Increase in Statutory Holiday Entitlement Still Leaves UK at Bottom of EU League Table." (2007, August 14). *Workplace Law.* Retrieved from www.workplacelaw.net/services/news/8964/UK-bottom-of-the-eu-holiday-entitlement-league

Index Foundation & Praxis Centre for Policy Studies. (2007). *Hospital Reform in Bulgaria and Estonia: What is Rational and What Not? Final Report.* Budapest, Hungary: Local Government and Public Service Reform Initiative of the Open Society Institute in Budapest.

Informe sobre las condiciones de empleo y de trabajo en el marco de las reformas del sector de la salud [Report on the employment and work conditions in health sector reforms]. (1999). Geneva, Switzerland: International Labor Organization.

"INO-PNA (Irish Nurses Organisation-Psychiatric Nurses Association) Submission to the Benchmarking Body on Major Pay Claims." (2007). *World of Irish Nursing,* 15(8 Special Suppl.). Retrieved from www.ino.ie/6403

Institute of Medicine of the National Academies. (2004). *Keeping Patients Safe: Transforming the Work Environment of Nurses.* Washington, DC: National Academies Press.

Institute of Medicine of the National Academies. (2011). *The Future of Nursing: Leading Change, Advancing Health.* Washington, DC: National Academies Press.

"Intentional Rounding: What Is the Evidence?" (2012, April). *Policy +,* Issue 35.

International Centre for Human Resources in Nursing. (2007a). *An Ageing Nursing Workforce.* Retrieved from www.icn.ch

International Centre for Human Resources in Nursing. (2007b). *Positive Practice Environments.* Retrieved from www.icn.ch

International Centre for Human Resources in Nursing. (2007c). *Workplace Bullying in the Health Sector.* Retrieved from www.icn.ch

International Centre for Human Resources in Nursing. (2009a). *Nursing Personnel Pensions.* Retrieved from www.icn.ch

International Centre for Human Resources in Nursing. (2009b). *Skill Mix Decision-Making for Nursing.* Retrieved from www.icn.ch

International Centre for Human Resources in Nursing. (2010). *An Ageing Nursing Workforce.* Retrieved from www.icn.ch

International Council of Nurses. (1999). *Position Statement: Strike Policy.* Retrieved from www.icn.ch

International Council of Nurses. (2006). *Position Statement: Abuse and Violence Against Nursing Personnel.* Retrieved from www.icn.ch

International Council of Nurses. (2007a). *Nursing Workforce Profile 2006.* Retrieved from www.icn.ch

International Council of Nurses. (2007b). *Position Statement: Nurses and Shift Work.* Retrieved from www.icn.ch

International Council of Nurses. (2008a). *Position Statement: Participation of Nurses in Health Services Decision Making and Policy Development.* Retrieved from www.icn.ch

International Council of Nurses. (2008b). "Qualità del lavoro = cure di qualità (Influenze positive negli ambienti di lavoro) [Quality work = quality care (Positive influences on work environments)]." *Professioni Infermieristiche* 61(1):1–32.

International Council of Nurses. (2010). *Nurse Practitioner/Advanced Practice Nurse: Definition and Characteristics.* Retrieved from www.icn.ch

International Council of Nurses. (2011). *Position Statement: Industrial Action.* Retrieved from www.icn.ch

International Council of Nurses, International Pharmaceutical Federation, World Dental Federation, World Medical Association, International Hospital Federation, and World Confederation for Physical Therapy. (2008a). *Guidelines: Incentives for Health Care Professionals.* Retrieved from www.icn.ch

International Council of Nurses, International Pharmaceutical Federation, World Dental Federation, World Medical Association, International Hospital Federation, & World Confederation for Physical Therapy. (2008b). *Positive Practice Environments for Health Care Professionals.* Retrieved from www.icn.ch

International Council of Nurses Workforce Forum. (2013). *Nursing Workforce Profile-Database Summary 2013.* Retrieved from www.icn.ch

International Labour Office. (2010). *Update of Sectoral Aspects Regarding the Global Economic Crisis: Tourism, Public Services, Education and Health.* Geneva, Switzerland: Author.

International Labour Office, International Council of Nurses, World Health Organisation, & Public Services International. (2002). *Framework Guidelines for Addressing Workplace Violence in the Health Sector.* Geneva, Switzerland: International Labour Office.

International Labour Office, International Council of Nurses, World Health Organisation, & Public Services International Joint Programme on Workplace Violence in the Health Sector. (2003). *Workplace Violence in the Health Sector: Case Study Bulgaria.* Geneva, Switzerland: International Council of Nurses.

International Labour Organization. (2002, October 24). "International Labour Organization Joint Programme Launches New Initiative Against Workplace Violence in the Health Sector." (Press release--ILO/02/49).

International Labour Organization Sectoral Activities Programme. (1998). *Terms of Employment and Working Conditions in Health Sector Reforms.* Geneva, Switzerland: International Labour Office.

Irish Nurses Organisation. (2005). *Annual Report 2005.* Dublin, Ireland: Author.

Irish Nurses Organisation. (2006). *Getting Started – The Public Health Nurses Guide to Commencing the Process of Developing an Advanced Nurse Practitioner Role Within the Community.* Dublin, Ireland: Author.

Irish Nurses Organisation. (2007). *Forming EU Healthcare Policy: A Showcase of Irish Involvement.* Dublin, Ireland: Author.

Irish Nurses and Midwives Organisation. (2013). *ICN Workforce Forum 2013, Dublin, Ireland, September 23–25, 2013: Overview Paper.* Retrieved from www.icn.ch

Jacobs, A. T. J. M. (2005). "The Netherlands: In the Tradition of Intersectoral Parts." *Bulletin of Comparative Labour Relations* 56:89–115.

Jesse, M., Habicht, J., Aavikson, A., Koppel, A., Irs, A., & Thompson, S. (2004). *Health Care Systems in Transition: Estonia.* Copenhagen, Denmark: WHO Regional Office for Europe on behalf of the European Observatory on Health Systems and Policies.

Joel, L. A. (2011). *Kelly's Dimensions of Professional Nursing* (10th ed.). New York: McGraw Hill.

Johnson, B. (2011). "UK Telehealth Initiatives in Palliative Care: A Review." *International Journal of Palliative Nursing* 17(6):301–308.

Johnson, S. L. (2009). "International Perspectives on Workplace Bullying Among Nurses: A Review." *International Nursing Review* 56(1):34–40.

Jokivuori, P. (2007). *Nurses' Union Rejects Pay Offer and Calls for Industrial Action.* Retrieved from www.eurofound.europa.eu/eiro/2007/10/articles/fi0710039i.htm

Jones, R. A. P. (2007). *Nursing Leadership and Management: Theories, Processes and Practice.* Philadelphia, PA: F. A. Davis Company.

Josefsson, K., Sonde, L., & Wahlin, T.-B. R. (2007). "Registered Nurses' Education and Their Views on Competence Development in Municipal Elderly Care in Sweden: A Questionnaire Survey." *International Journal of Nursing Studies* 44(2):245–258.

Josefsson, K., Sonde, L., & Wahlin, T.-B. R. (2008). "Competence Development of Registered Nurses in Municipal Elderly Care in Sweden: A Questionnaire Survey." *International Journal of Nursing Studies* 45(3):428–441.

Josefsson, K., Sonde, L., Winblad, B., & Wahlin, T.-B. R. (2007). "Work Situation of Registered Nurses in Municipal Elderly Care in Sweden: A Questionnaire Survey." *International Journal of Nursing Studies* 44(1):71–82.

Josephson, M., Lindberg, P., Fochsen, G., & Vingard, E. (2003). "Sustainable Health Among Swedish Nurses." In H.-M. Hasselhorn, P. Tackenberg, & B. H. Müller, (Eds.), *Working Conditions and Intent to Leave the Profession Among Nursing Staff in Europe* (pp. 213–219). (SALTA-JOINT PROGRAMME FOR WORKING LIFE RESEARCH IN EUROPE, Report No. 7). Retrieved January 5, 2007, from www.arbetslivsinstitutet.se

Jung, L. (2001). *National Labour Law Profile: Federal Republic of Germany.* Retrieved June 2, 2007, from www.ilo.org/public/english/dialogue/.../ger.htm

Kaarna, M., Põlluste, K., Lepnurm, R., & Thetloff, M. (2004). "The Progress of Reforms: Job Satisfaction in a Typical Hospital in Estonia." *International Journal for Quality in Health Care* 16(3):253–261.

Kalafati, M., Bellah, T., Kontodimopoulos, N., & Niakas, D. (2005). "Quality of Life and Burnout in Critical and Non-Critical Care Unit Nurses: Nursing Abstracts from the 2nd Conference of the World Federation of Critical Care Nurses." *Connect: The World of Critical Care Nursing* 4(3):117.

Kalnins, I. (2002). "Latvian Community Nurses Practising in a Time of Turmoil: A Thin Line of Defence for Children at Risk." *International Nursing Review* 49(2):111–121.

Kalnins, I. (2006). "Caring for the Terminally Ill: Experiences of Latvian Family Caregivers." *International Nursing Review* 53(2):129–135.

Känd, M., & Rekor, M. (2005). *Perceived Involvement in Decision Making and Job Satisfaction: The Evidence from a Job Satisfaction Survey Among Nurses in Estonia* (SSE Riga Working Papers 2005:6(74)). Riga, Latvia: Stockholm School of Economics in Riga.

Kangas, O., & Rostgaard, T. (2007). "Preferences or Institutions? Work-Family Life Opportunities in Seven European Countries." *Journal of European Social Policy* 17(3):240–256.

Kapborg, I. (2000). "The Nursing Education Programme in Lithuania: Voices of Student Nurses." *Journal of Advanced Nursing* 32(4):857–863.

Karasek, R.A. Jr. (1979). "Job Demands, Job Decision Latitude, and Mental Strain: Implications for Job Redesign." *Administrative Science Quarterly* 24:285–308.

Karnite, R. (2005, April 14). *Medical Workers' Pay Protests Accelerate Reform of Healthcare System.* Retrieved from www.eurofound.europa.eu/eiro/2005/02/feature/lv0502101f.htm

Karnite, R. (2007. September 17). *Low Salaries Lead to Illegal Payments in the Healthcare Sector.* Retrieved from www.eurofound.europa.eu

Karnite, R.(2008, September 2). *Healthcare Workers Prepare to Strike Again.* Retrieved from www.eurofound.europa.eu

Kasearu, K. (2009). "The Effect of Union Type on Work-Life Conflict in Five European Countries." *Social Indicators Research* 93(3):549–567.

Kauppinen, T. (n.d.). *Industrial Relations in the New European Member States (EU 10).* Retrieved from www.ser.nl/~/media/files/internet/publicaties/overige/2000_2009/2004/b23574_5.ashx

Kautoch, M., & Czabanowska, K. (2011). "When the Grass Gets Greener at Home: Poland's Changing Incentives for Health Professional Mobility." In M. Wismar, C. B. Maier, I. A. Glinos, G. Dussault, & J. Figueras (Eds.), *Health Professional Mobility and Health Systems: Evidence from 17 European Countries* (pp. 419–448). Copenhagen, Denmark: World Health Organization on behalf of European Observatory on Health Systems and Policies.

Keller, S.M. (2009). "Effects of Extended Work Shifts and Shift Work on Patient Safety, Productivity, and Employee Health." *AAOHN Journal* 57(12):497–502.

Kelly, B. (1996). "Hospital Nursing: 'It's a Battle!' – A Follow-Up Study of English Graduate Nurses." *Journal of Advanced Nursing* 24(5):1063–1069.

Kerkstra, A., & Hutten, J. B. F. (1996). "Organization and Financing of Home Nursing in the European Union." *Journal of Advanced Nursing* 24(5):1023 1032.

Keune, M. (2008). *EU Enlargement and Social Standards: Exporting the European Social Model.* Brussels, Belgium: European Trade Union Institute for Research, Education and Health and Safety.

Kiik, R., & Sirotkina, R. (2006). "Hospice – The Ideology and Perspectives in Estonia." *International Nursing Review* 53(2):136–142.

Kingma, M. (1999). "Discrimination in Nursing." *International Nursing Review* 46(3):87–90.

Kingma, M. (2001). "Workplace Violence in the Health Sector. A Problem of Epidemic Proportion." *International Nursing Review* 48(3):129–130.

Kingma, M. (2003). "Economic Incentive in Community Nursing: Attraction, Rejection or Indifference?" *Human Resources for Health* 1:2. Retrieved from www.human-resources-health.com/content/1/1/2

Kirpal, S. (2003). *Nurses in Europe: Work Identities of Nurses Across 4 European Countries*. Bremen, Germany: University of Bremen.

Kleitsa, E. (2003, November 5). "Greece: Strike Rocks Government." Retrieved from www.socialistworld.net/mob/view/29

Kloster, T., Høie, M., & Skarr, R. (2007). "Nursing Students' Career Preferences: A Norwegian Study." *Journal of Advanced Nursing* 59(2):155–162.

Kohl, H., & Platzer, H. W. (2003). "Labour Relations in Central and Eastern Europe and the European Social Model." *Transfer* 9(4):11–30.

Köhler, H-D., & Begega, S. G. (2007). "Consequences of Enlargement for the Old Periphery of Europe: Observations from the Spanish Experience with European Works Councils." In P. Leisink, B. Steijn, & U. Veersma (Eds.), *Industrial Relations in the New Europe: Enlargement, Integration and Reform* (pp. 99–114). Cheltenham, England: Edgar Elgar.

Kopel, A., Kahur, K., Habicht, T., Saar, P., Habicht, J., & van Ginneken, E. (2008). "Estonia: Health System Review." *Health Systems in Transition* 10(1):1–230.

Korkut, U. (2006). "Entrenched Elitism in Trade Unions in Poland and Romania: An Explanation for the Lack of Union Strength and Success?" *Economic and Industrial Democracy* 27(1):67–104.

Korompeli, A., Sourtzi, P., Tzavara, C., & Velonakis, E. (2009). "Rotating Shift-Related Changes in Hormonal Levels in Intensive Care Unit Nurses." *Journal of Advanced Nursing* 65(6):1274–1282.

Kovács, B. (2009). *Parental Leave in Romania and Hungary and European Accession: Welfare State Untransformed*. Retrieved from www.science.gov

Kovarova, M., Hanzlikova, A., Rimarcik, M., & Jurkovic, M. (2003). "Intent to Leave Nursing in Slovakia." In H.-M. Hasselhorn, P. Tackenberg, & B. H. Müller (Eds.), *Working Conditions and Intent to Leave the Profession Among Nursing Staff in Europe* (pp. 220–229). (SALTA-JOINT PROGRAMME FOR WORKING LIFE RESEARCH IN EUROPE, Report No. 7). Retrieved January 5, 2007, from www.arbetslivsinstitutet.se

Kowalska, I. (2007, October). "Working Time of Health Professionals." *Health Policy Monitor*. Retrieved February 15, 2008, from www.hpm.org/survey/pl/a10/5

Krajewski-Siuda, K., & Romaniuk, P. (2006). "Wanted Nurses." *European Journal of Public Health* 16(4):447.

Kritsantonis, N. D. (1998). "Greece: The Maturing of the System." In A. Ferner, & R. Hyman (Eds.), *Changing Industrial Relations in Europe* (pp. 504–528). Oxford: Blackwell.

Lado, M., & Vaughan-Whitehead, D. (2003). "Social Dialogue in Candidate Countries: What for?" *Transfer* 9(1):364–387.

Lai, T., Habicht, T., Kahur, K., Reinap, M., Kiivet, R., & van Ginneken, E. (2013). "Estonia: Health System Review." *Health Systems in Transition* 15(6):1–196.

Laine, M., & the NEXT-Study Group. (2003). "Job Insecurity in the Nursing Profession in Europe." In H.-M. Hasselhorn, P. Tackenberg, & B. H. Müller (Eds.), *Working Conditions and Intent to Leave the Profession Among Nursing Staff in Europe* (pp. 70–75). (SALTA-JOINT PROGRAMME FOR WORKING LIFE RESEARCH IN EUROPE, Report No. 7). Retrieved January 5, 2007, from www. arbetslivsinstitutet.se

Lambrinou, E., Sourtzi, P., Kalokerinou, A., & Lemonidou, C. (2009). "Attitudes and Knowledge of the Greek Nursing Students Towards Older People." *Nurse Education Today* 29(6):617–622.

Lamond, D. (2000). "The Information Content of the Nurse Change of Shift Report: A Comparative Study." *Journal of Advanced Nursing* 31(4):794–804.

Lane, C., Antunes, A. F., & Kingma, M. (2009). *The Nursing Community, Macro-Economic and Public Finance Policies: Towards a Better Understanding.* Geneva, Switzerland: World Health Organization & International Council of Nurses.

Legido-Quigley, H., McKee, M., Nolte, E., & Glinos, I. A. (2008). *Assuring the Quality of Health Care in the European Union: A Case for Action.* Copenhagen, Denmark: World Health Organization on behalf of the European Observatory on Health Systems and Policies.

Leisink, P., Steijn, B., & Veersma. U. (2007a). "Concluding Analysis." In P. Leisink, B. Steijn, & U. Veersma (Eds.), *Industrial Relations in the New Europe: Enlargement, Integration and Reform* (pp. 235–256). Cheltenham, England: Edward Elgar.

Leisink, P., Steijn, B., & Veersma, U. (2007b). "Industrial Relations in the New Europe: Introduction." In P. Leisink, B. Steijn, & U. Veersma (Eds.), *Industrial Relations in the New Europe: Enlargement, Integration and Reform* (pp. 1–19). Cheltenham, England: Edward Elgar.

LeLan, R. (2004, août). *Les conditions de travail perçues par les professionnels des établissements do santé [Work conditions as perceived by professionals in health-care establishments]* (No. 335). Paris: Observatoire National de la Démographie des Professions de Santé (ONDPS).

LeLan, R. (2006, mars). *La reduction du temps de travail vue par les salaries hospitaliers en 2003 [Reduced working time as seen in 2003 by salaried hospital employees]* (No. 469). Paris: Observatoire National de la Démographie des Professions de Santé (ONDPS).

Lethbridge, J. (2004). "Public Health Sector Unions and Deregulation in Europe." *International Journal of Health Services* 34(3):435–452.

Lewis, M.A. (2006). "Nurse Bullying: Organizational Considerations in the Maintenance and Perpetration of Health Care Bullying Cultures." *Journal of Nursing Management* 14(1):52–58.

Li, J., Galatsch, M., Siegrist, J., Müller, B. H., & Hasselhorn, H.-M. (2011). "Reward Frustration at Work and Intention to Leave the Nursing Profession – Prospective Results from the European Longitudinal NEXT Study." *International Journal of Nursing Studies* 48(5):628–635.

Liaropoulos, L., Siskou, O., Kaitelidou, D., Theodorou, M., & Katostaras, T. (2008). "Informal Payments in Public Hospitals in Greece." *Health Policy* 87(1):72–81.

Lilja, K. (1998). "Finland: Continuity and Modest Moves Towards Company-Level Corporatism." In A. Ferner, & R. Hyman (Eds.), *Changing Industrial Relations in Europe* (pp. 171–189). Oxford: Blackwell.

Lipsky, M. (1975). "Protest as a Political Resource." In S. Welch, & J. Comer (Eds.), *Public Opinion: Its Information, Measurement, and Impact* (pp. 478–503). Palo Alto, CA: Mayfield Publishing Company.

Lockley, S. W., Barger, L. K., Ayas, N. T., & Others. (2007). "Effects of Health Care Provider Work Hours and Sleep Deprivation on Safety and Performance." *Joint Commission Journal on Quality and Patient Safety* 33(11):7–18.

Longley, M., Riley, N., Davies, P., & Hernández-Quevedo, C. (2012). "United Kingdom (Wales): Health System Review." *Health Systems in Transition* 14(11):1–84.

López-Valcárcel, B. G., Pérez, P. B., & Quintana, C. D. D. (2011). "Opportunities in an Expanding Health Service: Spain Between Latin America and Europe." In M. Wismer, C. B. Maier, I. A. Glinos, G. Dussault, & J. Figueras (Eds.), *Health Professional Mobility and Health Systems: Evidence from 17 European Countries*(pp. 263–293). Copenhagen, Denmark: World Health Organization on behalf of the European Observatory on Health Systems and Policies.

López-Valcárcel, B. G., Quintana, C. D. D., & Socorro, E. R. (2006). "Spain." In B. Rechel, C.-A. Dubois, & M. McKee (Eds.), *The Health Care Workforce in Europe: Learning from Experience* (pp. 115–127). Copenhagen, Denmark: WHO Regional Office for Europe on behalf of the European Observatory for Health Systems and Policies.

Lovén, K. (2009). *Sweden: Industrial Relations: Profile.* n.p.: Oxford Research.

Lucio, M. M. (1998). "Spain: Regulating Employment and Social Fragmentation." In A. Ferner, & R. Hyman (Eds.), *Changing Industrial Relations in Europe* (pp. 426–458). Oxford: Blackwell.

Lum, L., Kervin, J., Clark, K., Reid, F., & Sirola, W. (1998). "Explaining Nursing Turnover Intent: Job Satisfaction, Pay Satisfaction or Organizational Commitment." *Journal of Organizational Behavior* 19(3):305–320.

Luminita, C. (2007, February 26). *Trade Unions in Health Care Threaten General Strike.* Retrieved from www.eurofound.europa.eu/eiro/2006/11/articles/ro0611039i.htm

Magnavita, N., & Hepaniemi, I. (2011). "Workplace Violence Against Nursing Students and Nurses: An Italian Experience." *Journal of Nursing Scholarship* 43(2):203–210.

Mahon, A., & Young, R. (2006). "Health Care Managers As a Critical Component of the Health Care Workforce." In C.-A. Dubois, M. McKee, & E. Nolte (Eds.), *Human Resources for Health in Europe* (pp. 116–139). Maidenhead, Berkshire, England: Open University Press.

Malhotra, G. (2006). *Grow Your Own: Creating the Conditions for Sustainable Workforce Development.* London: King's Fund.

Malta: Council for Nurses and Midwives. (2002). *The Scope of Professional Practice.* Retrieved from https://ehealth.gov.mt/healthportal/others/regulatory_councils/council_for_nurses_and_midwives/councils_for_nurses_midwives.aspx.

"Maltese Nurses Successfully Reach Agreement After Long Dispute." (2001). *SEW News,* No. 2. Retrieved December 12, 2006, from www.icn.ch/sewmay-july01.htm

Manion, J. (2009). *Managing the Multi-Generational Nursing Workforce: Managerial and Policy Implications.* Geneva, Switzerland: International Centre for Human Resources in Nursing.

Marion. (2007, April 27). *Occupational (dis-)Continuity of Graduate Nursing Staff.* Retrieved from www.eurofound.europa.eu

Marquier, R. (2005, avril). *Les cinq premières années de carrière des infirmiers sortis de formation initiale [The first five years of a nurse's career after initial training]* (No. 393). Paris: Observatoire National de la Démographie des Professions de Santé (ONDPS).

Marquier, R., & Idmachiche, S. (2006). "Les trois premières années de carrière des infirmiers de la generation 2001 [Nurses from the 2001 generation: The first three years of their careers]." *Dossiers solidarité et santé* No. 1: 35–50.

Martellotti, E. (2005). "La tecnologia della comunicazione per una nuova immagine degli infermieri [Communication technology for a new image of nurses]." *L'infermiere* 49(9):5–7.

Martinez, A., & Martinez, C. (2002). "Working in Spanish ICUs Compared with UK ICUs." *Connect: The World of Critical Care Nursing* 2(2):59–60.

Maslach, C. (1993). "Burnout: A Multi-Dimensional Perspective." In W. B. Schaufele, C. Maslach, & T. Marek (Eds.), *Professional Burnout: Recent Developments in Theory and Research* (pp. 19–32). Philadelphia, PA: Taylor & Francis.

"Maternity Leaves Around the World: Worst and Best Countries for Paid Maternity Leave." (2012, May 22). *The Huffington Post Canada*. Retrieved from www.huffingtonpost.ca

McCarthy, G. (2000). "Nursing in a Changing World." In J. Robins (Ed.), *Nursing and Midwifery in Ireland in the Twentieth Century: Fifty Years of An Bord Altranais (The Nursing Board) 1950–2000* (pp. 213–233). Dublin, Ireland: An Bord Altranais.

McCarthy, G., Tyrrell, M. P., & Cronin, C. (2002*). National Study of Turnover in Nursing and Midwifery* (Commissioned by the Department of Health and Children). Cork, Ireland: National University of Ireland, Department of Nursing Studies.

McConaghy, B. (2007). "EU Policy – The State Of Play." *World of Irish Nursing* 15(6). Retrieved from www.inmo.le/6379

McDaid, D., Wiley, M., Maresso, A., & Mossialos, E. (2009). "Ireland: Health System Review." *Health Systems in Transition* 11(4):1–268.

McDonald, R., Campbell, S., & Lester, H. (2009). "Practice Nurses and the Effects of the New General Practitioner Contract in the English National Health Service: The Extension of a Professional Project?" *Social Science and Medicine* 68(7):1206–1212.

McGillis-Hall, L. (1997). "Staff Mix Models: Complementary or Substitution Roles for Nurses." *Nursing Administration Quarterly* 21(2):31–39.

McHugh, M. D., Kelly, L. A., & Aiken, L. H. (2011). "Contradicting Fears, California's Nurse-to-Patient Mandate Did Not Reduce the Skill Level of the Nursing Workforce in Hospitals." *Health Affairs* 30(7):1299–1306.

McHugh, M. D., Kutney-Lee, A., Cimiotti, J. P., & Others. (2011). "Nurses' Widespread Dissatisfaction, Burnout and Frustration with Health Benefits Signals Problems for Patient Care." *Health Affairs* 30(2):202–210.

McKee, M., Dubois, C.-A., & Sibbald, B. (2006). "Changing Professional Boundaries." In C.-A. Dubois, M. McKee, & E. Nolte (Eds.), *Human Resources for Health in Europe* (pp. 63–78). Maidenhead, Berkshire, England: Open University Press.

Meadows, S., Levenson, R., & Baeza, J. (n.d.). *The Last Straw: Explaining the NHS Nursing Shortage.* n.p.: King's Fund.

Meisner, A., Hasselhorn, H.-M., Estryn-Behar, M., Nézet, O., Pokorski, J., & Gould, D. (2007). "Nurses' Perception of Shift Handovers in Europe – Results from the European Nurses' Early Exit Study." *Journal of Advanced Nursing* 57(5):535–542.

Mermet, E., & Lehndorff, S. (2001). *New Forces of Employment and Working Time in the Service Economy.* Brussels, Belgium: European Trade Union Institute.

Midy, F. (2003a, April). "Home Care and Nursing Roles Revisited." *Health Policy Monitor.* Retrieved January 4, 2007, from www.hpm.org

Midy, F. (2003b). *Les principaux changements dans la profession infirmière depuis vingt ans [Principal changes in the nursing profession over twenty years]*. Retrieved June 6, 2005, from www.irdes.fr

Miettinen, A. (2005, December 14). *Job Commitment in [the] Nursing Profession*. Retrieved from www.eurofound.europa.eu

Mihailova, T. (2007, July 30). *Medical Workers Threaten Strike in Emergency Hospital*. Retrieved from www.eurofound.europa.eu./eiro/2007/06/articles/bg0706049i.htm

Milosevic, M., Golubic, R., Knezevic, B., Golubic, K., Bubas, M., & Mustajbegovic, J. (2011). "Work Ability as a Major Determinant of Clinical Nurses' Quality of Life." *Journal of Clinical Nursing* 20(19–20):2931–2938.

Mischke, C., Schrader, C. F., & Schüssler, D. (2006). *Arguments and Strategies: Family Health Nursing and Midwifery in the Field of Prevention and Health Promotion*. Berlin, Germany: German Nurses Association.

Mladovsky, P., Srivastava, D., Cylus, J., Karanikolos, M., Evetovits, T., Thomson, S., et al. (2012). *Health Policy Responses to the Financial Crisis in Europe*. Copenhagen, Denmark: World Health Organization on behalf of the European Observatory on Health Systems and Policies.

Monecchi, E., & Peroni, A. (2007). "La persona e la motivazione: I sistemi premianti come strumenti di gestione del personale sanitario [The individual and motivation: Prize winning systems for managing health-care personnel]." *Professioni Infermieristiche* 60(2):94–98.

Mooney, M. (2007). "Facing Registration: The Expectations and the Unexpected." *Nurse Education Today* 27(8):840–847.

Moore, C. (2006). "The Transition from Student to Qualified Nurse: A Military Perspective." *British Journal of Nursing* 15(10):540–542.

Moreno-Casbas, T., Fuentelsaz-Gallego, C., González-María, E., & Contreras-Moreira, M. (2011). *RN4CAST Nurses' Reports of Working Conditions and Their Consequences for Retention and Quality*. Presentation at the ICN Conference Nurses Driving Access, Quality and Health, Valletta, Malta, 2–8 May 2011.

Morris, C. (2011). "A Global Update on the Development of Palliative Care Services." *International Journal of Palliative Nursing* 17(10):472–475.

Mosoiu, D., Andrews, C., & Perolls, G. (2000). "Palliative Care in Romania." *Palliative Medicine* 14(1):65–67.

Mossialos, E., & McKee, M. (2002). *EU Law and the Social Character of Health Care Systems*. Brussels, Belgium: Peter Lang.

Mrozowicki, A. (2013, January 24). *Nurses Protest Over Public Healthcare Policies*. Retrieved from www.eurofound.europa.eu

Mulholland, H. (2006, October 24). "Unions Threaten Strike Over Nurses' Pay." *The Guardian*. Retrieved from www.theguardian.com/politics/2006/oct/24/publicservices.uk

Müller-Mundt, G. (1997). "Trends in Hospital Restructuring and Impact on the Workforce in Germany." *Medical Care* 35(10):OS132–OS142.

Murray, S. A., Sallnou, L., & Aguiar, H. (2012). *Palliative Care in Primary Care: An Update from the Taskforce*. Milan, Italy: European Association for Palliative Care.

Murrells, T., Robins, S., & Griffiths, P. (2008). "Is Satisfaction a Direct Predictor of Nursing Turnover? Modelling the Relationship Between Satisfaction, Expressed

Intention and Behaviour in a Longitudinal Cohort Study." *Human Resources for Health* 6(22):1–12.

Muscat, N., Calleja, N., Calleja, A., & Cylus, J. (2014). "Malta: Health System Review." *Health Systems in Transition* 16(1):1–97.

Muscat, N. A., & Grech, K. (2006). "Malta." In B. Rechel, C.-A. Dubois, & M. McKee (Eds.), *The Health Care Workforce in Europe: Learning from Experience* (pp. 59–70). Copenhagen, Denmark: WHO Regional Office for Europe on behalf of the European Observatory and Health Systems and Policies.

Musques, J., & Naiditch, M. (2008, October). "Regulating Nurses-Follow Up." *Health Policy Monitor*. Retrieved March 3, 2010, from www.hpm.org

Naiditch, M. (2007, October). "New Nursing Regulation." *Health Policy Monitor*. Retrieved March 3, 2010, from www.hpm.org

National Council for the Professional Development of Nursing and Midwifery. (2004). *An Evaluation of the Effectiveness of the Role of the Clinical Nurse/ Midwife Specialist*. Dublin, Ireland: Author.

National Council for the Professional Development of Nursing and Midwifery. (2005). *A Preliminary Evaluation of the Role of the Advanced Nurse Practitioner*. Dublin, Ireland: Author.

National Council for the Professional Development of Nursing and Midwifery. (2007). *Framework for the Establishment of Advanced Nurse Practitioners and Advanced Midwife Practitioner Posts* (3rd ed.). Dublin, Ireland: Author.

Needleman, J., Buerhaus, P., Pankratz, S., & Others. (2011). "Nurse Staffing and Inpatient Hospital Mortality." *The New England Journal of Medicine* 364(11):1037–1045.

Neumann, G. T. F- L. (2004, February 12). *New Working Time Regulations for Healthcare Workers*. Retrieved from www.eurofound.europa.eu/observatories/ eurwork/articles/new-working-time-regulations-for-healthcare-workers

"New Report Makes Grim Reading for European Nurses and Midwives." (2012, August). *Queensland Nurse*, p. 18.

NHS (National Health Service) Staff Council. (2009). *Improving Working Lives in the NHS: A Framework Developed by the NHS Staff Council*. London: NHS Employers.

Nightingale, F. (1954a). "Subsidiary Notes as to the Introduction of Female Nursing into Military Hospitals in Peace and in War." In L. R. Seymer (Ed.), *Selected Writings of Florence Nightingale* (pp. 27–122). New York: The Macmillan Company.

Nightingale, F. (1954b). "Suggestions on the Subject of Providing Training and Organizing Nurses for the Sick Poor in Workhouse Infirmaries." In L. R. Seymer (Ed.), *Selected Writings of Florence Nightingale* (pp. 271–318). New York: The Macmillan Company.

Nightingale, F. (1954c). "Thoughts Submitted by Order Concerning I: Hospital-Nurses, II: Nurses in Civil Hospitals, III: Nurses in Her Majesty's Hospitals." In L. R. Seymer (Ed.), *Selected Writings of Florence Nightingale* (pp. 5–26). New York: The Macmillan Company.

Nolte, E., & McKee, M. (2008a). "Caring for People with Chronic Conditions: An Introduction." In E. Nolte, & M. McKee (Eds.), *Caring for People with Chronic Conditions: A Health System Perspective* (pp. 1–14). Maidenhead, Berkshire, England: Open University Press.

Nolte, E., & McKee, M. (2008b). "Integration and Chronic Care: A Review." In E. Nolte, & M. McKee (Eds.), *Caring for People with Chronic Conditions: A*

Health Systems Perspective (pp. 64–91). Maidenhead, Berkshire, England: Open University Press.

Nolte, E., McKee, M., & Knai, C. (2008). "Managing Chronic Conditions: An Introduction to the Experience in Eight Countries." In E. Nolte, C. Knai, & M. McKee (Eds.), *Managing Chronic Conditions: Experience in Eight Countries* (pp. 1–14). Copenhagen, Denmark: World Health Organization on behalf of the European Observatory on Health Systems and Policies.

"Nurses Fired for Strike in Poland." (2009, April 21). Retrieved from www.libcom.org

"Nurses Strike Against Austerity Measures." (2012, November 29). Retrieved December 1, 2012, from www.reuters.com/article/2012/11/29/us-croatia-strike-idUSBRE8AS0B020121129

"Nurses Vote to Strike Over Public Sector Cuts." (2009, November 10). *IRISHecho*. Retrieved from www.irishecho.com.au/2009/11/10/irish-nurses-vote-to-strike-over-public-sector-cuts/803

Nursing in Hungary. (n.d.). Retrieved July 24, 2009, from www.eti.hu/hce/nursing/NursingInHun.htm#2

Nystrom, P. (2009). *EPSU/UNI Europa Report: Policies, Strategies and Implementation: How Issues of Third Party Violence Have Been Tackled in Practice by Social Partners in the Commerce, Hospital, Private Security and Local and Regional Government Sectors.* Brussels, Belgium: UNI Europa & European Federation of Public Service Unions (EPSU).

O'Brien, T. (2007). "Overseas Nurses in the National Health Service: A Process of Deskilling." *Journal of Clinical Nursing* 16(12):2229–2236.

OECD (Organisation for Economic Co-Operation and Development). (2009). *Health at a Glance 2009: OECD Indicators.* Paris: OECD Publishing.

OECD (Organisation for Economic Co-Operation and Development). (2012). *Health at a Glance: Europe 2012.* Paris: OECD Publishing.

Ogińska, H., Camerino, D., Estryn-Beher, M., Pokorski, J., & the NEXT-Study Group. (2003). "Work Schedules of Nurses in Europe." In H.-M. Hasselhorn, P. Tackenberg, & B. H. Müller (Eds.), *Working Conditions and Intent to Leave the Profession Among Nursing Staff in Europe* (pp. 82–87). (SALTA-JOINT PROGRAMME FOR WORKING LIFE RESEARCH IN EUROPE, Report No. 7). Retrieved January 5, 2007, from www.arbetslivsinstitutet.se.

Oliver, D. (2005). "Palliative Care Education in Croatia." *International Journal of Palliative Nursing* 11(8):419.

Olzak, S., & Ryo, E. (2007). "Organizational Diversity, Vitality and Outcomes in the Civil Rights Movement." *Social Forces* 85(4):1561–1591.

Ordem dos Enfermeiros. (2011). *OEDATA em: 31-12-2011: membros activos [OEDATA em: 31-12-2011: Active Members].* Retrieved from www.ordemenfermeiros.pt

Padaiga, Z., Pukas, M., & Starkienė, L. (2011). "Awareness, Planning and Retention: Lithuania's Approach to Managing Health Professional Mobility." In M. Wismar, C. B. Maier, I. A. Glinos, G. Dussault, & J. Figueras (Eds.), *Health Professional Mobility and Health Systems: Evidence from 17 Countries* (pp. 395–417). Copenhagen, Denmark: World Health Organization on behalf of the European Observatory on Health Systems and Policies.

Padaiga, Z., Starkienė, L., Logminiene, Z., & Reamy, J. (2006). "Lithuania." In B. Rechel, C.-A. Dubois, & M. McKee (Eds.), *The Health Care Workforce in*

Europe: Learning from Experience (pp. 47–58). Copenhagen, Denmark: WHO Regional Office for Europe on behalf of the European Observatory on Health Systems and Policies.

Page, A. (Ed.). (2004). *Keeping Patients Safe: Transforming the Work Environment of Nurses*. Washington, DC: National Academies Press.

Palese, A., Tosatto, D., & Mesaglio, M. (2009). "Process and Factors Influencing Italian Nurse Graduates' First Choice of Employment: A Descriptive Study." *Journal for Nurses in Staff Development* 25(4):184–190.

Papageorgiou, D., Fouka, G., Plakas, S., Kelesi, M., Fasoi, G., & Vardaki, Z. (2012). "Private Duty Nurses in Greek Hospitals: A Literature Review." *International Nursing Review* 59(4):458–465.

Pearson, S., & Peels, S. (2001). "A Global View of Nursing in the New Millennium – 3: The Organization of Nursing." *International Journal of Nursing Practice* 7(3):S11–S13.

Peckover, S., & Chidlaw, R. G. (2007). "The (Un)-Certainties of District Nurses in the Context of Cultural Diversity." *Journal of Advanced Nursing* 58(4):377–385.

Pedersen, H. S., & Christiansen, R. H. (2005, September 19). *Violence in the Workplace*. Retrieved June 19, 2009, from www.eurofound.europa.eu/ewco/2005/09/DK0509NU03.htm

Peeters, M., McKee, M., & Merkur, S. (2010). "EU Law and Health Professionals." In E. Mossialos, G. Permanand, R. Baeten, & T. K. Hervey (Eds.), *Health Systems Governance in Europe: The Role of European Law and Policy* (pp. 589–634). New York: Cambridge University Press.

Peña-Casas, R., & Pochet, P. (2009). *Convergence and Divergence of Working Conditions in Europe: 1990–2005*. Retrieved from www.eurofound.europa.eu

Philips, K. (2006). *Capacity Building for Social Dialogue in Estonia*. Retrieved from www.eurofound.europa.eu

Picot, G. (2005). "Entre médecins et personnel infirmier à l'hôpital public: Un rapport social instable: Le cas de deux services hospitaliers [Between physicians and nursing personnel in the public hospital: An unstable social relationship: The case of two hospital services]." *Revue française des affaires sociales* 59(1):83–100.

Pike, G., & Ball, J. (2007). *Black and Minority Ethnic and Internationally Recruited Nurses: Results from RCN Employment/Working Well Surveys 2005 and 2002*. London: Royal College of Nursing.

Pike, G., & Williams, M. (2006). *Nurses and Public Sector Pay: Labour Force Survey Analysis 2006*. Hove, East Sussex, England: Employment Research Ltd.

Pike, G., & Williams, M. (2008). *Nurses Pay: Occupational Comparisons – Labour Force Survey Analysis 2008*. London: Royal College of Nursing.

Pikó, B. (1999). "Work-Related Stress Among Nurses: A Challenge For Institutions." *The Journal of the Royal Society for the Promotion of Health* 119(3):156–162.

Pillinger, J. (2000). *Working Time in Europe: A European Working Time Policy in the Public Services*. n.p.: European Trade Union Institute.

Plantenga, J., Remery, C., Siegel, M., & Sementini, L. (2008). "Childcare Services in 25 European Union Member States: The Barcelona Targets Revisited." *Comparative Social Research* 25:27–53.

"PM's Commission on the Future of Nursing at a Glance." (2010, March 2). *Nursing Times*. Retrieved from www.nursingtimes.net

Poghosyan, L., Aiken, L. H., & Stone, D. M. (2009). "Factor Structure of the Maslach Burnout Inventory: An Analysis of Data from Large Scale Cross-Sectional Surveys of Nurses from Eight Countries." *International Journal of Nursing Studies* 46(7):894–902.

Pokorski, J., van der Schoot, E., Wickström, G., Pokorska, J., Hasselhorn, H.-M., & the NEXT-Study Group. (2003). "Meaning of Work in the European Nursing Profession." In H.-M. Hasselhorn, P. Tackenberg, & B. H. Müller (Eds.), *Working Conditions and Intent to Leave the Profession Among Nursing Staff in Europe* (pp. 58–63). (SALTA-JOINT PROGRAMME FOR WORKING LIFE RESEARCH IN EUROPE, Report No. 7). Retrieved January 5, 2007, from www.arbetslivsinstitutet.se

"Polish Nurses Protest About Health Spending." (2007, August). *EPHA Newsletter.* Retrieved September 8, 2008, from www.epha.org/spip.php?mot171&debut_articles=20#pagination_articles

"Preserving the Nursing Workforce: The Importance of Job Satisfaction in Early Career." (2008, March 8). *Policy+*, Issue 8.

"Public Sector Spending Cuts Impact on Nurses Across Europe." (2011). *ICHRN eNewsletter* 5(2):3.

Purcell, J., Purcell, K., & Tailby, S. (2004). "Temporary Work Agencies: Here Today, Gone Tomorrow." *British Journal of Industrial Relations* 42(4):705–727.

Quintas, C., & Cristovam, M. L. (2002, September 16). *Public Sector Reforms Contested.* Retrieved from www.eurofound.europa.eu

Radulova, E. (2009). "The Construction of EU's Childcare Policy Through the Open Method of Coordination." In S. Kröger (Ed.), *What We have Learnt: Advances, Pitfalls and Remaining Questions in OMC Research* (European Integration Online Papers (EIoP). Special Issue 13(1), Article 13. Retrieved from www.eiop.or.at/eiop/texte/2009-013a.htm

Rafferty, A. M., & Clarke, S. P. (2009). "Nursing Work-Force: A Special Issue." *International Journal of Nursing Studies* 46(7):875–878.

Ray, R., & Schmitt, J. (2007). *No-Vacation Nation.* Washington, DC: Center for Economic and Policy Research.

Ray, R., & Schmitt, J. (2008). "The Right to Vacation: An International Perspective." *International Journal of Health Services* 38(1):21–45.

Rechel, B., Buchan, J., & McKee, M. (2009). "The Impact of Health Facilities on Healthcare Workers' Well-Being and Performance." *International Journal of Nursing Studies* 46(7):1025–1034.

Regulation (EC) No. 883/2004 of the European Parliament and of the Council of 29 April 2004 on the Coordination of Social Security Systems.

Report on the Second WHO Ministerial Conference on Nursing and Midwifery in Europe, Munich, Germany, 15–17 June 2000. (2001). Copenhagen, Denmark: World Health Organization Regional Office for Europe.

Review Body for Nursing and Other Health Professions. (2007). *Twenty-Second Report on Nursing and Other Health Professions: 2007.* n.p.: The Stationary Office.

Richardson, A., Turnock, C., Finley, A., Harris, L., & Carson, S. (2005). "Evaluating the Impact of 12 Hour Shifts in Critical Care: Nursing Abstracts from the 2nd Conference of the World Federation of Critical Care Nursing." *Connect: The World of Critical Care Nursing* 4(2):Article 7. Retrieved from www.connect-publishing.org

Rigoli, F., & Dussault, G. (2003). "The Interface Between Health Sector Reform and Human Resources in Health." *Human Resources for Health* 1(9). Retrieved from www.human-resources-health.com/content/1/1/9

Robinson, S., & Griffiths, P. (2009). *Scoping Review: Preceptorship for Newly Qualified Nurses: Impacts, Facilitators and Constraints.* London: King's College, National Research Unit.

Rocafort, J., & Centeno, C. (2008). *EAPC Review of Palliative Care in Europe.* Milan, Italy: European Association of Palliative Care in Europe.

Roche, M., Diers, D., Duffield, C., & Catling-Paull, C. (2010). "Violence Toward Nurses, the Work Environment and Patient Outcomes." *Journal of Nursing Scholarship* 42(1):13–22.

Rogers, A. E., Hwang, W.-T., Scott, L. D., Aiken, L. H., & Dinges, D. F. (2004). "The Working Hours of Hospital Staff Nurses and Patient Safety." *Health Affairs* 23(4):202–212.

Rose, E. (2005). "Ideas and Suggestions: Input for the German Debate." *Bulletin of Comparative Labour Relations* 56:145–157.

Rosskam, E., & Leather, A. (2006). *Failing Health Systems in Eastern Europe.* Ferney-Voltaire, France: Public Services International.

Royal College of Nursing. (2006). *Nurse Practitioners 2006: The Results of a Survey of Nurse Practitioners Conducted on Behalf of the RCN Nurse Practitioner Association.* London: Author.

Royal College of Nursing. (2007). *Black and Minority Ethnic and Internationally Recruited Nurses: Results from RCN Employment/Working Well Surveys 2005 and 2002.* London: Author.

Rudman, A., & Gustavsson, B. J. P. (2011). "Early-Career Burnout Among New Graduate Nurses: A Prospective Observational Study of Intra-Individual Change Trajectories." *International Journal of Nursing Studies* 48(3):292–306.

Ruzafa-Martinez, M., Madrigal-Torres, M., Velandrino-Nicolás, A., & López-Iborra, L. (2008). "Satisfacción laboral de los profesionales de enfermeria españoles que trabajan en hospitales ingleses [Work satisfaction of Spanish nurses working in English hospitals]." *Gaceta Sanitaria* 22(5):434–442.

Saar, P., & Habicht, J. (2011). "Migration and Attrition: Estonia's Health Sector and Cross-Border Mobility to Its Northern Neighbour." In M. Wismar, C. B. Maier, I. A. Glinos, G. Dussault, & J. Figueras (Eds.), *Health Professional Mobility and Health Systems: Evidence from 17 European Countries* (pp. 339–364). Copenhagen, Denmark: World Health Organization on behalf of the European Observatory on Health Systems and Policies.

Safuta, A., & Baeten, R. (2011). "Of Permeable Borders: Belgium as Both Source and Host Country." In M. Wismar, C. B. Maier, I. A. Glinos, G. Dussault, & J. Figueras (Eds.), *Health Professional Mobility and Health Systems: Evidence from 17 European Countries* (pp. 129–162). Copenhagen, Denmark: World Health Organization on behalf of the European Observatory on Health Systems and Policies.

Sagan, A., Panteli, D., Borkowski, W., Dmowski, M., Domański, F., Czyżewski, M., et al. (2011). "Poland: Health System Review." *Health Systems in Transition* 13(8):1–193.

Sala, R., & Usa, M. (1997). "Industrial Action by Nurses: The Italian Situation." *Nursing Ethics* 4(4):330–338.

Sandier, S., Paris, V., & Polton, D. (2004). *Healthcare Systems in Transition: France.* Copenhagen, Denmark: WHO Regional Office for Europe on behalf of the European Observatory on Health Systems and Policies.

Sandin, I., & Walldal, E. (2002). "The Latvian Nurses Education and Profession in a Changing Society." *VÅRD i NORDEN* 22(4):22–26.

Santry, C. (2010, January 12). "Nurses Say Patients at Risk Under Working Time Rules." *Nursing Times.* Retrieved from www.nursingtimes.net

Sarfati, H. (2010). *Decent Pensions for Nurses.* Geneva, Switzerland: International Council of Nurses.

Satterly, F. (2004). *Where Have All the Nurses Gone? The Impact of the Nursing Shortage on American Health Care.* Amherst, NY: Prometheus Books.

Savova, E. (2008, March 13). "Doctors, Nurses in Bulgaria Ready to Protest." *The Sofia Echo.* Retrieved from www.sofiaecho.com

Scappucci, G. (1998). "Social and Employment Policy." In G. Glöckler, L. Junius, G. Scappucci, S. Usherwood, & J. Vassallo (Eds.), *Guide to EU Policies* (pp. 249–262). London: Blackstone Press Limited.

Schlanger, J. (2003). "Health Care and Social Care Reforms in the Czech Republic." *TRANSFER, European Review of Labour and Research* 9(1):137–144.

Schober, M., & Affara, F. (2006). *International Council of Nurses: Advanced Nursing Practice.* Oxford: Blackwell Publishing Ltd.

Schoonhoven, L., Heinen, M., & van Achterberg, T. (2012). *Striking Variation in the International Results: Nurse Job Satisfaction, Burnout and Work Environment in the Netherlands.* Presentation at the International Conference Nursing Workforce and Quality of Care in European Hospitals, Basel, Switzerland, September 2012.

van der Schoot, E., & van der Heijden, B. (2003). "Intent to Leave Nursing in the Netherlands." In H.-M. Hasselhorn, P. Tackenberg, & B. H. Müller (Eds.), *Working Conditions and Intent to Leave the Profession Among Nursing Staff in Europe* (pp. 193–202). (SALTA-JOINT PROGRAMME FOR WORKING LIFE RESEARCH IN EUROPE, Report No. 7). Retrieved January 5, 2007, from www.arbetslivsinstitutet.se

van der Schoot, E., Ogińska, H., Estryn-Behar, M., & the NEXT-Study Group. (2003). "Burnout in the Nursing Profession in Europe." In H.-M. Hasselhorn, P. Tackenberg, & B. H. Müller (Eds.), *Working Conditions and Intent to Leave the Profession Among Nursing Staff in Europe* (pp. 53–57). (SALTA-JOINT PROGRAMME FOR WORKING LIFE RESEARCH IN EUROPE, Report No. 7). Retrieved January 5, 2007, from www.arbetslivsinstitutet.se

Scott, D., Rogers, A. E., Hwang, W.-T., & Zhang, Y. (2006). "Effects of Critical Care Nurses' Work Hours on Vigilance and Patients' Safety." *American Journal of Critical Care* 15(1):30–37.

Scott, P. A., Matthews, A., & Kirwan, M. (2012). *Work Environment and Nurse Reported Outcomes: Findings of Interest from Ireland, RN4CAST Study.* Presentation at International Conference NursingWorkforce and Quality of Care in European Hospitals, Basel, Switzerland, September 14, 2012.

Seago, J. A., & Ash, M. (2002). "Registered Nurse Unions and Patient Outcomes." *Journal of Nursing Administration* 32(3):143–151.

Seago, J. A., Spetz, M. A., & Others. (2011). "Hospital RN Job Satisfaction and Nurse Unions." *Journal of Nursing Administration* 41(3):109–114.

Segrestin, B., & Tonneau, D. (2002). *La reduction du temps de travail dans les établissements prives sanitaires, médico-sociaux et sociaux [Work time reduction in private health care, medical-social, and social structures]* (No. 171). Paris: Observatoire National de la Démographie des Professions de Santé (ONDPS).

Sermeus, W. (2012). *RN4CAST – Nurse Forecasting in Europe: Project Overview.* Presentation at Nursing Workforce and Quality of Care in European Hospitals International Conference, Basel, Switzerland, 14 September 2012.

Sermeus, W., Aiken, L. H., Van den Heede, K., Rafferty, A. M., Griffiths, P., Moreno-Casbas, M. T., et al. (2011). "Nurse Forecasting in Europe (RN4CAST): Rationale, Design and Methodology." *BMC Nursing* 10(6). Retrieved from www.biomedcentral.com/1472-6955/10/6

Shaw, C. (2006). "Managing the Performance of Health Professionals." In C.-A. Dubois, M. McKee, & E. Nolte (Eds.), *Human Resources for Health in Europe* (pp. 98–115). Maidenhead, Berkshire, England: Open University Press.

Shaw, J., Hunt, J., & Wallace, C. (2007). *Economic and Social Law of the European Union.* Houndmills, England: Palgrave Macmillan.

Sheehan, B. (2008). *Public Service Union Protests Against Recruitment Freeze in Health Service.* Retrieved from www.eurofound.europa.eu

Sicart, D. (2006). "Les evolutions démographiques des professions de santé [Demographic evolution of health-care professions]." *Dossiers solidarité et santé* No. 1:7–22.

Siebens, K., Dierckx de Casterlé, B., Abraham, I., Dierckx, K., Braes, T., Darras, E., et al. (2006). "The Professional Self-Image of Nurses in Belgian Hospitals: A Cross-Sectional Questionnaire Survey." *International Journal of Nursing Studies* 43(1):71–82.

Siering, U. (2008). "Germany." In E. Nolte, C. Knai, & M. McKee (Eds.), *Managing Chronic Conditions: Experience in Eight Countries* (pp. 75–96). Copenhagen, Denmark: World Health Organization on behalf of the European Observatory on Health Systems and Policies.

da Silva, A., & Fernandes, R. M. P. (2008). *Os enfermeiros estrangeiras em Portugal [Foreign nurses in Portugal].* Lisbon, Portugal: Ordem dos Enfermeiros.

de Silva, D., & Fahey, D. (2008). "England." In E. Nolte, C. Knai, & M. McKee (Eds.), *Managing Chronic Conditions: Experience in Eight Countries* (pp. 29–54). Copenhagen, Denmark: World Health Organization on behalf of the European Observatory on Health Systems and Policies.

de Silva, S.R. (1998). *Elements of a Sound Industrial Relations System.* n.p.: International Labour Organisation ACT/EMP Publications.

Silvestro, A. (2002). "La rabbia degli infermieri francesi [French nurses' anger]." *L'infermiere* 46(2):1–2.

Simoens, S., Villeneuve, M., & Hurst, J. (2005). *Tackling Nurse Shortages in OECD Countries.* Paris: Organisation for Economic Co-operation and Development.

Simon, M., Klimmerling, A., Hasselhorn, H.-M., & the NEXT-Study Group. (2004). "Work-Home Conflict in the European Nursing Profession." *International Journal of Occupational and Environmental Health* 10(4):384–391.

Simon, M., Tackenberg, P., Nienhaus, A., Estryn-Behar, M., Conway, P. M., & Hasselhorn, H.-M. (2008). "Back or Neck-Pain-Related Disability of Nursing Staff in Hospitals, Nursing Homes and Home Care in Seven Countries – Results from the European NEXT-Study." *International Journal of Nursing Studies* 45(1):24–34.

Singh, D. (2008). *How Can Chronic Disease Management Programmes Operate Across Care Settings and Providers?* Copenhagen, Denmark: WHO Regional Office for Europe.

313

Sironi, C. (2004). "Relazione su: 26° incontro annuale del WENR 26–27 settembre 2003, Utrecht, Paesi Bassi [Presentation at the 26th annual WENR meeting, 26–27 September, 2003, Utrecht, Netherlands]." *Professioni Infermieristiche* 57(1):61–64.

Sjögren. K., Fochsen, G., Josephson, M., & Lagerström, M. (2005). "Reasons for Leaving Nursing Care and Improvements Needed for Considering a Return: A Study Among Swedish Nursing Personnel." *International Journal of Nursing Studies* 42(7):751–758.

Skela, S. B., & Pagon, M. (2008). "Relationship Between Nurses and Physicians in Terms of Organizational Culture: Who is Responsible for Subordination of Nurses?" *Croatian Medical Journal* 49(3):334–343.

Slovakia: The Manifesto of the Government of the Slovak Republic. (2006, August). Retrieved from www.mosr.sk/data/files/793.pdf

Social Partners Report on Workplace Stress Agreement. (2008, December 15). Retrieved February 2, 2009, from www.ec.europa.eu

"Social Security – Family & Maternity Benefits." (2010). *Angloinfo.* Retrieved December 12, 2010, from www.bulgaria.angloinfo.com

Somma, N.M. (2010). "How Do Voluntary Organizations Foster Protest? The Role of Organizational Involvement on Individual Protest Participation." *The Sociological Quarterly* 51(3):384–407.

Spain. (2003). *Ley 55/2003 de 16 de diciembre del Estatuto Marco del personal estatutario de los servicios de salud.[Law 55/2003 of December 16 on the Marco Regulation of statutory personnel in health-care services].*

Speroff, T., Nwosu, S., Greery, R. A., & Others. (2010). "Organizational Culture: Variation Across Hospitals and Connection to Patient Safety Climate." *Quality & Safety in Health Care* 19(6):592–596.

Spetz, J. (2011). *Unemployed and Underemployed Nurses.* Geneva, Switzerland: International Council of Nurses.

Spitzer, A., Camus,D., Desaulles, C., & Kuhne, N. (2006). "The Changing Context of Western European Healthcare Systems: Convergence Versus Divergence in Nursing Problematics." *Social Science & Medicine* 63(7):1796–1810.

Sroka, J. (2006, July 3). *Polish Hospital Dispute Drags On.* Retrieved from www.eurofound.europa.eu

Stanley, D. J. (2008). "Celluloid Angels: A Research Study of Nurses in Feature Films: 1900–2007." *Journal of Advanced Nursing* 64(1):84–95.

Stanojovic, M., & Vehovar, U. (2007). "Slovenia's Integration into the European Market Economy: Gradualism and its 'Rigidities.' " In P. Leisink, B. Steijn, & U. Veersma (Eds.), *Industrial Relations in the New Europe: Enlargement, Integration and Reform* (pp. 81–98). Cheltenham, England: Edgar Elgar.

Stavrou, P. (2007, September 17). *New Code of Practice to Prevent Sexual Harassment at Work.* Retrieved from www.eurofound.europa.eu/ewco/2007/06/CY070601/9I.htm

Steel, D., & Cylus, J. (2012). "United Kingdom (Scotland): Health System Review." *Health Systems in Transition* 14(9):1–150.

Stevens, F. C. J., & Diederiks, J. P. M. (1995). "Health Culture in Europe: An Exploration of National and Social Differences in Health-Related Values." In G. Lüschen, W. Cockerham, J. van der Zee, F. Stevens, J. Diederiks, M. Garcia, et al. (Eds.), *Health Systems in the European Union: Diversity, Convergence and Integration* (pp. 75–88). Munich, Germany: Oldenbourg.

Stone, P. W., Clarke, S., Cimiotti, J., & Correa-de-Araujo, R. (2004). "Nurses' Working Conditions: Implications for Infectious Disease." *Emerging Infectious Diseases* 10(11):1984–1989.

Stordeur, S., D'Hoore, W. D., van der Heijden, B., Dibisceglie, M., Laine, M., van der Schoot, E., et al. (2003a). "Leadership, Job Satisfaction and Nurses' Commitment." In H.-M. Hasselhorn, P. Tackenberg, & B. H. Müller (Eds.), *Working Conditions and Intent to Leave the Profession Among Nursing Staff in Europe* (pp. 28–45). (SALTA-JOINT PROGRAMME FOR WORKING LIFE RESEARCH IN EUROPE, Report No. 7). Retrieved January 5, 2007, from www.arbetslivsinstitutet.se

Stordeur, S., D'Hoore, W., & the NEXT Study Group. (2007). "Organizational Configuration of Hospitals Succeeding in Attracting and Retaining Nurses." *Journal of Advanced Nursing* 57(1):45–58.

Stordeur, S., Kiss, P., Verpraet, R., De Meester, M., Braeckman, L., & D'Hoore, W. (2003b). "Intent to Leave Nursing in Belgium." In H.-M. Hasselhorn, P. Tackenberg, & B. H. Müller (Eds.), *Working Conditions and Intent to Leave the Profession Among Nursing Staff in Europe* (pp. 125–135). (SALTA-JOINT PROGRAMME FOR WORKING LIFE RESEARCH IN EUROPE, Report No. 7). Retrieved January 5, 2007, from www.arbetslivsinstitutet.se

Strauss, A. L. (with Bucher, R.). (2001a). "Professions in Process." In A. L. Strauss, *Professions, Work and Careers* (pp. 9–23). New Brunswick, NJ: Transaction, Inc.

Strauss, A. L. (with Schatzman, L., Bucher, R., Ehrlich, D., & Sabshin, M.). (2001b). "The Nurses at PPI." In A. L. Strauss, *Professions, Work and Careers* (pp. 203–228). New Brunswick, NJ: Transaction, Inc.

Strople, B., & Hani, P. O. (2006). "Can Technology Improve Intershift Report? What the Research Reveals." *Journal of Professional Nursing* 22(3):197–204.

Strózik, M. (2006). "Poland." In B. Rechel, C.-A. Dubois, & M. McKee (Eds.), *The Health Care Workforce in Europe: Learning from Experience* (pp. 87–99). Copenhagen, Denmark: WHO Regional Office for Europe on behalf of the European Observatory on Health Systems and Policies.

Suhrcke, M., Fahey, D. K., & McKee, M. (2008). "Economic Aspects of Chronic Disease and Chronic Disease Management." In E. Nolte, & M. McKee (Eds.), *Caring for People with Chronic Conditions: A Health System Perspective* (pp. 43–63). Maidenhead, Berkshire, England: Open University Press.

Sula, P. (2004, July 7). *Protest by Silesian Healthcare Workers*. Retrieved from www.eurofound.europa.eu/ciro/2004/07/inbrief/pl0407101n.htm

Sundin, L., Hochwälder, J., Bildt, C., & Lisspers, J. (2007). "The Relationship Between Different Work-Related Sources of Social Support and Burnout Among Registered and Assistant Nurses in Sweden: A Questionnaire Survey." *International Journal of Nursing Studies* 44(5):758–769.

Surplus of Spanish Nurses Explained by Myriam Ovalle, Spanish General Council of Nursing. (n.d.). Retrieved from www.epha.org

Svensson, R. (1996). "The Interplay Between Doctors and Nurses: A Negotiated Order Perspective." *Sociology of Health & Illness* 18(3):379–398.

Swedish Association of Health Professionals. (2008, April 22). *Mediation Failed*. Retrieved May 10, 2008, from www.vardforbundet.se

Szende, A., & Culyer, A. J. (2006). "The Inequity of Informal Payments for Health Care: The Case of Hungary." *Health Policy* 75:262–271.

Tang, C. J., Chan, S. W., Zhou, W. T., & Liaw, S. Y. (2013). "Collaboration Between Hospital Physicians and Nurses: An Integrated Literature Review." *International Nursing Review* 60(3):291–302.

"Tensions Rise in Athens as Nurses and Students Fight Reforms." (2008, December 4). Retrieved December 6, 2008, from www.libcom.org

Theodorou, M., Charalambous, C., Petrou, C., & Cylus, J. (2012). "Cyprus: Health System Review." *Health Systems in Transition* 14(6):1–128.

Thompson, R., & Witter, S. (2000). "Informal Payments in Transitional Economies: Implications for Health Sector Reform." *International Journal of Health Planning and Management* 15(3):169–187.

Thomson, S., Figueras, J., Evetovits, T., Jowett, M., Mladovsky, P., Maresso, A., et al. (2014). *Economic Crisis, Health Systems and Health in Europe: Impact and Implications for Policy.* Copenhagen, Denmark: World Health Organization.

Tomev, L., Daskalova, N., & Ivanova, V. (2003). *Workplace Violence in the Health Sector: Case Study – Bulgaria.* Geneva, Switzerland: ILO, WHO, PSI Workplace Violence in the Health Sector Project.

Tomev, L., Daskalova, N., & Mihailova, T. (2005). *Social Dialogue in the Health Sector: Case Study Bulgaria* (WP235). Geneva, Switzerland: International Labour Office.

Tomev, L., Michailova, T., & Daskalova, N. (2003). "Health Reform in Bulgaria and Its Impact on Industrial Relations in the Health Sector." *TRANSFER European Review of Labour and Research* 9(1):145–152.

Tountas, Y., Karnaki, P., Pavi, E., & Souliotis, K. (2005). "The 'Unexpected' Growth of the Private Health Sector in Greece." *Health Policy* 74:167–180.

Tovey, E. J., & Adams, A. E. (1999). "The Changing Nature of Nurses' Job Satisfaction: An Exploration of Sources of Satisfaction in the 1990s." *Journal of Advanced Nursing* 30(1):150–158.

Tragakes, E. (with Brigis, G., Karaskevica, J., Rurane, A., Stuburs, A., & Zusmane, E.). (2008). "Latvia: Health System Review." *Health Systems in Transition* 10(2):1–253.

Trbanc, M. (2008, April 30). *Spotlight on Harassment in the Workplace.* Retrieved from www.eurofound.europa.eu/ewco/2007/07/SI0707019I.htm

Trif, A. (2007). "Collective Bargaining in Eastern Europe: Case Study Evidence from Romania." *European Journal of Industrial Relations* 13(2):237–256.

Triggle, N. (2007, April 17). "Nurses Ready for Action Over Pay." *BBC News.*

Tunsch, G. (1998). "Luxembourg: A Small Success Story." In A. Ferner, & R. Hyman (Eds.), *Changing Industrial Relations in Europe* (pp. 348–356). Oxford: Blackwell.

"UK Workers Get Least Paid Leave." (2007, August 13). *BBC News.*

Utriainen, K., Kyngäs, H., & Nikkilä, J. (2009). "Well-Being at Work Among Ageing Hospital Nurses in Northern Finland: A Grounded Theory Study." *International Journal of Circumpolar Health* 68(2):145–157.

Vandenbrande, T., Van Gyes, G., Lehndorff, S., Schilling, G., Schief, S., & Kohl. H. (2007). *Industrial Relations in EU Member States 2000–2004.* Retrieved from www.eurofound.europa.eu

Vandenbroeck, S., Vanbelle, E., De Witte, H., Moerenhout, E., Sercu, M., De Man, H., et al. (2012). *An Investigation into Burn-Out and Enthusiasm Among Doctors and Nurses in Belgian Hospitals.* Leuven, Belgium: Katholieke Universiteit Leuven.

Van den Heede, K., Florquin, M., Bruyneel, L., Aiken, L., Diya, L., Lesaffre, E., et al. (2011). "Effective Strategies for Nurse Retention in Acute Hospitals: A Mixed Method Study." *International Journal of Nursing Studies* 50(2):185–194.

Vašková, R. (2006, September 25). *Sexual Harassment in the Workforce.* Retrieved from www.eurofound.europa.eu/ewco/2006/07/CZ0607019I.htm

Vaughan-Whitehead, D. (2007). "Work and Employment Conditions in New EU Member States: A Different Reality." In P. Leisink, B. Steijn, & U. Veersma (Eds.), *Industrial Relations in the New Europe: Enlargement, Integration and Reform* (pp. 41–62). Cheltenham, England: Edward Elgar.

Venema, A., & van der Klauw, M. (2012, September 7). *Impact of Workplace Violence on Employees.* Retrieved from www.eurofound.europa.eu

Vere-Jones, E. (2008, March 3). "UK Second in Euro League of Violence Against Nurses." *Nursing Times.* Retrieved from www.nursingtimes.net

Verhaeghe, R., Vlerick, P., Gemmel, P., Van Maele, G., & De Backer, G. (2006). "Impact of Recurrent Changes in the Work Environment on Nurses' Psychological Well-Being and Sickness Absence." *Journal of Advanced Nursing* 56(6):646–656.

Vermandere, C. (2014, March 10). *Risk of Burn-Out Among Medical Staff.* Retrieved from www.eurofound.europa.eu/ewco/2014/01/BE1401021I.htm

Versieck, K., Bouten, R., & Pacolet, J. (1995). *Manpower Problems in the Nursing/Midwifery Profession in the EC.* Leuven, Belgium: Katholieke Universiteit Leuven & Hoger Instituut voor de Arbeid.

Vigneau, C., & Sobczak, A. (2005). "France: The Helping Hand of the State." *Bulletin of Comparative Labour Relations* No. 56:31–48.

Vilain, A., & Niel, X. (1999). *Les infirmiers en activité: Croissance des effectifs à un rythme moins élevé dans les vingt prochaines années [Nurses in action: Increase in numbers at a lesser rate in the last twenty years]* (No. 12). Paris: Observatoire National de la Démographie des Professions de Santé (ONDPS).

Vilbrod, A., & Douguet, F. (2007). *Les infirmières liberals et les autres professionnels du secteur sanitaire et social: Une cooperation jamais acquise, toujours à construire et à reconstruire [Free lance nurses and other professionals in the health and social sector: A cooperation never acquired, always to build and rebuild].* Paris: DRESS.

Vlădescu, C., Scintee, G., Olsavszky, V., Allin, S., & Mladovsky, P. (2008). "Romania: Health System Review." *Health Systems in Transition* 10(3):1–172.

Vŏncina, L., Jemiai, N., Merkur, S., Golna, C., Maeda, A., Chao, S., et al. (2006). "Croatia: Health System Review." *Health Systems in Transition* 8(7):1–108.

Vŏrk, A., Priinits, M., & Kallaste, E. (2004). *Migration of Healthcare Workers from Estonia: The Potential Extent of Migration, Its Influence on the Needs of Healthcare Workers and Political Choices. Summary.* Tallinn, Estonia: PRAXIS Centre for Policy Studies.

Vuorenkoski, L., Mladovsky, P., & Mossialos, E. (2008). "Finland: Health System Review." *Health Systems in Transition* 10(4):1–168.

Waddington, J. (2005). *Trade Union Membership in Europe: The Extent of the Problem and the Range of Trade Union Responses.* Brussels, Belgium: ETUI-REHS.

von Wahl, A. (2005). "Liberal, Conservative, Social Democratic, or European: The European Union as Equal Employment Regime." *Social Politics* 12(1):67–95.

Wahlberg, A. C., Cederound, E., & Wredling, R. (2003). "Telephone Nurses' Experience of Problems with Telephone Advice in Sweden." *Journal of Clinical Nursing* 12(1):37–45.

Wait, S. (2006). "France." In B. Rechel, C.-A. Dubois, & M. McKee (Eds.), *The Health Care Workforce in Europe: Learning from the Experience* (pp. 19–32). Copenhagen, Denmark: WHO Regional Office for Europe on behalf of the European Observatory on Health Systems and Policies.

Walters, D. (2002). "The Framework Directive." In D. Walters (Ed.), *Regulating Health and Safety Management in the European Union: A Study of the Dynamics of Change* (pp. 39–57). Brussels, Belgium: P.I.E. – Peter Lang.

Wanberg, C. R. (2012). "Facilitating Organizational Socialization: An Introduction." In C. R. Wanberg (Ed.), *The Oxford Handbook of Organizational Socialization* (pp. 17–21). New York: Oxford University Press.

Warneck, W. (2007). *Strike Rules in the EU27 and Beyond*. Brussels, Belgium: European Trade Union Institute for Research, Education and Health and Safety.

Watson, R., Hoogbruin, A. L., Rumeu, C., Beunza, M., Barbarin, B., Macdonald, J., et al. (2003). "Differences and Similarities in the Perception of Caring Between Spanish and UK Nurses." *Journal of Clinical Nursing* 12(1):85–92.

Weiler, A. (2005, September 12). *Sexual Harassment in the Workplace*. Retrieved from www.eurofound.europa.eu

Weiler, A., Newell, H., & Carley, M. (2007). *Industrial Relations Developments in Europe: 2006*. Retrieved from www.eurofound.europa.eu

Weinberg, D. B. (2003). *Code Green: Money-Driven Hospitals and the Dismantling of Nursing*. Ithaca, NY and London: Cornell University Press.

Weinbrenner, S., & Busse, R. (2006). "Germany." In B. Rechel, C.-A. Dubois, & M. McKee (Eds.), *The Health Care Workforce in Europe: Learning from Experience* (pp. 33–46). Copenhagen, Denmark: WHO Regional Office for Europe, on behalf of the European Observatory on Health Systems and Policies.

Welz, C., & Kauppinen, T. (2004). *Social Dialogue and Conflict Resolution in the Acceding Countries*. Dublin, Ireland: European Foundation for the Improvement of Living and Working Conditions.

"What are the Benefits and Challenges of 'Bedside' Nursing Handovers?" (2012). *Policy+*, Issue 36.

"What are 12-Hour Shifts Good for?" (2013). *Policy+*, Issue 38.

Whitehead, J. (2001). "Newly Qualified and Staff Nurses' Perceptions of the Role Transition." *British Journal of Nursing* 10(5):330–332, 334–339.

Widerszal-Bazyl, M., Radkiewicz, P., Hasselhorn, H.-M., Conway, P., & the NEXT-Study Group. (2003a). "The Job Demand-Control-Support Model Applied to Analysis of Nursing Work in Ten European Countries." In H.-M. Hasselhorn, P. Tackenberg, & B. H. Müller (Eds.), *Working Conditions and Intent to Leave the Profession Among Nursing Staff in Europe* (pp. 101–107). (SALTA-JOINT PROGRAMME FOR WORKING LIFE RESEARCH IN EUROPE, Report No. 7). Retrieved January 5, 2007, from www.arbetslivsinstitutet.se

Widerszal-Bazyl, M., Radkiewicz, P., Pokorski, J., Pokorska, J., Ogińska, H., & Pietsch, E. (2003b). "Who Wants to Leave Nursing in Poland." In H.-M. Hasselhorn, P. Tackenberg, & B. H. Müller (Eds.), *Working Conditions and Intent to Leave the Profession Among Nursing Staff in Europe* (pp. 203–212). (SALTA-JOINT PROGRAMME FOR WORKING LIFE RESEARCH IN EUROPE, Report N° 7). Retrieved January 5, 2007, from www.arbetslivsinstitutet.se

Willem, A., Buelens M., & De Jonghe, I. (2007). "Impact of Organizational Structure on Nurses' Job Satisfaction: A Questionnaire Survey." *International Journal of Nursing Studies* 44(6):1011–1020.

Wiskow, C., Albreht, T., & de Pietro, C. (2010). *How to Create an Attractive and Supportive Working Environment for Health Professionals.* Geneva, Switzerland: World Health Organization on behalf of the European Observatory on Health Systems and Policies.

"Working Without Limits? Re-Organising Work and Reconsidering Workers' Health." (2001). *Newsletter of the European Trade Union Technical Bureau for Health and Safety,* Nos. 15–16. Special Issue for the TUTB-SALTSA Conference.

World Health Organization: Europe. (2006). *Human Resources for Health in the WHO European Region.* Copenhagen, Denmark: WHO Regional Office for Europe.

World Health Organization Regional Committee for Europe. (2007, June 30). *Health Workforce Policies in the European Region* (EUR/RC57/Conf. Doc./3. 30 June 2007). Copenhagen, Denmark: Author.

World Health Organization: Regional Office for Europe. (2013). *European Health for all Database.* Retrieved from www.euro.who.int

Wright, M., Clark, J., Greenwood, A., Callaway, M., & Clark, D. (2003). *Palliative Care Policy Development In Central and Eastern Europe and Central Asia: An Open Society Institute Initiative.* Retrieved August 10, 2007, from www.health. osf.lt/downloads/news/CWPublicationonBudapestConference.doc

Zabarauskaite, R. (2013, May 7). *Job Satisfaction among Community Nurses.* Retrieved from www.eurofound.europa.eu.

Zander, B. (2012). *Implementation of DRGs in Germany: Are There Any Effects on Outcomes?* Presentation at the International Conference on the Nursing Workforce and Quality of Care in European Hospitals, Basel, Switzerland, 14 September 2012.

Websites

www.cancervard.se. Cancer Services-Sweden.

www.dbfk.de. Deutscher Berufsverband für Pflegeberufe (German Organization of Nursing Professionals).

www.eapc-taskforce-development.eu. EAPC (European Association for Palliative Care) Taskforce on the Development of Palliative Care.

www.eapcnet.org. European Association for Palliative Care.

www.eski.hu. Directorate General of IT and Health System Analysis-Hungary.

www.euro.who.int/nursingmidwifery. World Health Organization Regional Office for Europe: Nursing and Midwifery.

www.hospice.hu. Hungarian Hospice-Palliative Association.

www.hums.hr. Croatian Nurses Association.

www.infirmiers.com. French Nurses Website.

www.mumn.org. Malta Union of Midwives and Nurses.

www.regos.hr. Central Registry of Affiliates-Croatia.

www.rn4cast.eu. Human Resources Management for Nursing in Europe: A Study on the Impact of Nurse Deployment on Patient Safety or Nurse Forecasting in Europe.

www.sahha.gov.mt. Ministry for Energy and Health-Malta.

Index